KAPLAN

MCAT®

Critical Analysis and Reasoning Skills Review

2027–2028

Edited by Alexander Stone Macnow, MD

ACKNOWLEDGMENTS

Editor-in-Chief, 2027–2028 Edition
M. Dominic Eggert

Contributing Editor, 2027–2028 Edition
Ae-Ri Kim, PhD; Elizabeth Minten, MD PhD; Gregory J. Riviello, MA; Christopher Vestuto

Prior Edition Editorial Staff: Elisabeth Fassas, MD MSc

Published by Kaplan North America, LLC
1515 West Cypress Creek Road
Fort Lauderdale, Florida 33309

Printed in India.

ISBN: 979-8-3497-0117-7

10 9 8 7 6 5 4 3 2 1

TABLE OF CONTENTS

The *Kaplan MCAT CARS Review* Team. viii
Getting Started Checklist. ix
Preface x
About the MCAT xi
How This Book Was Created xxiii
Using This Book xxiv
Studying for the MCAT xxvi

UNIT 1: CARS STRATEGY 1

CHAPTER 1: ABOUT CARS 3
Introduction 3
1.1 Section Format 4
1.2 What Does CARS Test? 5
1.3 Using This Book to Prepare for CARS. 7
Conclusion. 8
Skill and Strategy Summary 8

CHAPTER 2: PASSAGE STRATEGY 9
Introduction 9
2.1 Preview and Choose. 10
2.2 Read and Distill 12
Conclusion. 15
Skill and Strategy Summary 15

CHAPTER 3: KEYWORDS. 17
Introduction 17
3.1 Connection Keywords. 18
3.2 Logic Keywords 22
3.3 Author Keywords 25
Conclusion. 28
Skill and Strategy Summary 28

TABLE OF CONTENTS

CHAPTER 4: INTERROGATING PASSAGES 31

Introduction 31

4.1 Passive vs. Active Reading 32

4.2 Chunking and Passage Architecture 35

4.3 Chatting and Author Perspective 37

Conclusion 40

Skill and Strategy Summary 41

CHAPTER 5: TEST DAY TOOLS: OUTLINING AND HIGHLIGHTING 43

Introduction 43

5.1 Outlining 44

5.2 Highlighting 50

5.3 Choosing Your Tool 55

5.4 Practice Passage 57

Conclusion 64

Skill and Strategy Summary 64

CHAPTER 6: QUESTION STRATEGY, TYPES, AND SKILLS 67

Introduction 68

6.1 The Kaplan Method for CARS Questions 68

6.2 Question Types and Skills 75

6.3 Wrong Answer Pathologies 79

6.4 Practice Question Set 81

6.5 Answers and Explanations 84

Conclusion 90

Skill and Strategy Summary 90

CHAPTER 7: PRACTICING AND REVIEWING CARS 93

Introduction 93

7.1 Structuring Your CARS Prep 94

7.2 Effective Review of CARS 98

Conclusion 104

Skill and Strategy Summary 104

UNIT 2: FOUNDATIONS OF COMPREHENSION SKILLS 105

CHAPTER 8: INTERPRET MEANING 107

8.1 Skill Description 108

8.2 Question Variations and Examples 111

8.3 Applying the Kaplan Method 113

8.4 Skillbuilder 115
Skill and Strategy Summary 123

CHAPTER 9: RECOGNIZE OPINION 125
9.1 Skill Description 126
9.2 Question Variations and Examples 129
9.3 Applying the Kaplan Method 132
9.4 Skillbuilder 135
Skill and Strategy Summary 141

CHAPTER 10: PARAPHRASE DETAIL 143
10.1 Skill Description 144
10.2 Question Variations and Examples 148
10.3 Applying the Kaplan Method 153
10.4 Skillbuilder 155
Skill and Strategy Summary 161

CHAPTER 11: SUMMARIZE TEXT 163
11.1 Skill Description 164
11.2 Question Variations and Examples 167
11.3 Applying the Kaplan Method 169
11.4 Skillbuilder 171
Skill and Strategy Summary 178

CHAPTER 12: FOUNDATIONS OF COMPREHENSION PRACTICE 179
How to Use This Chapter 179
Passage 1 (Questions 1–6) 179
Passage 2 (Questions 7–13) 182
Answers and Explanations 184

UNIT 3: REASONING WITHIN THE TEXT SKILLS 189

CHAPTER 13: DESCRIBE PURPOSE 191
13.1 Skill Description 192
13.2 Question Variations and Examples 194
13.3 Applying the Kaplan Method 197
13.4 Skillbuilder 201
Skill and Strategy Summary 207

CHAPTER 14: EVALUATE REASONING . . . 209
14.1 Skill Description . . . 210
14.2 Question Variations and Examples . . . 216
14.3 Applying the Kaplan Method . . . 219
14.4 Skillbuilder . . . 222
Skill and Strategy Summary . . . 230

CHAPTER 15: MAKE DEDUCTION . . . 231
15.1 Skill Description . . . 232
15.2 Question Variations and Examples . . . 236
15.3 Applying the Kaplan Method . . . 238
15.4 Skillbuilder . . . 241
Skill and Strategy Summary . . . 249

CHAPTER 16: REASONING WITHIN THE TEXT PRACTICE . . . 251
How to Use This Chapter . . . 251
Passage 1 (Questions 1–6) . . . 251
Passage 2 (Questions 7–12) . . . 254
Answers and Explanations . . . 256

UNIT 4: REASONING BEYOND THE TEXT SKILLS . . . 261

CHAPTER 17: ANTICIPATE RESPONSE . . . 263
17.1 Skill Description . . . 264
17.2 Question Variations and Examples . . . 267
17.3 Applying the Kaplan Method . . . 270
17.4 Skillbuilder . . . 274
Skill and Strategy Summary . . . 281

CHAPTER 18: PREDICT OUTCOME/EXPLANATION . . . 283
18.1 Skill Description . . . 284
18.2 Question Variations and Examples . . . 286
18.3 Applying the Kaplan Method . . . 289
18.4 Skillbuilder . . . 291
Skill and Strategy Summary . . . 299

CHAPTER 19: STRENGTHEN/WEAKEN ARGUMENT . . . 301
19.1 Skill Description . . . 302
19.2 Question Variations and Examples . . . 308
19.3 Applying the Kaplan Method . . . 312

19.4 Skillbuilder 314
Skill and Strategy Summary 321

CHAPTER 20: IMAGINE EXAMPLE/ANALOGY 323
20.1 Skill Description 324
20.2 Question Variations and Examples 328
20.3 Applying the Kaplan Method 330
20.4 Skillbuilder 333
Skill and Strategy Summary 339

CHAPTER 21: REASONING BEYOND THE TEXT PRACTICE 341
How to Use This Chapter 341
Passage 1 (Questions 1–6) 341
Passage 2 (Questions 7–12) 344
Answers and Explanations 346

UNIT 5: ADDITIONAL PRACTICE 353

CHAPTER 22: MIXED PRACTICE 355
How to Use This Chapter 355
Passage 1 (Questions 1–7) 355
Passage 2 (Questions 8–13) 358
Passage 3 (Questions 14–20) 360
Answers and Explanations 362

APPENDIX: THE MCAT INTERFACE 369
Interface Shortcuts 370
Navigating the Test 371
Leveraging Interface Features 374
Conclusion 377
Skill and Strategy Summary 378

GLOSSARY 381

INDEX 387

THE *KAPLAN MCAT CARS REVIEW* TEAM

M. Dominic Eggert
CARS Curriculum Architect, Lead Author, Editor-in-Chief

Gregory J. Riviello, MA
Senior Author, Editor

Jennifer M. Kindy, MS
Author, Contributing Editor

Christopher Vestuto
Author

Ryan G. Davis, MD, MPH
Author

Ae-Ri Kim, PhD
Author

Paula L. Fleming, MBA, MA
Author

Thanks to Chrystal Akor; Kevin Anderson; Mark Badovinac; Jeff Batzli; Alvin Bisarya, MD; Hari Priya Chandran; Dana D'Agostino; Deepika Devan; Logan Emlet; Thomas Faiella; Elisabeth Fassas, MD, MSc; Rita Garthaffner; John Giordano; Jessica Gleicher; Joanna Graham; Luke Graham; Rohit Gupta, MD; Andrew Kula; Nirmala Kumari; Andrew La Voy; Wes Madison; Rich Maraggio; Brandon McKenzie; Elizabeth Minten, MD, PhD; Madhura Naik; Nicholas Nguyen, MPH; Beena P V; Kevin Pierce; Andrea Repole; Christine Ricketts; Srividhya Sankar; Rebecca Stover; Dori Surdis; Todd Tedesco; Nic Turek; Mike Wolff; Kristen Workman; Amy Zarkos; and the countless others who made this book possible.

GETTING STARTED CHECKLIST

Getting Started Checklist

- [ ] Register for your free online assets: if you bought this book new as part of a set, scan the QR code on the front of the book set's slipcase and enter the unique code there; if you bought this book separately, instead go to **www.kaptest.com/booksonline**.
- [ ] Create a study calendar that ensures you complete content review and sufficient practice by Test Day!
- [ ] As you finish a chapter and the online practice for that chapter, check it off on the table of contents.
- [ ] Register to take the MCAT at **www.aamc.org/mcat.**
- [ ] Set aside time during your prep to make sure the rest of your application—personal statement, recommendations, and other materials—is ready to go!
- [ ] Take a moment to admire your completed checklist, then get back to the business of prepping for this exam!

PREFACE

And now it starts: your long, yet fruitful journey toward wearing a white coat. Proudly wearing that white coat, though, is hopefully only part of your motivation. You are reading this book because you want to be a healer.

If you're serious about going to medical school, then you are likely already familiar with the importance of the MCAT in medical school admissions. While the holistic review process puts additional weight on your experiences, extracurricular activities, and personal attributes, the fact remains: along with your GPA, your MCAT score remains one of the two most important components of your application portfolio—at least early in the admissions process. Each additional point you score on the MCAT pushes you in front of thousands of other students and makes you an even more attractive applicant. But the MCAT is not simply an obstacle to overcome; it is an opportunity to show schools that you will be a strong student and a future leader in medicine.

We at Kaplan take our jobs very seriously and aim to help students see success not only on the MCAT, but as future physicians. We work with our learning science experts to ensure that we're using the most up-to-date teaching techniques in our resources. Multiple members of our team hold advanced degrees in medicine or associated biomedical sciences, and are committed to the highest level of medical education. Kaplan has been working with the MCAT for over 50 years and our commitment to premed students is unflagging; in fact, Stanley Kaplan created this company when he had difficulty being accepted to medical school due to unfair quota systems that existed at the time.

We stand now at the beginning of a new era in medical education. As citizens of this 21st-century world of healthcare, we are charged with creating a patient-oriented, culturally competent, cost-conscious, universally available, technically advanced, and research-focused healthcare system, run by compassionate providers. Suffice it to say, this is no easy task. Problem-based learning, integrated curricula, and classes in interpersonal skills are some of the responses to this demand for an excellent workforce—a workforce of which you'll soon be a part.

We're thrilled that you've chosen us to help you on this journey. Please reach out to us to share your challenges, concerns, and successes. Together, we will shape the future of medicine in the United States and abroad; we look forward to helping you become the doctor you deserve to be.

Good luck!

Alexander Stone Macnow, MD
Editor-in-Chief
Department of Pathology and Laboratory Medicine
Hospital of the University of Pennsylvania

BA, Musicology—Boston University, 2008
MD—Perelman School of Medicine at the University of Pennsylvania, 2013

ABOUT THE MCAT

Anatomy of the MCAT

Here is a general overview of the structure of Test Day:

Section	Number of Questions	Time Allotted
Test Day Certification		4 minutes
Tutorial (optional)		10 minutes
Chemical and Physical Foundations of Biological Systems	59	95 minutes
Break (optional)		10 minutes
Critical Analysis and Reasoning Skills (CARS)	53	90 minutes
Lunch Break (optional)		30 minutes
Biological and Biochemical Foundations of Living Systems	59	95 minutes
Break (optional)		10 minutes
Psychological, Social, and Biological Foundations of Behavior	59	95 minutes
Void Question		3 minutes
Satisfaction Survey (optional)		5 minutes

The structure of the four sections of the MCAT is shown below.

Chemical and Physical Foundations of Biological Systems	
Time	95 minutes
Format	• *59 questions* • *10 passages* • *44 questions are passage-based, and 15 are discrete (stand-alone) questions* • *Score between 118 and 132*
What It Tests	• *Biochemistry: 25%* • *Biology: 5%* • *General Chemistry: 30%* • *Organic Chemistry: 15%* • *Physics: 25%*

Critical Analysis and Reasoning Skills (CARS)	
Time	90 minutes
Format	• *53 questions* • *9 passages* • *All questions are passage-based. There are no discrete (stand-alone) questions.* • *Score between 118 and 132*
What It Tests	Disciplines: • *Humanities: 50%* • *Social Sciences: 50%* Skills: • *Foundations of Comprehension: 30%* • *Reasoning Within the Text: 30%* • *Reasoning Beyond the Text: 40%*
Biological and Biochemical Foundations of Living Systems	
Time	95 minutes
Format	• *59 questions* • *10 passages* • *44 questions are passage-based, and 15 are discrete (stand-alone) questions.* • *Score between 118 and 132*
What It Tests	• *Biochemistry: 25%* • *Biology: 65%* • *General Chemistry: 5%* • *Organic Chemistry: 5%*
Psychological, Social, and Biological Foundations of Behavior	
Time	95 minutes
Format	• *59 questions* • *10 passages* • *44 questions are passage-based, and 15 are discrete (stand-alone) questions* • *Score between 118 and 132*
What It Tests	• *Biology: 5%* • *Psychology: 65%* • *Sociology: 30%*
Total	
Testing Time	375 minutes (6 hours, 15 minutes)
Total Seat Time	447 minutes (7 hours, 27 minutes)
Questions	230
Score	472 to 528

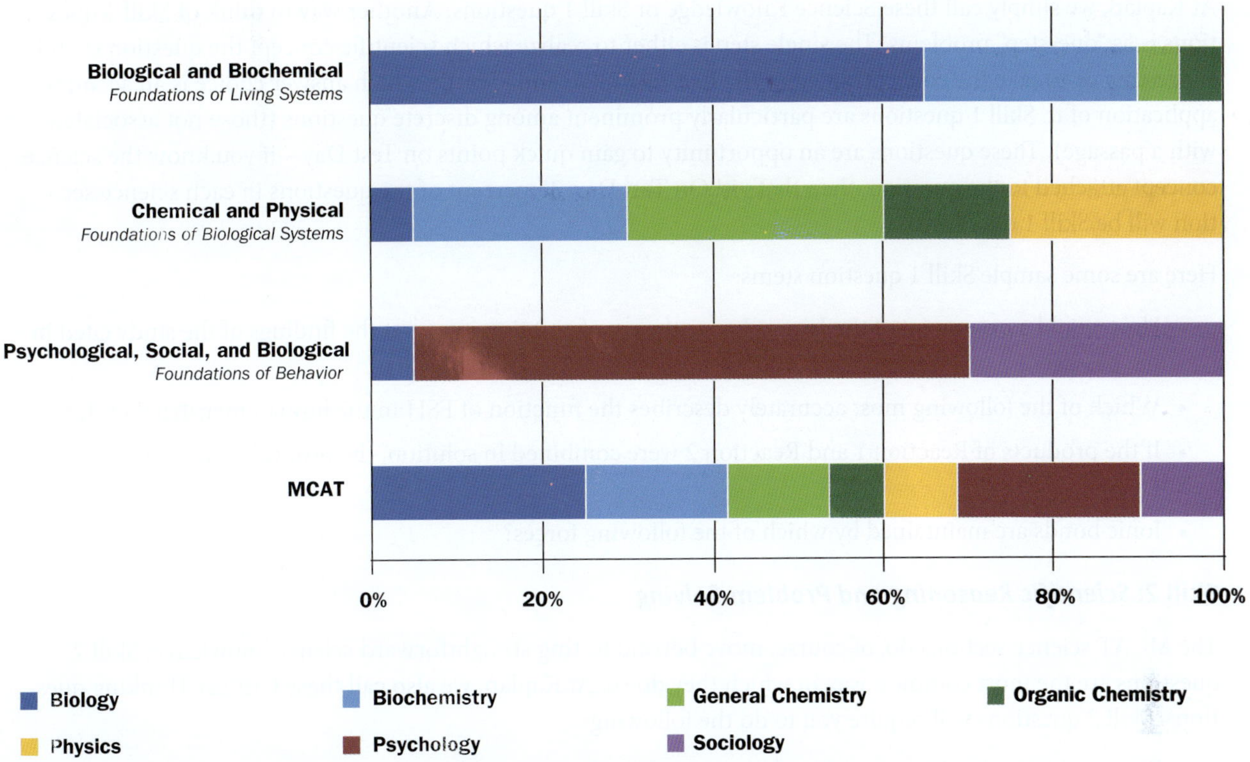

Scientific Inquiry and Reasoning Skills (SIRS)

The AAMC has defined four *Scientific Inquiry and Reasoning Skills* (SIRS) that will be tested in the three science sections of the MCAT:

1. *Knowledge of Scientific Concepts and Principles* (35 percent of questions)
2. *Scientific Reasoning and Problem-Solving* (45 percent of questions)
3. *Reasoning About the Design and Execution of Research* (10 percent of questions)
4. *Data-Based and Statistical Reasoning* (10 percent of questions)

Let's see how each one breaks down into more specific Test Day behaviors. Note that the bullet points of specific objectives for each of the SIRS are taken directly from the *Official Guide to the MCAT Exam*; the descriptions of what these behaviors mean and sample question stems, however, are written by Kaplan.

Skill 1: *Knowledge of Scientific Concepts and Principles*

This is probably the least surprising of the four SIRS; the testing of science knowledge is, after all, one of the signature qualities of the MCAT. Skill 1 questions will require you to do the following:

- Recognize correct scientific principles
- Identify the relationships among closely related concepts
- Identify the relationships between different representations of concepts (verbal, symbolic, graphic)
- Identify examples of observations that illustrate scientific principles
- Use mathematical equations to solve problems

At Kaplan, we simply call these Science Knowledge or Skill 1 questions. Another way to think of Skill 1 questions is as "one-step" problems. The single step is either to realize which scientific concept the question stem is suggesting or to take the concept stated in the question stem and identify which answer choice is an accurate application of it. Skill 1 questions are particularly prominent among discrete questions (those not associated with a passage). These questions are an opportunity to gain quick points on Test Day—if you know the science concept attached to the question, then that's it! On Test Day, 35 percent of the questions in each science section will be Skill 1 questions.

Here are some sample Skill 1 question stems:

- How would a proponent of the James–Lange theory of emotion interpret the findings of the study cited in the passage?
- Which of the following most accurately describes the function of FSH in the human menstrual cycle?
- If the products of Reaction 1 and Reaction 2 were combined in solution, the resulting reaction would form:
- Ionic bonds are maintained by which of the following forces?

Skill 2: *Scientific Reasoning and Problem-Solving*

The MCAT science sections do, of course, move beyond testing straightforward science knowledge; Skill 2 questions are the most common way in which they do so. At Kaplan, we also call these Critical Thinking questions. Skill 2 questions will require you to do the following:

- Reason about scientific principles, theories, and models
- Analyze and evaluate scientific explanations and predictions
- Evaluate arguments about causes and consequences
- Bring together theory, observations, and evidence to draw conclusions
- Recognize scientific findings that challenge or invalidate a scientific theory or model
- Determine and use scientific formulas to solve problems

Just as Skill 1 questions can be thought of as "one-step" problems, many Skill 2 questions are "two-step" problems, and more difficult Skill 2 questions may require three or more steps. These questions can require a wide spectrum of reasoning skills, including integration of multiple facts from a passage, combination of multiple science content areas, and prediction of an experiment's results. Skill 2 questions also tend to ask about science content without actually mentioning it by name. For example, a question might describe the results of one experiment and ask you to predict the results of a second experiment without actually telling you what underlying scientific principles are at work—part of the question's difficulty will be figuring out which principles to apply in order to get the correct answer. On Test Day, 45 percent of the questions in each science section will be Skill 2 questions.

Here are some sample Skill 2 question stems:

- Which of the following experimental conditions would most likely yield results similar to those in Figure 2?
- All of the following conclusions are supported by the information in the passage EXCEPT:
- The most likely cause of the anomalous results found by the experimenter is:
- An impact to a person's chest quickly reduces the volume of one of the lungs to 70% of its initial value while not allowing any air to escape from the mouth. By what percentage is the force of outward air pressure increased on a 2 cm^2 portion of the inner surface of the compressed lung?

Skill 3: *Reasoning About the Design and Execution of Research*

The MCAT is interested in your ability to critically appraise and analyze research, as this is an important day-to-day task of a physician. We call these questions Skill 3 or Experimental and Research Design questions. Skill 3 questions will require you to do the following:

- Identify the role of theory, past findings, and observations in scientific questioning
- Identify testable research questions and hypotheses
- Distinguish between samples and populations and distinguish results that support generalizations about populations
- Identify independent and dependent variables
- Reason about the features of research studies that suggest associations between variables or causal relationships between them (such as temporality and random assignment)
- Identify conclusions that are supported by research results
- Determine the implications of results for real-world situations
- Reason about ethical issues in scientific research

Over the years, the AAMC has received input from medical schools to require more practical research skills of MCAT test takers, and Skill 3 questions are the response to these demands. This skill is unique in that the outside knowledge you need to answer Skill 3 questions is not taught in any one undergraduate course; instead, the research design principles needed to answer these questions are learned gradually throughout your science classes and especially through any laboratory work you have completed. It should be noted that Skill 3 comprises 10 percent of the questions in each science section on Test Day.

Here are some sample Skill 3 question stems:

- What is the dependent variable in the study described in the passage?
- The major flaw in the method used to measure disease susceptibility in Experiment 1 is:
- Which of the following procedures is most important for the experimenters to follow in order for their study to maintain a proper randomized sample of research subjects?
- A researcher would like to test the hypothesis that individuals who move to an urban area during adulthood are more likely to own a car than are those who have lived in an urban area since birth. Which of the following studies would best test this hypothesis?

Skill 4: *Data-Based and Statistical Reasoning*

Lastly, the science sections of the MCAT test your ability to analyze the visual and numerical results of experiments and studies. We call these Data and Statistical Analysis questions. Skill 4 questions will require you to do the following:

- Use, analyze, and interpret data in figures, graphs, and tables
- Evaluate whether representations make sense for particular scientific observations and data
- Use measures of central tendency (mean, median, and mode) and measures of dispersion (range, interquartile range, and standard deviation) to describe data
- Reason about random and systematic error

- Reason about statistical significance and uncertainty (interpreting statistical significance levels and interpreting a confidence interval)
- Use data to explain relationships between variables or make predictions
- Use data to answer research questions and draw conclusions

Skill 4 is included in the MCAT because physicians and researchers spend much of their time examining the results of their own studies and the studies of others, and it's very important for them to make legitimate conclusions and sound judgments based on that data. The MCAT tests Skill 4 on all three science sections with graphical representations of data (charts and bar graphs), as well as numerical ones (tables, lists, and results summarized in sentence or paragraph form). On Test Day, 10 percent of the questions in each science section will be Skill 4 questions.

Here are some sample Skill 4 question stems:

- According to the information in the passage, there is an inverse correlation between:
- What conclusion is best supported by the findings displayed in Figure 2?
- A medical test for a rare type of heavy metal poisoning returns a positive result for 98% of affected individuals and 13% of unaffected individuals. Which of the following types of error is most prevalent in this test?
- If a fourth trial of Experiment 1 was run and yielded a result of 54% compliance, which of the following would be true?

SIRS Summary

Discussing the SIRS tested on the MCAT is a daunting prospect given that the very nature of the skills tends to make the conversation rather abstract. Nevertheless, with enough practice you'll be able to identify each of the four skills quickly, and you'll also be able to apply the proper strategies to solve those problems on Test Day. If you need a quick reference to remind you of the four SIRS, these guidelines may help:

Skill 1 (**Science Knowledge**) questions ask:

- Do you remember this science content?

Skill 2 (**Critical Thinking**) questions ask:

- Do you remember this science content? And if you do, could you please apply it to this novel situation?
- Could you answer this question that cleverly combines multiple content areas at the same time?

Skill 3 (**Experimental and Research Design**) questions ask:

- Let's forget about the science content for a while. Could you give some insight into the experimental or research methods involved in this situation?

Skill 4 (**Data and Statistical Analysis**) questions ask:

- Let's forget about the science content for a while. Could you accurately read some graphs and tables for a moment? Could you make some conclusions or extrapolations based on the information presented?

Critical Analysis and Reasoning Skills (CARS)

The *Critical Analysis and Reasoning Skills* (CARS) section of the MCAT tests three discrete families of textual reasoning skills; each of these families requires a higher level of reasoning than the last. Those three skills are as follows:

1. *Foundations of Comprehension* (30 percent of questions)
2. *Reasoning Within the Text* (30 percent of questions)
3. *Reasoning Beyond the Text* (40 percent of questions)

These three categories of skills are tested through nine humanities- and social sciences-themed passages, with approximately 5 to 7 questions per passage. Let's take a more in-depth look into these three types. Again, the bullet points of specific objectives for each of the CARS are taken directly from the *Official Guide to the MCAT Exam*; the descriptions of what these behaviors mean and sample question stems, however, are written by Kaplan.

Foundations of Comprehension

Questions in this category will ask for basic facts and simple inferences about the passage; the questions themselves will be similar to those seen on reading comprehension sections of other standardized exams like the SAT® and ACT®. *Foundations of Comprehension* questions will require you to do the following:

- Understand the basic components of the text
- Infer meaning from rhetorical devices, word choice, and text structure

This covers a wide range of question skills (Summarize Text, Recognize Opinion, Paraphrase Detail, and Interpret Meaning) but finding the correct answer to all *Foundations of Comprehension* questions will follow from a basic understanding of the passage and the point of view of its author (and occasionally that of other voices in the passage). Because these questions tend to avoid digging too deeply into the passage, Kaplan calls these *surface* questions.

Here are some sample *Foundations of Comprehension* question stems:

- **Summarize Text**—The author's primary thesis in this passage is:
- **Recognize Opinion**—Based on the information in the second paragraph, which of the following is the most accurate summary of the opinion held by Schubert's critics?
- **Paraphrase Detail**—According to the passage, which of the following is FALSE about literary reviews in the 1920s?
- **Interpret Meaning**—The word "obscure" (paragraph 3), when used in reference to the historian's actions, most nearly means:

Reasoning Within the Text

While *Foundations of Comprehension* questions will usually depend on interpreting a single piece of information in the passage or understanding the passage as a whole, *Reasoning Within the Text* questions will typically require you to infer unstated parts of arguments or bring together two disparate pieces of the passage. *Reasoning Within the Text* questions will require you to:

- Integrate different components of the text to draw relevant conclusions

In other words, questions in this type often ask either *How do these two details relate to one another?* or *What else must be true that the author didn't say?* The CARS section will also ask you to judge certain parts of the passage or even judge the author. These questions, which fall under the *Reasoning Within the Text* skill, can ask you to identify authorial bias, evaluate the credibility of cited sources, determine the logical soundness of an argument, or search for relevant evidence in the passage to support a given conclusion. In all, this category includes Inference and Strengthen–Weaken (Within the Passage) questions, as well as a smattering of related—but rare—question types. This category, which Kaplan refers to as *deep* questions because of their tendency to venture into the deep reasoning of the passage, encompasses the following skills: Describe Purpose, Evaluate Reasoning, and Make Deduction.

Here are some sample *Reasoning Within the Text* question stems:

- **Describe Purpose**—The author's discussion of the effect of socioeconomic status on social mobility primarily serves which of the following functions?
- **Evaluate Reasoning**—Which of the following facts is used in the passage as the most prominent piece of evidence in favor of the author's conclusions?
- **Make Deduction**—In putting together the argument in the passage, the author most likely assumes:

Reasoning Beyond the Text

The distinguishing factor of *Reasoning Beyond the Text* questions is in the title of the category: the word *Beyond*. Questions of this type, which make up a larger share of the CARS section than questions from either of the other two types, will always introduce a completely new situation that was not present in the passage itself; these questions will ask you to determine how one influences the other. *Reasoning Beyond the Text* questions will require you to:

- Apply or extrapolate ideas from the passage to new contexts
- Assess the impact of introducing new factors, information, or conditions to ideas from the passage

Because they always introduce ideas not discussed in the passage, Kaplan refers to these as *new info* questions. They test the following skills: Anticipate Response, Predict Outcome/Explanation, Imagine Example/Analogy, and Strengthen/Weaken Argument.

Here are some sample *Reasoning Beyond the Text* question stems:

- **Anticipate Response**—If a document were located that demonstrated Berlioz intended to include a chorus of at least 700 in his *Grande Messe des Mortes*, how would the author likely respond?
- **Imagine Example/Analogy**—Which of the following is the best example of a "virtuous rebellion," as it is defined in the passage?
- **Predict Outcome/Explanation**—Extending the author's discussion of ancient Greek history, a conflict between a democracy and an oligarchy would most likely result in:
- **Strengthen/Weaken Argument**—Which of the following sentences, if added to the end of the passage, would most WEAKEN the author's conclusions in the last paragraph?

CARS Summary

Through the *Foundations of Comprehension* category of skills, the CARS section tests many of the reading skills you have been building on since grade school, albeit in the context of very challenging doctorate-level passages. But through the two other categories (*Reasoning Within the Text* and *Reasoning Beyond the Text*), the MCAT demands that you understand the deep structure of passages and the arguments within them at an advanced level. And, of course, all of this is tested under very tight timing restrictions: only 102 seconds per question—and that doesn't even include the time spent reading the passages.

Here's a quick reference guide to the three categories and 11 skills tested in CARS:

Foundations of Comprehension skills:

- Interpret Meaning: Use context to determine what a word/phrase from the passage is intended to communicate.
- Recognize Opinion: Identify what the author or someone else feels about a passage idea based on word choice or other context clues.
- Paraphrase Detail: Recognize a specific piece of information that is stated or strongly implied at one location in the passage.
- Summarize Text: Articulate the main idea of the passage or of a part of it.

Reasoning Within the Text skills:

- Describe Purpose: Identify why the author wrote the passage or a part of it.
- Evaluate Reasoning: Characterize logical connections between ideas in the passage.
- Make Deduction: Infer a claim that follows from multiple parts of the passage, such as an assumption in an argument.

Reasoning Beyond the Text skills:

- Anticipate Response: Identify what the author or someone else would feel/say/do about a new situation based on its similarities to passage ideas.
- Predict Outcome/Explanation: Apply causal reasoning or another connection from the passage to a new situation.
- Strengthen/Weaken Argument: Characterize the logical relationship between a new claim and arguments from the passage.
- Imagine Example/Analogy: Identify new examples of categories defined in the passage or analogies of passage concepts.

Scoring

Each of the four sections of the MCAT is scored between 118 and 132, with the median at approximately 125. This means the total score ranges from 472 to 528, with the median at about 500. Why such peculiar numbers? The AAMC stresses that this scale emphasizes the importance of the central portion of the score distribution, where most students score (around 125 per section, or 500 total), rather than putting undue focus on the high end of the scale.

Note that there is no wrong answer penalty on the MCAT, so you should select an answer for every question—even if it is only a guess.

The AAMC has released the 2022–2024 correlation between scaled score and percentile, as shown on the following page. It should be noted that the percentile scale is adjusted and renormalized over time and thus can shift slightly from year to year. Percentile rank updates are released by the AAMC around May 1 of each year.

Total Score	Percentile	Total Score	Percentile
528	100	499	46
527	100	498	42
526	100	497	39
525	100	496	36
524	100	495	34
523	99	494	31
522	99	493	28
521	98	492	25
520	97	491	23
519	96	490	21
518	95	489	18
517	94	488	16
516	92	487	14
515	91	486	12
514	89	485	11
513	87	484	9
512	84	483	8
511	82	482	6
510	79	481	5
509	77	480	4
508	74	479	3
507	71	478	2
506	68	477	2
505	65	476	1
504	62	475	1
503	58	474	<1
502	55	473	<1
501	52	472	<1
500	49		

Source: AAMC. 2025. Summary of MCAT Total and Section Scores. Accessed October 2025.
https://students-residents.aamc.org/mcat-research-and-data/percentile-ranks-mcat-exam

Further information on score reporting is included at the end of the next section (see *After Your Test*).

MCAT Policies and Procedures

We strongly encourage you to download the latest copy of *MCAT® Essentials*, available on the AAMC's website, to ensure that you have the latest information about registration and Test Day policies and procedures; this document is updated annually. A brief summary of some of the most important rules is provided here.

MCAT Registration

The only way to register for the MCAT is online. You can access AAMC's registration system at **www.aamc.org/mcat**.

The AAMC posts the schedule of testing, registration, and score release dates in the fall before the MCAT testing year, which runs from January into September. See the AAMC's website for the exact dates that registration opens each year. There is one standard registration fee, but the fee for changing your test date or test center increases the closer you get to your MCAT.

Fees and the Fee Assistance Program (FAP)

Payment for test registration must be made by American Express, Discover, MasterCard, or VISA. As described earlier, the fee for rescheduling your exam or changing your testing center increases as one approaches Test Day. In addition, it is not uncommon for test centers to fill up well in advance of the registration deadline. For these reasons, we recommend identifying your preferred Test Day as soon as possible and registering. There are ancillary benefits to having a set Test Day, as well: when you know the date you're working toward, you'll study harder and are less likely to keep pushing back the exam. The AAMC offers a Fee Assistance Program (FAP) for students with financial hardship to help reduce the cost of taking the MCAT, as well as for the American Medical College Application Service (AMCAS®) application. Further information on the FAP can be found at **www.aamc.org/students/applying/fap**.

Testing Security

On Test Day, you will be required to present a qualifying form of ID. Generally, a current driver's license or United States passport will be sufficient (consult the AAMC website for the full list of qualifying criteria). When registering, take care to spell your first and last names (middle names, suffixes, and prefixes are not required and will not be verified on Test Day) precisely the same as they appear on this ID; failure to provide this ID at the test center or differences in spelling between your registration and ID will be considered a "no-show," and you will not receive a refund for the exam.

During Test Day registration, other identity data collected may include: a digital palm vein scan, a Test Day photo, a digitization of your valid ID, and signatures. Some testing centers may use a metal detection wand to ensure that no prohibited items are brought into the testing room. Prohibited items include all electronic devices, including watches and timers, calculators, cell phones, and any and all forms of recording equipment; food, drinks (including water), and cigarettes or other smoking paraphernalia; hats and scarves (except for religious purposes); and books, notes, or other study materials. If you require a medical device, such as an insulin pump or pacemaker, you must apply for accommodated testing. During breaks, you are allowed access to food and drink, but not to electronic devices, including cell phones.

Testing centers are under video surveillance and the AAMC does not take potential violations of testing security lightly. The bottom line: *know the rules and don't break them.*

Accommodations

Students with disabilities or medical conditions can apply for accommodated testing. Documentation of the disability or condition is required, and requests may take two months—or more—to be approved. For this reason, it is recommended that you begin the process of applying for accommodated testing as early as possible. More information on applying for accommodated testing can be found at **www.aamc.org/students/applying/mcat/accommodations**.

After Your Test

When your MCAT is all over, no matter how you feel you did, be good to yourself when you leave the test center. Celebrate! Take a nap. Watch a movie. Get some exercise. Plan a trip or outing. Call up all of your neglected friends or message them on social media. Go out for snacks or drinks with people you like. Whatever you do, make sure that it has absolutely nothing to do with thinking too hard—you deserve some rest and relaxation.

Perhaps most importantly, do not discuss specific details about the test with anyone. For one, it is important to let go of the stress of Test Day, and reliving your exam only inhibits you from being able to do so. But more significantly, the Examinee Agreement you sign at the beginning of your exam specifically prohibits you from discussing or disclosing exam content. The AAMC is known to seek out individuals who violate this agreement and retains the right to prosecute these individuals at their discretion. This means that you should not, under any circumstances, discuss the exam in person or over the phone with other individuals—including us at Kaplan—or post information or questions about exam content to Facebook, Student Doctor Network, or other online social media. You are permitted to comment on your "general exam experience," including how you felt about the exam overall or an individual section, but this is a fine line. In summary: *if you're not certain whether you can discuss an aspect of the test or not, just don't do it!* Do not let a silly Facebook post stop you from becoming the doctor you deserve to be.

Scores are typically released approximately one month after Test Day. The release is staggered during the afternoon and evening, ending at 5 p.m. Eastern Standard Time. This means that not all examinees receive their scores at exactly the same time. Your score report will include a scaled score for each section between 118 and 132, as well as your total combined score between 472 and 528. These scores are given as confidence intervals. For each section, the confidence interval is approximately the given score ± 1; for the total score, it is approximately the given score ± 2. You will also be given the corresponding percentile rank for each of these section scores and the total score.

AAMC Contact Information

For further questions, contact the MCAT team at the Association of American Medical Colleges:

MCAT Resource Center
Association of American Medical Colleges
www.aamc.org/mcat
(202) 828-0600
www.aamc.org/contactmcat

HOW THIS BOOK WAS CREATED

The *Kaplan MCAT Review* project began shortly after the release of the *Preview Guide for the MCAT 2015 Exam*, 2nd edition. Through thorough analysis by our staff psychometricians, we were able to analyze the relative yield of the different topics on the MCAT, and we began constructing tables of contents for the books of the *Kaplan MCAT Review* series. A dedicated staff of 30 writers, 7 editors, and 32 proofreaders worked over 5,000 combined hours to produce these books. The format of the books was heavily influenced by weekly meetings with Kaplan's learning-science team.

In the years since this book was created, a number of opportunities for expansion and improvement have occurred. This edition is the product of our largest revision since the series' creation more than a decade ago.

To better accommodate students who prefer learning visually, our six science titles have added more than 500 new images and updated more than a hundred existing figures. All of these new images were chosen by an expert team of MCAT faculty members, led by veteran teachers and tutors with advanced science or medical degrees. Our objective with these new images was not to add visual flair but to enhance student learning outcomes. Toward that end, our team of medical illustrators partnered with our MCAT experts to ensure scientific accuracy and relevance for the exam.

On top of this extensive science image expansion, we completely rewrote *Critical Analysis and Reasoning Skills Review* based on what we've learned from more than ten years of helping students improve on the CARS section in our classrooms. In addition to this collective experience, internal data suggests that our new approach is more effective at helping students get higher CARS scores. Our streamlined and simplified CARS strategies accompany an extended focus on the critical thinking skills tested on the exam, best embodied by our new Skillbuilder activities that enable targeted skill practice in a lower pressure setting.

These books were submitted for publication in April 2026. For any updates after this date, please visit www.kaptest.com/pages/retail-book-corrections-and-updates.

If you have any questions about the content presented here, email KaplanMCATfeedback@kaplan.com. For other questions not related to content, email booksupport@kaplan.com.

Each book has been vetted through at least ten rounds of review. To that end, the information presented in these books is true and accurate to the best of our knowledge. Still, your feedback helps us improve our prep materials. Please notify us of any inaccuracies or errors in the books by sending an email to KaplanMCAT-feedback@kaplan.com.

USING THIS BOOK

Kaplan MCAT Critical Analysis and Reasoning Skills Review, and the other six books in the *Kaplan MCAT Review* series, bring the Kaplan classroom experience to you—right in your home, at your convenience. This book offers the same Kaplan strategies and practice that make Kaplan the #1 choice for MCAT prep.

This book is designed to help you review the *Critical Analysis and Reasoning Skills* section of the MCAT. Unlike other books in this MCAT series, there is no content to review for the *Critical Analysis and Reasoning Skills* section. The questions are written in such a way that they do not presume any prior fund of knowledge. Instead, CARS is a test of skill and strategy. This book will help you build your critical thinking skills with targeted practice drills and passages. It will also help you develop a strategic toolkit to manage passages, questions, and every aspect of the CARS section.

Learning Objectives

At the beginning of each chapter, you'll find a short list of objectives describing the skills and strategies covered within that chapter. Learning objectives for these texts were developed in conjunction with Kaplan's learning science team. They have been designed specifically to focus your attention on tasks and concepts that are likely to be relevant to your MCAT testing experience. These learning objectives will function as a means to guide your review of the chapter and indicate what information and relationships you should be focused on within each chapter. Before starting each chapter, read these learning objectives carefully. They will not only allow you to assess your existing familiarity with the content of the chapter, but also provide a goal-oriented focus for your studying experience.

Sidebars

The following is a guide to the four types of sidebars you'll find in *Kaplan MCAT Critical Analysis and Reasoning Skills Review*:

- **Bridge:** These sidebars create connections between CARS topics that appear in multiple chapters throughout the book.
- **Key Concept:** These sidebars draw attention to the most important takeaways in a given topic, and they sometimes offer synopses or overviews of complex information.
- **MCAT Expertise:** These sidebars point out how skills may be tested on the MCAT or offer key strategy points and test-taking tips that you should apply on Test Day.
- **Real World:** These sidebars illustrate how a concept in the text relates to the practice of medicine or the world at large.

Additional guidance on how to use the different chapters of this book can be found in Chapter 1. In the end, this is your book, so write in the margins, draw diagrams, highlight the key points—do whatever is necessary to help you get that higher score. We look forward to working with you as you achieve your dreams and become the doctor you deserve to be!

Online Resources

In addition to the resources located within this text, you also have online resources awaiting you. If you purchased this book as part of a 7-book set, scan the QR code that appears on your slipcase (the illustrated box that originally contained the books) and enter your unique access code, which appears on a sticker on the front of that slipcase. If you purchased this book separately, book-specific resources are available at **www.kaptest.com/booksonline**. Make sure to log on and take advantage of free practice and other resources!

Please note that access to the online resources is limited to the original owner of this book.

STUDYING FOR THE MCAT

The first year of medical school is a frenzied experience for most students. To meet the requirements of a rigorous work schedule, students either learn to prioritize their time or else fall hopelessly behind. It's no surprise, then, that the MCAT, the test specifically designed to predict success in medical school, is a high-speed, time-intensive test. The MCAT demands excellent time-management skills, endurance, and grace under pressure both during the test as well as while preparing for it. Having a solid plan of attack and sticking with it are key to giving you the confidence and structure you need to succeed.

Creating a Study Plan

The best time to create a study plan is at the beginning of your MCAT preparation. If you don't already use a calendar, you will want to start. You can purchase a planner, print out a free calendar from the Internet, use a built-in calendar or app on one of your smart devices, or keep track using an interactive online calendar. Pick the option that is most practical for you and that you are most likely to use consistently. If you purchased this book new as part of a set, your online resources come with a study plan to space out your readings, chapter quizzes, full-length practice tests, and other study materials (see the previous page for how to log on).

Once you have a calendar, you'll be able to start planning your study schedule with the following steps:

1. **Fill in your obligations and choose a day off.**

   Write in all your school, extracurricular, and work obligations first: class sessions, work shifts, and meetings that you must attend. Then add in your personal obligations: appointments, lunch dates, family and social time, etc. Making an appointment in your calendar for hanging out with friends or going to the movies may seem strange at first, but planning social activities in advance will help you achieve a balance between personal and professional obligations even as life gets busy. Having a happy balance allows you to be more focused and productive when it comes time to study, so stay well-rounded and don't neglect anything that is important to you.

   In addition to scheduling your personal and professional obligations, you should also plan your time off. Taking some time off is just as important as studying. Kaplan recommends taking at least one full day off per week, ideally from all your study obligations but at minimum from studying for the MCAT.

2. **Add in study blocks around your obligations.**

   Once you have established your calendar's framework, add in study blocks around your obligations, keeping your study schedule as consistent as possible across days and across weeks. Studying at the same time of day as your official test is ideal for promoting recall, but if that's not possible, then fit in study blocks wherever you can.

   To make your studying as efficient as possible, block out short, frequent periods of study time throughout the week. From a learning perspective, studying one hour per day for six days per week is much more valuable than studying for six hours all at once one day per week. Specifically, Kaplan recommends studying for no longer than three hours in one sitting. Within those three-hour blocks, also plan to take ten-minute breaks every hour. Use these breaks to get up from your seat, do some quick stretches, get a snack and drink, and clear your mind. Although ten minutes of break for every 50 minutes of studying may sound like a lot, these breaks will allow you to deal with distractions and rest your brain so that, during the 50-minute study blocks, you can remain fully engaged and completely focused.

3. **Add in your full-length practice tests.**

   Next, you'll want to add in full-length practice tests. You'll want to take one test very early in your prep and then spread your remaining full-length practice tests evenly between now and your test date. Staggering tests in this way allows you to form a baseline for comparison and to determine which areas to focus on right away, while also providing realistic feedback throughout your prep as to how you will perform on Test Day.

When planning your calendar, aim to finish your full-length practice tests and the majority of your studying by one week before Test Day, which will allow you to spend that final week completing a final review of what you already know. In your online resources, you'll find sample study calendars for several different Test Day timelines to use as a starting point. The sample calendars may include more focus than you need in some areas, and less in others, and it may not fit your timeline to Test Day. You will need to customize your study calendar to your needs using the steps above.

The total amount of time you spend studying each week will depend on your schedule, your personal prep needs, and your time to Test Day, but it is recommended that you spend somewhere in the range of 300–350 hours preparing before taking the official MCAT. One way you could break this down is to study for three hours per day, six days per week, for four months, but this is just one approach. You might study six days per week for more than three hours per day. You might study over a longer period of time if you don't have much time to study each week. No matter what your plan is, ensure you complete enough practice to feel completely comfortable with the MCAT and its content. A good sign you're ready for Test Day is when you begin to earn your goal score consistently in practice.

How to Study

The MCAT covers a large amount of material and studying for Test Day can initially seem daunting. To combat this, we have some tips for how to take control of your studying and make the most of your time.

Goal Setting

To take control of the amount of content and practice required to do well on the MCAT, break the content down into specific goals for each week instead of attempting to approach the test as a whole. A goal of "I want to increase my overall score by 5 points" is too big, abstract, and difficult to measure on the small scale. More reasonable goals are "I will read two chapters each day this week." Goals like this are much less overwhelming and help break studying into manageable pieces.

Active Reading

Don't just passively read this book. Instead, read actively. Highlighting can be an excellent tool, but use it sparingly: highlighting every sentence isn't active reading, it's coloring. Frequently stop and ask yourself questions while you read (e.g., *What is the main point? How does this fit into the overall scheme of things? Could I thoroughly explain this to someone else?*). By making connections and focusing on the grander scheme, not only will you ensure you know the essential content, but you also prepare yourself for the level of critical thinking required by the MCAT. See Chapter 4 of this book for more on active reading.

Focus on Areas of Greatest Opportunity

If you are limited by only having a minimal amount of time to prepare before Test Day, focus on your biggest areas of opportunity first. Areas of opportunity are topic areas that are highly tested and that you have not yet mastered. You likely won't have time to take detailed notes for every page of these books; instead, use your results from practice materials to determine which areas are your biggest opportunities and seek those out. After you've taken a full-length test, make sure you are using your performance report to best identify areas of opportunity. Skim over content matter for which you are already demonstrating proficiency, pausing to read more thoroughly when something looks unfamiliar or particularly difficult.

Practice, Review, and Tracking

Leave time to review your practice questions and full-length tests. You may be tempted, after practicing, to push ahead and cover new material as quickly as possible, but failing to schedule ample time for review will actually throw away your greatest opportunity to improve your performance. The brain rarely remembers anything it sees or does only once. When you carefully review the questions you've solved (and the explanations for them), the process of retrieving that information reopens and reinforces the connections you've built in your brain. This builds long-term retention and repeatable skill sets—exactly what you need to beat the MCAT!

For more on practice and review, including how to construct powerful review tools like Why I Missed It (WIMI) and How I'll Fix It (HIFI) sheets, see Chapter 7 of this book.

Where to Study

One often-overlooked aspect of studying is the environment where the learning actually occurs. Although studying at home is many students' first choice, several problems can arise in this environment, chief of which are distractions. Studying can be a mentally draining process, so as time passes, these distractions become ever more tempting as escape routes. Although you may have considerable willpower, there's no reason to make staying focused harder than it needs to be. Instead of studying at home, head to a library, quiet coffee shop, or another new location whenever possible. This will eliminate many of the usual distractions and also promote efficient studying; instead of studying off and on at home over the course of an entire day, you can stay at the library for three hours of effective studying and enjoy the rest of the day off from the MCAT.

No matter where you study, make your practice as much like Test Day as possible. Just as is required during the official test, don't have snacks or chew gum during your study blocks. Turn off your music, television, and phone. Practice on the computer with your online resources to simulate the computer-based test environment. When completing practice questions, do your work on scratch paper or noteboard sheets rather than writing directly on any printed materials since you won't have that option on Test Day. Because memory is tied to all of your senses, the more test-like you can make your studying environment, the easier it will be on Test Day to recall the information you're putting in so much work to learn.

UNIT 1

CARS STRATEGY

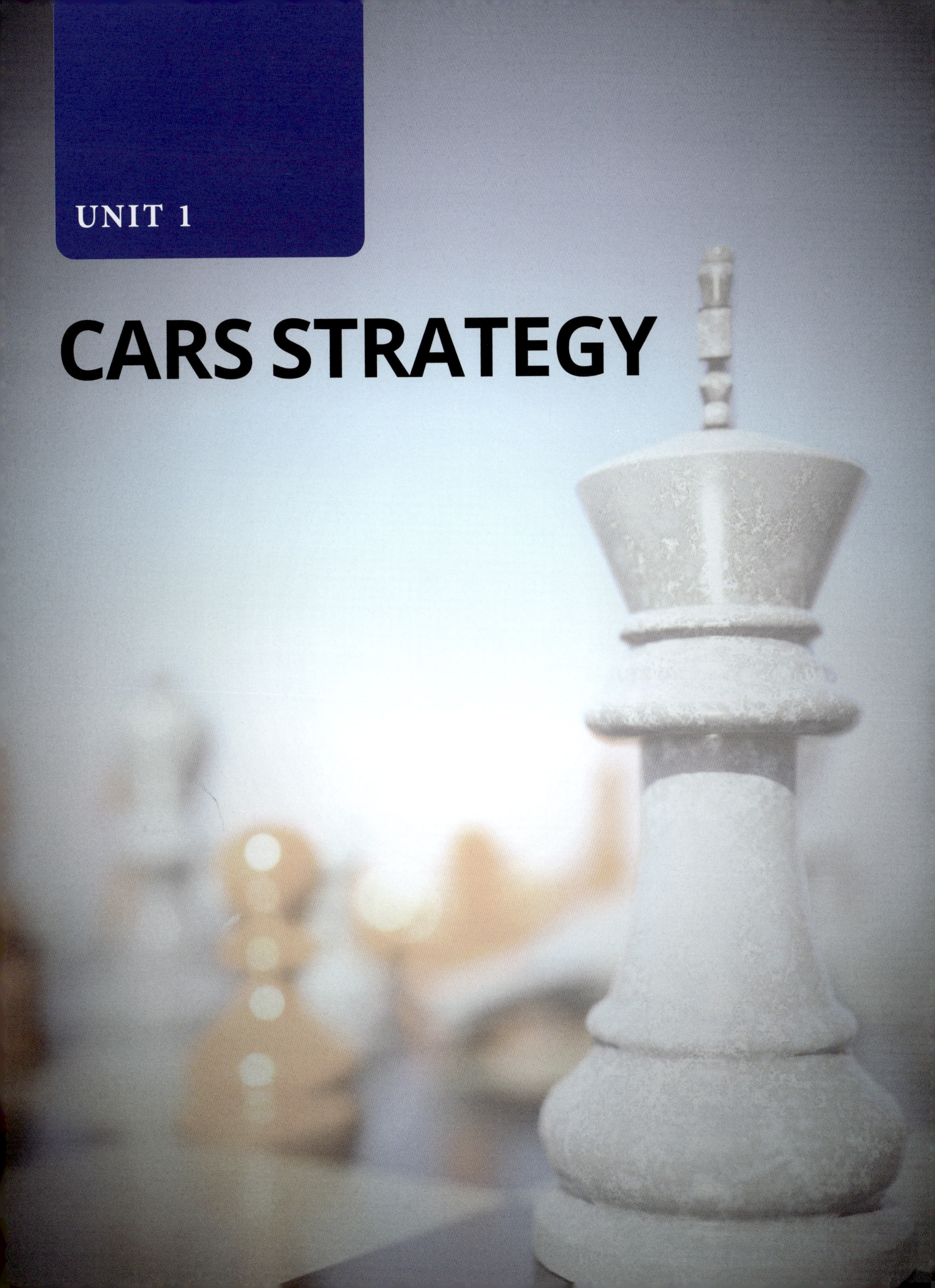

CHAPTER 1

ABOUT CARS

In This Chapter

Introduction 3
1.1 Section Format 4
1.2 What Does CARS Test? 5
Foundations of Comprehension 5
Reasoning Within the Text 6
Reasoning Beyond the Text 6
1.3 Using This Book to Prepare for CARS 7
Conclusion 8
Skill and Strategy Summary 8

LEARNING OBJECTIVES

After Chapter 1, you will be able to:

- Recognize the standardized and predictable features of the CARS section
- Identify the official categories of CARS passages and questions
- Appreciate what CARS tests and why it is included on the MCAT
- Devise a plan for using this book to prepare for the CARS section

Introduction

You enter the examination room to find your first patient of the day, a middle-aged woman who glances uneasily in your direction when you come through the door. Before you can even introduce yourself, she tells you, "Doc, I've been feeling so tired lately."

As a physician, your mind immediately clicks into a mode that goes far beyond those simple words. "Tired" could mean a thousand things, so you begin to "read" the situation, much like a detective sifting through clues. "Tell me more about this fatigue," you begin. "Is it worse in the morning or evening? Does it prevent you from doing things you normally enjoy? Have you noticed any other changes? Anything at all?"

You intently observe not just what she says in response, but how she says it: the slight hesitation before mentioning a nearly overlooked detail, the way her eyes flick away when discussing a particular stressor. You notice her complexion, the tone of her voice, her energy level while speaking, the subtle cues that words alone don't convey. Is her "tiredness" accompanied by shortness of breath? A recent, unexplained weight loss? A low mood that colors her every response?

Each question, each observation, adds a layer to your understanding, helping you piece together a complex puzzle. You're looking for patterns, for underlying causes, for the story hidden beneath the surface complaint.

This deep, analytical "reading"—the kind that separates surface-level impressions from true understanding—isn't just for the clinic. It's a skill you'll actively use when you encounter the Critical Analysis and Reasoning Skills, or CARS, section of the MCAT. Here, your "patients" are passages, complex texts excerpted from academic journals and books in the humanities and social sciences. And just like the physician in the exam room, your task is to uncover the deeper issues that lie beneath the surface presentation.

The CARS section rewards the same type of interrogation that physicians use to uncover patient pathologies. What is the author truly arguing, beyond their explicit statements? What assumptions are they making? What evidence do they present, and how strong is it? What is their tone, and how does it shape their message?

This book will help you learn to "listen" to the author's voice, identify the nuances in their arguments, and see how different pieces of information connect to form a larger picture. The CARS section, at its heart, tests your ability to critically analyze information, reason through complex arguments, and comprehend meaning that isn't always immediately obvious—skills that are directly involved in the diagnostic reasoning of an insightful physician.

1.1 Section Format

The journey to master the CARS section begins with understanding what you're up against. Like all of the other sections on the MCAT, CARS scores are scaled to values ranging from 118 to 132. However, CARS has consistently had the lowest average score (below 125) of any section on the test for more than a decade, according to data from the Association of American Medical Colleges (AAMC), the maker of the MCAT. On top of that, CARS also has the smallest standard deviation, meaning that fewer students are reaching top scores of 130+. In short, CARS is statistically the most difficult section on the MCAT.

Fortunately, this difficulty means that a high score on the CARS section can really distinguish you as a med school applicant. And contrary to naysayers who contend that critical thinking ability is just something you're born with (or not), you can improve at CARS with the right mindset and preparation.

For one thing, CARS is predictable. While every passage and question is unique, CARS is nevertheless a standardized test that uses the same basic format every time. There are always nine passages and 53 questions, and you always have 90 minutes to complete them. Passages are always about the same length, usually between 500 and 600 words. The number of questions varies per passage, but that number is usually between five and seven. Table 1.1 summarizes these basic facts about CARS.

Time Limit	90 minutes
Total Number of Passages	9 passages
Passage Length	500–600 words
Total Number of Questions	53 questions
Number of Questions per Passage	5–7 questions

Table 1.1 CARS Section Basic Facts

Every passage in the CARS section is different, but they are always taken from the same set of academic fields. About half of the passages are excerpts from journal articles or books in **humanities** disciplines, while the other half come from sources in **social sciences**. Table 1.2 reproduces the official list of CARS passage disciplines provided by the AAMC.

Humanities	Social Sciences
Architecture	Anthropology
Art	Archaeology
Dance	Economics
Ethics	Education
Literature	Geography
Music	History
Philosophy	Linguistics
Popular Culture	Political Science
Religion	Population Health
Theater	Psychology
Studies of Diverse Cultures	Sociology
	Studies of Diverse Cultures

Table 1.2 Humanities and Social Sciences Disciplines in the CARS Section
Source: AAMC. 2020. *What's on the MCAT® Exam?* Accessed June 2025.
https://students-residents.aamc.org/media/9261/download

1.2 What Does CARS Test?

So the AAMC does not expect you to be an expert at everything to succeed in the CARS section. Instead, the situation is more like the story at the beginning of this chapter: rather than merely recalling facts from a textbook, the skilled physician interprets and analyzes information in real time.

As the name "Critical Analysis and Reasoning Skills" suggests, the CARS section is ultimately a test of your critical thinking abilities. In fact, the test maker has identified three broad categories of abilities, which Kaplan has further subdivided into 11 specific skills. These skills are covered in depth in later chapters of this book, but for now it's worth previewing the AAMC's official three skill types: Foundations of Comprehension, Reasoning Within the Text, and Reasoning Beyond the Text.

Foundations of Comprehension

Foundations of Comprehension (**FOC**) is about understanding the basic meaning of the passage. Can you grasp what the author is saying, identify the main topics, and understand how different ideas are connected at a fundamental level? FOC questions measure whether you can accurately summarize key points, define terms as they are used in the passage, and generally demonstrate that you've understood the author's direct message. Questions testing this skill category will be similar to ones you've likely encountered in other standardized

MCAT EXPERTISE

Don't be intimidated by the wide range of topics! The variety ensures that no single educational background gives an unfair advantage. Whether you're reading about ancient philosophy or modern economic policy, your ability to comprehend, analyze, and reason is still being tested in the same way. Your focus should be on honing those critical reading skills, not on trying to become an expert in every field appearing in CARS passages.

tests of reading comprehension, such as the Reading sections of the SAT and ACT.

Because the vast majority of FOC questions involve paraphrasing stated details or other more straightforward tasks, Kaplan describes these as **surface questions**. In fairness, some of these questions may require you to dig a little more deeply into the passage, but they generally lack the complexity found in the other two types. Consequently, when you see these questions on Test Day, you will generally want to tackle them right away.

Reasoning Within the Text

The skills in this category involve a more subtle analysis of the passage. It's not just about what the author says, but how they say it and why. **Reasoning Within the Text** (**RWT**) includes analyzing the arguments presented, evaluating the evidence offered, and understanding the relationships between different passage ideas. You'll be asked to make connections between disparate parts of the passage, analyze the structure and strength of passage arguments, and uncover the author's motivations for including different pieces of information.

RWT questions are generally more complex than FOC questions, and answering them often involves a more elaborate process, so Kaplan characterizes these as **deep questions**. Many of these questions are better to save for later in a question set, but the Kaplan strategies can empower you to tackle some of these with less struggle. For example, if you use the Kaplan Method for CARS Passages to uncover the author's intentions as you actively read the passage, then you'll be empowered on Test Day to answer RWT questions about author purpose right away.

Reasoning Beyond the Text

While the first two skill types focus exclusively on the content of the passage, the third and final skill category measures how well you can handle something unexpected: **Reasoning Beyond the Text** (**RBT**) questions always include some kind of new information. About half of these questions ask you about how the new information affects the passage as written, while the other half require you to go in the opposite direction, analyzing how passage ideas would apply in a new scenario. The new information can appear in the question stem, answer choices, or both.

Unlike FOC and RWT, each of which comprises about 30% of CARS questions, RBT accounts for 40%. This skill category is the most tested one in CARS because it best represents how physicians apply their critical thinking skills, integrating new information that comes from patients (first-hand reports, clinical observations, lab test results, etc.) with the vast body of knowledge that comes from medical education and training.

BRIDGE

Kaplan has identified four specific skills within Foundations of Comprehension, and this book devotes a chapter to each of them:

- Chapter 8: Interpret Meaning
- Chapter 9: Recognize Opinion
- Chapter 10: Paraphrase Detail
- Chapter 11: Summarize Text

In addition, if you'd like to practice the whole range of FOC skills, check out the targeted passage sets provided in Chapter 12.

BRIDGE

For Reasoning Within the Text, Kaplan has uncovered three key skills, discussed later in this book:

- Chapter 13: Describe Purpose
- Chapter 14: Evaluate Reasoning
- Chapter 15: Make Deduction

For practice in all three of these skills, check out the passage sets in Chapter 16.

In many ways, RBT is the easiest skill type to recognize in a question because it always involves ideas that aren't directly mentioned in the passage. That's why Kaplan characterizes these as **new info questions**. More than the other categories, RBT questions are usually best saved for later in a question set. Making connections between a new idea addressed in the question and the existing ideas in the passage is often tricky, requiring you to identify points of similarity that aren't always obvious.

BRIDGE

Reasoning Beyond the Text contains four skills, which can be found in the following chapters:

- Chapter 17: Anticipate Response
- Chapter 18: Predict Outcome/Explanation
- Chapter 19: Strengthen/ Weaken Argument
- Chapter 20: Imagine Example/Analogy

Finally, Chapter 21 contains passages that exclusively test these four skills for targeted RBT practice.

1.3 Using This Book to Prepare for CARS

So now that you have a more comprehensive picture of what's tested in CARS, you might be wondering what you have to do to prepare and how this book can help. *CARS Review* is divided into five units, as summarized in Table 1.3.

Humanities	Social Sciences
Unit 1	CARS Strategy
Unit 2	Foundations of Comprehension Skills
Unit 3	Reasoning Within the Text Skills
Unit 4	Reasoning Beyond the Text Skills
Unit 5	Additional Practice

Table 1.3 Units in *Critical Analysis and Reasoning Skills Review*

For most students, especially those just beginning CARS prep, you should start with Unit 1. This first chapter in Unit 1 has provided some basic information on the test to get you started.

Chapters 2–5 focus on the different facets of reading strategy: Chapter 2 provides an overview of the Kaplan Method for CARS Passages, Chapter 3 takes a deeper dive into keywords, Chapter 4 details the reading process known as elaborative interrogation, and Chapter 5 discusses the strategic options of outlining and highlighting.

The last two chapters in Unit 1 cover other aspects of CARS strategy. Chapter 6 shifts gears from passages to questions, giving an overview of the Kaplan Method for CARS Questions, a preview of the different question skills discussed later in the book, and an analysis of patterns in wrong answers. Chapter 7 discusses how to improve your CARS score, emphasizing the importance of practice and review.

Units 2–4 cover the real content tested on the CARS section—the skills. Most of the chapters in these units target a specific skill, defining it, providing examples, and giving you a chance to practice that skill in a targeted way, using a specially designed activity called a **Skillbuilder**. These Skillbuilders present a lower-stress way to practice the skill, using shorter passages and unique **active reading checks** that let you test your comprehension of each paragraph as you go, while serving up a set of test-like questions focusing on the targeted skill. Each unit concludes with a practice chapter with specially curated passage sets that exclusively test that unit's skills.

Finally, Unit 5 consists of additional test-like practice, spanning the full range of skills tested on the CARS section. Everyone, even more experienced CARS testers, will find value in the practice provided there.

Conclusion

Yes, CARS is weird compared to the rest of the MCAT, and yes, it's harder than the science sections, at least for most premeds. But, as outlined in this chapter, CARS is ultimately a predictable test, one whose patterns you can learn and master. On top of that, CARS is highly relevant for aspiring physicians because it models the type of critical thinking that doctors use every day. Most importantly, you too can succeed on the CARS section with the right guidance, the appropriate mindset, and a lot of practice, all of which this book aims to provide.

Skill and Strategy Summary

Section Format

- CARS is statistically the most difficult section of the MCAT, so a high score can significantly distinguish you as a med school applicant.
- CARS follows a predictable, standardized format.
  - You always have 90 minutes to complete 9 passages and 53 questions.
  - Passages are 500–600 words and include 5–7 questions.
- Passage topics are drawn from academic journals and books in the **humanities** and **social sciences**.

What Does CARS Test?

- CARS is a test of your critical thinking skills, many of which physicians use on a daily basis.
- The **Association of American Medical Colleges** (**AAMC**), the maker of the MCAT, defines three broad categories of skills in CARS.
  - **Foundations of Comprehension** (**FOC**): Account for 30% of CARS questions and test surface-level understanding of the passage and its author.
  - **Reasoning Within the Text** (**RWT**): Account for 30% of CARS questions and test deeper understanding of passage structure and argumentation.
  - **Reasoning Beyond the Text** (**RBT**): Account for 40% of CARS questions and test the ability to make connections between the passage and new information.

Using This Book to Prepare for CARS

- This book is organized into five units to systematically guide your CARS preparation.
  - Unit 1 covers CARS strategy, including passage strategy (Chapters 2–5), question strategy (Chapter 6), and strategies for improving your CARS score through practice and review (Chapter 7).
  - Units 2, 3, and 4 cover the specific AAMC skills, with a discussion of what the skills are, how they're tested, and how to approach questions on these skills strategically. Each skill chapter ends with a special **Skillbuilder** activity that includes **active reading checks** and test-like questions to help you train the skill. Each unit also contains one chapter of test-like practice that focuses on unit skills.
  - Unit 5 contains additional test-like practice targeting the full range of CARS skills.

CHAPTER 2

PASSAGE STRATEGY

In This Chapter

Introduction 9

2.1 Preview and Choose 10

Choice Factors 12

2.2 Read and Distill 12

Reading the Passage 13

Distilling the Passage 13

Conclusion 15

Skill and Strategy Summary 15

LEARNING OBJECTIVES

After Chapter 2, you will be able to:

- Distinguish the steps of Kaplan's PCRD method
- Deploy the Preview and Choose steps to use your time more efficiently and maximize point-scoring potential on the CARS section
- Follow the Read and Distill steps to enhance your comprehension of the passage and actively prepare to attack CARS questions

Introduction

You stand scrubbed in, gloved and gowned, beneath the bright lights of an operating room. On the table before you is a patient who needs a complex cardiac procedure. Do you simply pick up a scalpel and begin?

Of course not. Hours before you ever entered the OR, you were devising a precise strategy. You reviewed the patient's entire history, analyzed every angle of the CT scans and echocardiograms, and mapped out each step of the surgery, anticipating potential complications and preparing for them. In medicine, a successful outcome is rarely accidental; it is the result of a deliberate, well-executed plan.

Your approach to the CARS section demands the same level of strategic preparation. Walking into this 90-minute marathon of complex passages without a plan is like a surgeon walking into the OR without reviewing the patient's chart. You might make it through, but you're leaving the outcome to chance. The key to unlocking a higher CARS score is to trade that uncertainty for a systematic method—a reliable strategy that you can deploy on every passage, every time.

This chapter introduces the **Kaplan Method for CARS Passages**, a four-step strategy designed to give you that control. The method, which we abbreviate **PCRD**, stands for **P**review, **C**hoose, **R**ead, and **D**istill (see Figure 2.1). Think of it as your surgical plan for Test Day. It transforms you from a passive reader into an active, strategic test-taker, giving you a customized approach for the unique challenges of the MCAT.

The Kaplan Method for CARS Passages

PREVIEW for difficulty

Estimate difficulty based on topic and structure

CHOOSE when to read it

Decide whether to read the passage *now* or *later*

READ each paragraph actively

Use keywords to interrogate the text and identify the most important ideas in each paragraph

DISTILL the meaning of the passage

Capture the most important info from each paragraph in your own words or the author's words and determine why the passage was written

Figure 2.1 The Kaplan Method for CARS Passages

2.1 Preview and Choose

The timing on the CARS section is tight. With only 90 minutes for nine passages, you have 10 minutes per passage. Keep in mind, though, that this is just an average. If every passage and question set took exactly 10 minutes, then it really wouldn't matter what order you complete them in. You'd finish everything in 90 minutes regardless of what strategy you used.

Unfortunately, things aren't quite so simple. You may already recognize that some passages take you more time than others. Some passages are more challenging for just about everyone, and your personal comfort with a topic can also influence its difficulty for you. So what's the best approach when not every passage is equal?

To answer this question, consider a scenario with just two passages and a time limit of 20 minutes. Each of these passages has seven questions. One of the passages is hard, with difficult vocabulary, convoluted sentences, and a tough set of reasoning-heavy questions, while the other passage is shorter and more straightforward with questions of easy to moderate difficulty. How many more points is the hard passage worth than the easy passage?

The answer is zero. Both passages contain the same number of questions, so they're worth the same number of points. Even if you spent twice as much time on the harder passage, it would still be worth exactly the same as the easier one. But the situation is even worse than that: because you're likely to get fewer questions correct on the hard passage, you end up spending more time to get fewer points.

If that hard passage showed up before the easy passage, you'd lose a lot of time on it, potentially spending all 20 minutes before getting to the passage that offers quicker points. Even if you had some time left over, it likely wouldn't be enough to read the full passage and fully attempt each question (see Figure 2.2). Starting with the easier passage instead is the better

MCAT EXPERTISE

Even though every passage doesn't take exactly 10 minutes, that's actually a helpful guideline for managing your pacing on Test Day. Our recommendation is to check your timing after every other passage set, completing easier passages first to try to get ahead on the timing curve early in the section. Use the following guideposts:

- 2 passages complete: 70 minutes left
- 4 passages complete: 50 minutes left
- 6 passages complete: 30 minutes left
- 8 passages complete: 10 minutes left

If you find yourself behind at any point, you know you'll need to speed up on the next passage or two to get back on track.

option. You'll likely have 10 minutes or more left over after finishing it, letting you make some headway on the harder passage.

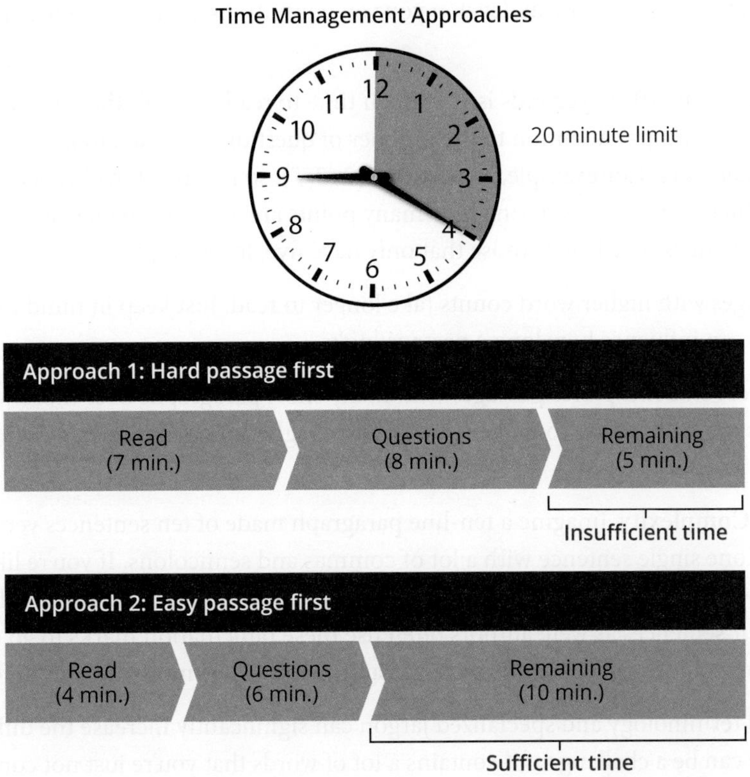

Figure 2.2 The Advantage of Triaging Hard Passages

The same considerations apply when you're dealing with nine passages as with two. Instead of just completing passages in order, you want to adopt a strategic approach: invest a small amount of time to decide whether each passage is likely to be a time-killer.

You might be familiar with the medical principle of **triage**, in which doctors prioritize which patients to help based on what will save the most lives. When applied to the MCAT, triage is the attempt to save as many points as possible to maximize your score. Triaging will empower you to save time-wasting passages for the end, where you can guess on them if you absolutely must. In fact, many students even find that, with their hardest passages, they wouldn't lose that many points just making wild guesses compared to how they'd do if they invested all the time necessary to understand them.

This is why the Preview and Choose steps of the Kaplan Method for CARS Passages are so essential. These steps put you in the driver's seat of the CARS section, so that you're completing passages in the order that makes the most sense to you, the one that maximizes your potential for points.

Here's how it works: when you first encounter a CARS passage, you want to spend about 10–15 seconds looking it over, getting a sense of its topic and difficulty level for you. That's the **Preview** step. Based on that impression, you answer one question: should I attempt this passage *now* or come back to it *later*? That's the **Choose** step.

Choice Factors

It can take a lot of practice before you get good at recognizing which passages will waste your time. Everyone has unique strengths and weaknesses, so watch out for patterns in passages that you struggle with as you continue your CARS prep. Based on Kaplan's extensive experience with MCAT students, the following factors are worth paying attention to, at least until you develop your own intuitions about which passages you're better off saving for later.

Number of Questions. While 10–15 seconds isn't enough time to read through the question stems and assess their difficulty, you can at least pay attention to the number of questions attached to a passage. Every passage lists the questions attached to it (for example, "Questions 32–37"), so if you're torn between doing a passage now and saving it for later, start by considering how many points are at stake: you'll generally want to complete passages with seven questions before those that only have five, for example.

Passage Length. Passages with higher word counts take longer to read. Just keep in mind that factors like the number of paragraphs can influence how long a passage looks.

Paragraph Length. Most students prefer passages with many short paragraphs over those with fewer long ones. Long paragraphs are both harder to make sense of and tougher to navigate when doing research for a question.

Sentence Length and Complexity. Imagine a ten-line paragraph made of ten sentences versus a ten-line paragraph made up of one single sentence with a lot of commas and semicolons. If you're like most students, you'll find it easier to work with shorter, less complex sentences. Watch out for passages with a lot of dashes and parentheses in their sentences as well: authors often use these punctuation marks to go off on tangents, so a large number of them would suggest that the passage's argument will be more difficult to follow.

Vocabulary. Technical terminology and specialized jargon can significantly increase the difficulty of a passage. Even a shorter passage can be a challenge if it contains a lot of words that you're just not comfortable with.

Topic. Many students find abstract topics like philosophy and political science more challenging, but ultimately the difficulty of a particular topic will come down to your own experiences and preferences. You might already have a sense of what topics you like and which you dislike, but this is another place where practice can improve your ability to diagnose tough passages. Review CARS passage sets you've completed and look out for topics where you miss more questions than normal: save those for later on Test Day.

Some of these factors, like the topic, can be difficult to evaluate in just 10 or 15 seconds, but it's essential that you practice until you can consistently make these decisions quickly. The number of passages you triage for later can vary, but we generally recommend that you try to limit it to fewer than half: in a full CARS section, that would be at most four passages. Triaging any more than that could end up being counterproductive for managing your time.

2.2 Read and Distill

The first two steps of the Kaplan Method for CARS Passages are all about planning and setting yourself up for success. Turning to the last two steps, the focus is now on execution.

The Read and Distill steps are distinct but complementary. You want to organize your reading in a way that maximizes your comprehension and minimizes the need for rereading. That's the **Read** step. At the same time, you want to prepare yourself for tackling the questions, building a mental model of the passage that will let you find any answer you need. That's the **Distill** step. Let's break these down.

Reading the Passage

Once you commit to a passage, you should aim to read it the same way that CARS experts read: actively, asking the author questions that you answer with the passage. This process is known in cognitive psychology as **elaborative interrogation**.

At its core, elaborative interrogation is the process of asking "how" and "why" questions to understand something more deeply. This technique can be applied more broadly than just in the CARS section. For example, while studying MCAT science content, instead of just memorizing facts, you can ask yourself "why is this true?" or "how does this make sense in the context of what I already know?"

Research shows that interrogation is effective because it forces you to engage in a deeper, more active level of processing. Instead of passively reading words on a page, you are actively making connections between the new ideas in the passage and your existing knowledge. This creates a richer, more interconnected "web" of knowledge in your brain, which makes information easier to comprehend and recall later. Interrogation is extremely effective in CARS, as long as you ensure this web sticks strictly to what the passage states or implies; outside information can lead to wrong answer traps in questions.

Applying interrogation to CARS, you'll ask yourself questions like the following:

- Why is the author telling us this?
- Why does the author believe this?
- How does this connect to what the author said before?
- Where is the author going with this?

This process of interrogation is made easier by paying close attention to **keywords**. These are words and short phrases that reveal a passage's structure and its author's intentions. For example, *Contrast keywords* like "however" and "but" signal a change in direction, while *Logic keywords* like "therefore" and "because" help you identify conclusions and evidence in the author's arguments.

BRIDGE

For more on elaborative interrogation, check out Chapter 4.

BRIDGE

For more on keywords, including distinct types and lists of examples, turn to Chapter 3.

Distilling the Passage

Practicing the Read step of the Kaplan Method, with its focus on keywords and interrogation, gives you the best shot at understanding the passage as you read it. But understanding the passage is only useful if it helps you answer more questions correctly. This is where the Distill step comes in.

In the typical distillation you do in a general chemistry lab, you separate a mixture by heating it until the most volatile components boil away, leaving behind a purer, more concentrated substance. The Distill step in the PCRD method works in precisely the same way. A CARS passage is a complex mixture of main ideas, supporting details, examples, and rhetorical flourishes. Your goal is not to memorize this entire mixture, but to mentally "boil off" the less important details to isolate the passage's essence: its core logic and purpose.

The distillation that results after you distill a passage is a powerful tool, providing a simplified map of the passage that you will use to answer the questions efficiently. Instead of rereading the entire dense text for every question, you can refer to your distillation to quickly locate the relevant information in the passage.

You have a choice between two tools when you distill the passage:

- **Highlighting** (Distilling in the Author's Words): The MCAT interface includes a built-in highlighting tool. Use this functionality to highlight the most important terms in each paragraph, so you can glance at your highlights and get a sense of the general structure of the passage. If you've highlighted well, you'll be able to look at these highlights to find the information needed to answer many questions.
- **Outlining** (Distilling in Your Own Words): On Test Day, you'll receive a laminated booklet and a wet-erase marker, or a similar note-taking device. Whatever form it takes, you can use these notes to build a paragraph-by-paragraph outline of the passage. When answering the questions, you'll start with this outline to identify the relevant paragraph to research, allowing you to more quickly narrow down your search for answers. In some cases, you'll even find that your outline can answer questions directly, reducing your need to reread the passage itself.

Regardless of whether you distill in your own words or in the author's, you'll be creating a guide that reinforces your mental model of the passage. Both tools can enhance your understanding of passage and author, making question research more streamlined.

Distill the Big Picture

At the end of the Distill step, take a moment after finishing the last paragraph of the passage to reflect on the big picture. Look over the labels in your outline or the terms that you highlighted on screen and try to take the whole passage in at a glance. This reflection will reinforce your understanding of the passage and better prepare you to answer broad questions about it, as well as eliminate answer choices that depart too far from the author's intentions.

The best way to grasp the big picture is to try to state the author's **overall goal**, the reason they wrote the passage, in your own words. Try to answer one of the following questions:

- Why did the author write this?
- What is the author trying to accomplish?
- What question is the author trying to answer?
- What effect does the author intend to have on the reader?

While not identical, answering any one of these questions gives you a stronger grasp of the author's purpose and intentions, which will pay off in points on Test Day.

The goal of the passage is the gold standard for big-picture distillation, but it may not always be feasible to uncover with a tough passage under timed conditions. If figuring out the purpose is too hard, you can instead just aim for the passage's **main idea**. The main idea can describe the author's thesis (the idea that the author most wants the audience to believe after reading the passage) or the passage's major theme (the idea that connects all the paragraphs together). Answer one of the following questions for the main idea:

- What does the author want the audience to believe?
- What's the common thread running through all these paragraphs?
- What topic is the author most interested in?

Each of these questions will work better with some passages than others. If the first question you pose to yourself doesn't have a clear answer, try another one until you find one you can answer confidently.

MCAT EXPERTISE

Why do so many CARS passages lack clear thesis statements? The primary reason is that every passage you see on Test Day is an excerpt from a larger article or book chapter. The original sources may very well contain clear topic sentences, but the AAMC leaves these out of most excerpts. They don't do this to be tricky, but because they're trying to test if you can use critical thinking to figure out the big picture when the passage doesn't directly state it.

Once you have that overall goal or main idea in your own words, jot it down in your notes in an abbreviated form. If you prefer using the highlighting tool, you might be able to highlight part of this idea, but CARS passages are infamous for not having clear statements of their theses. Either way, be sure to have a clear idea of this big picture before moving on to the questions.

Conclusion

The PCRD method—Preview, Choose, Read, and Distill—is your comprehensive plan of attack for CARS passages. The Preview and Choose steps empower you to take control by triaging passages strategically. The Read and Distill steps ensure that you engage with every text like an expert, using interrogation to understand its purpose and a distillation tool to capture its major ideas.

Like any skill, this method requires practice to become second nature. By turning PCRD into a consistent habit, you will build the confidence and control needed to master the CARS section. The next three chapters in this book go into greater depth on this reading method, explaining keywords, elaborative interrogation, and the tools of outlining and highlighting.

Skill and Strategy Summary

Preview and Choose

- The **Kaplan Method for CARS Passages**, also known as the **PCRD method**, consists of the following steps:
  - **P**review for difficulty
  - **C**hoose when to read it
  - **R**ead each paragraph actively
  - **D**istill the meaning of the passage
- **Triaging** on the MCAT refers to completing passages or questions out of numerical order for the sake of optimizing your score. On the CARS section, triaging means saving harder passages or questions for later but completing easier ones as you see them.
- During the **Preview** step of the PCRD method, you spend 10 to 15 seconds glancing over the passage to get a sense of its topic and difficulty.
- During the **Choose** step, you decide whether to attempt the passage **now** or **later**, based on several possible choice factors:
  - Number of Questions: Passages with more questions are worth more points, so tackle them sooner if possible.
  - Passage Length: You may wish to save especially long passages for later.
  - Paragraph Length: Longer paragraphs are usually harder to read, so a passage with multiple of these should be attempted later.
  - Sentence Length and Complexity: A passage that's full of convoluted sentences should usually be triaged for later.
  - Vocabulary: Judge vocabulary based on your own familiarity; a passage with a lot of terminology you don't grasp should be saved for later.
  - Topic: Triage passages for later if they come from disciplines you struggle with or cover subjects you dislike.

Read and Distill

- During the **Read** step of the PCRD method, you read each paragraph of the passage actively.
  - Ask "how" and "why" questions of the author as you read, and answer them with the passage, a process called **elaborative interrogation**.
  - Rely on clues like **keywords**, words and short phrases that reveal passage structure and author intentions.
- During the **Distill** step, you build a mental map of the passage using one of two tools:
  - **Highlight** the passage, using the built-in highlighting function in the MCAT interface, to distill the passage in the author's words.
  - **Outline** the passage in your notes, using the pen and pages provided on Test Day, to distill the passage in your own words.
- Regardless of which tool you use, always distill the **big picture** of the passage by finding one of the following:
  - The **overall goal** is the author's reason for writing the passage, typically to accomplish something, such as answering a question or affecting their audience in some specific way.
  - The **main idea** is the passage's thesis, what the author is trying to convince their audience to believe, or theme, the thread that connects all paragraphs.

CHAPTER 3

KEYWORDS

In This Chapter

Introduction 17

3.1 Connection Keywords 18

Continuity 18

Contrast 19

Cause and Effect 20

Examples of Connection Keywords 21

3.2 Logic Keywords 22

Evidence and Conclusion 22

Counterpoint and Target 23

Examples of Logic Keywords 25

3.3 Author Keywords 25

Positive and Negative 26

Amplifying and Limiting 26

Determining Word Charge 27

Examples of Author Keywords 28

Conclusion 28

Skill and Strategy Summary 28

LEARNING OBJECTIVES

After Chapter 3, you will be able to:

- Recognize relationships between ideas as revealed by Connection keywords
- Uncover argumentative structures using Logic keywords
- Infer writers' beliefs and attitudes from their choice of Author keywords

Introduction

Your first clinical rotation has been challenging, and you find yourself briefly zoning out as your attending physician describes a patient's situation. You snap back to attention just in time to hear her say, "... the patient meticulously followed the prescribed diet and exercise regimen, his blood sugar levels remained dangerously high."

In your distraction, you missed the very first word of that sentence.

Your attending turns to you. "So, what does that tell us about our initial plan?"

You pause. Your mind races, trying to reconstruct the sentence. You realize you can't possibly answer her question without knowing that first word. The entire meaning of the situation hinges on it.

If she said, "*Although* the patient followed the regimen, his blood sugar remained high," it would mean the plan was appropriate but failed. It suggests the patient's condition is more complex than initially thought, and a more aggressive treatment may be needed. The plan was probably a step in the right direction, just not enough by itself.

But if she said instead, "*Because* the patient followed the regimen, his blood sugar remained high," the implication is completely different, and frankly, alarming. It would mean the prescribed plan was fundamentally flawed and actually caused the negative outcome. The plan was definitely a step in the wrong direction.

One interpretation suggests a medical puzzle; the other suggests a medical error. The difference between a helpful plan and a harmful one is contained in that single missing word.

Words like "although" and "because" might seem pretty unremarkable, but they're actually some of the most important words that appear in CARS passages. We call them "keywords" because they're the key to unlocking greater comprehension of the passage and its author.

More precisely, **keywords** are words and short phrases that reveal a passage's structure and its author's intentions. They do not include the major ideas in a passage but tend to be common words that many readers pay little attention to. Noticing these frequently overlooked words can give you an advantage on Test Day by enhancing your understanding of even the most difficult passages.

In this chapter, you'll learn all about the different variations of keywords, what they tell you, and how you can leverage keywords to get a higher CARS score.

Kaplan has identified three broad categories of keywords: Connection, Logic, and Author. Each category reveals essential information: relationships between passage ideas, the structure of passage arguments, and the author's beliefs and feelings, respectively. Let's dive into the first of these before turning to the other two.

3.1 Connection Keywords

When tackling a CARS passage, it is essential to recognize how what you're reading at any point fits into the text as a whole. **Connection keywords** are words and phrases that reveal specific kinds of relationships between ideas. While there are many ways in which ideas can be connected, the vast majority of Connection keywords will fall into one of two subtypes: Continuity or Contrast.

Continuity

Continuity keywords signal that the author is discussing more of the same material. Prominent examples include *and*, *also*, *moreover*, and *furthermore*. Other common examples are words used to point back to something that was just said (the demonstrative pronouns *this*, *that*, *these*, and *those*). Additionally, Continuity keywords include words that suggest continuous sequences of events, such as *next* and *first*, *second*, *third*, etc.

Generally speaking, when a sentence or phrase begins with a Continuity keyword like *also*, it will continue in the same vein as what came before. In other words, it won't be saying anything particularly new. You can take advantage of this tendency in two ways:

- If you understood what the author was saying before the Continuity keyword, then you can trust that what follows it will be more of the same. This allows you to pick up the pace of your reading a bit, at least until you come across a different keyword that suggests you should slow down.
- If you didn't understand what the author was saying, you can now figure it out by paying more attention to what follows the Continuity keyword. Instead of going back and rereading the difficult text you didn't understand, you can just read after the keyword to find what is often a simpler restatement of the same ideas.

The metaphor of a traffic light helps to describe how you should respond to different types of keywords. Continuity keywords are best thought of as green lights, signals for you to keep going without slowing down.

In addition to words and phrases, some punctuation marks function like Continuity keywords. Colons (:) and semicolons (;) are the most common examples, acting like verbal versions of the equals sign (=). The use of dashes—such as the ones surrounding this phrase—or parentheses (the marks enclosing this phrase) also commonly indicate elaboration on the same theme. Finally, quotation marks ("") have a variety of functions, but one common use is for authors to cite other writers who agree with them. In some cases, you'll see the passage author make a claim in their own words and then follow it up with a quotation from someone else that means the exact same thing, just stated more eloquently.

Contrast

Contrast keywords indicate the passage is about to discuss something new or different. The simplest example is *but*, with many others also commonly appearing in CARS: *however*, *on the other hand*, *yet*, *although*, etc. Like Continuity keywords, Contrast keywords serve as transitions between sentences, but they can also indicate deeper conceptual relationships, such as the incompatibility between two solutions to a political problem, or a point of disagreement between two literary critics who both dislike the same novel but differ on the reasons why.

Other Contrast keywords include words that indicate the passage of time, often used in pairs. *Historically*, *traditionally*, *used to*, *originally*, *initially*, and *before* are frequently coupled with another Contrast keyword like *now*, *currently*, *modern*, *later*, and *after* to create a time-based contrast. One other common example includes words of comparison (*more*, *most*, *less*, *least*, and words ending in *-er* or *-est*). With a comparison, the contrast is usually made with respect to a particular characteristic, such as quantity or quality.

On the traffic light analogy, Contrast keywords are yellow lights, signals for you to slow down your reading. That said, not all contrasts are equally important. A paragraph that begins with "But" is more likely to suggest a significant shift in passage direction than a "but" near the end of a sentence in the middle of a paragraph, which is more likely a minor point of contrast. These minor points will still show up in questions sometimes, but not as commonly as the major shifts. The upshot of this is that your default approach should be to slow down when encountering Contrast keywords, but be willing to pick your pace back up as soon as you recognize that a contrast is only a minor one that's less likely to be tested.

In the discussion of Continuity keywords, we noted that many punctuation marks can function like Continuity keywords. Be aware, however, that the inclusion of a Contrast keyword with one of these punctuation marks generally overrides that continuity. For example, a semicolon followed by "yet" will indicate a point of difference rather than a point of similarity.

MCAT EXPERTISE

The **traffic light system** is a simplified way of thinking about keywords that's especially useful for students who feel less comfortable reading CARS passages. With a typical traffic light or stoplight, green means go, yellow means slow down, and red means stop. Here's how these directives apply to CARS keywords:

- **Green Light: Continuity and Evidence keywords.** These indicate more of the same or supporting details, so they're usually less important if you already understand what you're reading.
- **Yellow Light: Contrast, Cause and Effect, and all Author keywords.** Points of contrast, causal relationships, and author perspective are all moderately high yield for CARS questions, so you should slow down to make sure you understand exactly what these keywords indicate before moving on.
- **Red Light: Conclusion, Counterpoint, and Target keywords.** Conclusions and counterarguments are both very high yield for CARS, though counterarguments are relatively rare. With any of these keyword types, not only should you slow down to ensure your understanding, but you should often include these particular details in your distillation of the passage (what you highlight on screen or outline in your notes). Distillation is explained in Chapter 5.

Cause and Effect

Another pair of Connection keywords appears less commonly, but they're still important because they point to testable content. **Cause keywords** and **Effect keywords** are used to show causal relationships in passages. Cause keywords include *caused by*, *due to*, and *as a result of*, while Effect keywords include *consequently*, *leading to*, and *resulting in*.

The word *because* is a special case. It can serve as a Cause keyword, but it also commonly functions as an Evidence keyword, so you'll need to pay attention to context. Ask yourself: Is the thing that follows "because" an event that could have produced the result that preceded "because"? If it is, you're dealing with a causal relationship, but otherwise "because" is an Evidence keyword that indicates a supporting reason in an argument, as discussed below. Other Cause and Effect keywords are sometimes used in arguments, but "because" is the most common word to serve both purposes.

You may sometimes see both types together, but more commonly you'll just be given one of the two keywords, with the context determining what the missing piece is. For example, in the sentence, "Firefighters were unable to contain the blaze, culminating in widespread deforestation," *culminating in* is an Effect keyword. That single term reveals both the cause (lack of containment of the fire) and the effect (deforestation).

One potential difficulty with cause-effect connections is that they are relative. Consider a chain of causality, which you'll sometimes see in CARS passages, with one cause leading to an effect, which in turn causes a different effect, and so on. For this to be possible, the same event is a cause in relation to one thing but an effect in relation to another.

For example, in a loose sense, you could say that your mother is an effect of your maternal grandmother (because your grandmother caused your mother to be born) but also a cause of you (because she caused you to be born). So mothers can be thought of as causes or effects, depending on who we're relating them to, as depicted in Figure 3.1. Ultimately, nothing by itself is a cause or an effect, but only in relation to something else. When you see Cause or Effect keywords, always ask: which cause is producing which effect?

BRIDGE

One common way that cause-effect relationships are tested is with the Predict Outcome/Explanation skill. Many of the questions testing this skill bring in a piece of new information and ask you for its expected effect or its probable cause. While the new information won't appear in the passage directly, it will be similar to a cause or effect discussed in the passage. To answer such a question, find the corresponding part (the cause if given the effect, or the effect if given the cause) in the passage, and then match it to something analogous in the answer choices. For more on Predict Outcome/Explanation, see Chapter 18.

KEY CONCEPT

Like the logical relationships discussed in the next section, cause-effect relationships are one-way: the cause always happens before the effect. Reversing the direction could lead you to fall into a wrong answer trap.

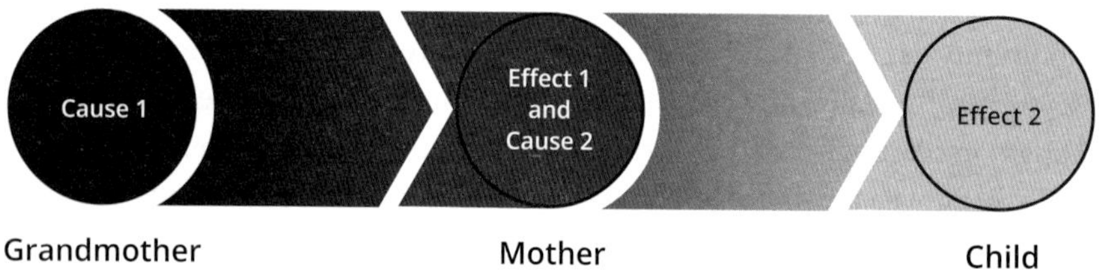

Figure 3.1 Chain of Causality

Cause keywords and Effect keywords are yellow lights because causal relationships are a common topic for CARS questions. Some questions simply ask you to identify a specific cause or effect, usually testing the

Paraphrase Detail skill, discussed in Chapter 10. In other cases, you'll find causal relationships inside passage arguments, which makes them subject to questions testing the skills Evaluate Reasoning (discussed in Chapter 14) and Strengthen/Weaken Argument (Chapter 19). The Predict Outcome/Explanation skill (Chapter 18) almost always requires connecting new information to causal relations described in the passage.

Examples of Connection Keywords

Table 3.1 lists examples of Connection keywords in each of the four categories. Remember that Continuity and Contrast are more common than Cause and Effect.

Continuity Keywords	Contrast Keywords
and	but
also	yet
moreover	however
furthermore	although
like	(even) though
such as	rather (than)
including	instead (of)
same/similar	in contrast
that is	on the other hand
in other words	otherwise
in addition	nevertheless
plus	whereas
as well as	while
equally	different
this/that/these/those	unlike
: [colon]	notwithstanding
; [semicolon]	another
— [dash]	still
( ) [parentheses]	despite
“ ” [quotation marks]	alternatively
Cause Keywords	unless
as a result of	not
due to	conversely
caused by	as opposed to
because	before + after
Effect Keywords	historically + currently
resulting in	traditional + modern
leading to	less/least
with the effect that	more/most
consequently	words ending in -er or -est [comparisons]

Table 3.1 Common Connection Keywords

3.2 Logic Keywords

In addition to the conceptual relationships discussed in the last section, there is one other type of connection that's so important for the CARS section that it deserves a separate category. **Logic keywords** reveal argumentative relations.

These relationships fall into two basic kinds: arguments (evidence-conclusion) and counterarguments (counterpoint-target). Just as we saw with cause-effect connections, which have distinctive Cause keywords and Effect keywords, there are actually two variations of keywords for each of these relationships, corresponding to the distinct parts in these one-way connections.

Evidence and Conclusion

Arguments are logical structures made up of two parts: a **conclusion**, which is just some statement that an author wants you to believe, and **evidence**, the reason or reasons that the author gives for believing that conclusion. Like cause and effect, this is a one-way relationship: the evidence gives you reason to believe the conclusion, but not vice versa. Also like cause and effect, this connection is relative: the same claim could be evidence in one argument but the conclusion in a different argument.

Let's consider an example to see all this in action. Take the claim, "Chronic sleep deprivation impairs immune function." When that claim appears by itself, it is neither evidence nor a conclusion, because those terms only exist in relation to each other. An unsupported claim is not an argument because it gives you no independent reason to believe it.

How could this claim function in an argument? As suggested, there are two ways, but let's start by treating it like a conclusion. What reasons do you have to believe "Chronic sleep deprivation impairs immune function?" The following argument presents one answer:

> **Evidence:** Studies show that sleep-deprived individuals have lower circulating levels of T-cells, which are critical for fighting off infection.
>
> **Conclusion:** Chronic sleep deprivation impairs immune function.

This argument has one piece of evidence for its conclusion, citing sleep deprivation studies that show lower levels of T-cells. This is a one-way relationship: the studies give us reason to believe the claim about sleep deprivation, but not vice versa. A general claim about sleep deprivation gives you no reason to believe that specific studies about it have been conducted. Just because a phenomenon is real doesn't mean there have been studies conducted investigating it.

Many arguments actually have multiple pieces of evidence. For example, the conclusion here would be further supported by this evidence: "During deep sleep, the body increases its production of cytokines, a type of protein that targets infection and inflammation." The connection is not as straightforward because the evidence here discusses normal sleep as opposed to sleep deprivation, but it nonetheless provides a reason to believe the conclusion: sleep-deprived individuals will have lower levels of cytokines because they'll be getting less deep sleep. Note that this new piece of evidence is independent of the original evidence; they give unique reasons for believing the conclusion, one connected to T-cells and one connected to cytokines.

Now let's take that same claim and look at how it can serve as evidence in a completely different argument:

> **Evidence:** Chronic sleep deprivation impairs immune function.
>
> **Evidence:** Overworked medical residents often suffer from chronic sleep deprivation.

Conclusion: Overworked medical residents are more susceptible to getting sick.

Here we have an argument with two pieces of evidence, and in this case, the pieces of evidence are actually connected. The first piece of evidence connects sleep deprivation to impaired immunity, while the second connects overworked medical residents to sleep deprivation. The conclusion just puts these pieces together: residents get sicker (because they're more likely to be sleep deprived, resulting in impaired immunity).

These two arguments could be combined into one larger argument, which uses the study results to support the sub-conclusion about sleep deprivation and immunity, which in turn supports the ultimate conclusion about sicker medical residents.

BRIDGE

For more on argumentation, see Chapter 14 on the Evaluate Reasoning skill and Chapter 15 on the Make Deduction skill.

So where do keywords come in? **Evidence keywords** appear before a piece of evidence in an argument, while **Conclusion keywords** appear before conclusions. Evidence keywords include *because, since, if, why, the reason is, on account of, is justified by*, and *after all*. Examples are often used as evidence in arguments, so Evidence keywords also include phrases such as *for example* and *for instance*. Conclusion keywords include *therefore, thus, then, so, argue for, argue that*, and *conclude*.

While sometimes appearing in pairs, more often you'll see just one of the two, with Evidence keywords being significantly more common than Conclusion because, as noted, pieces of evidence tend to outnumber conclusions in a CARS passage. So just as with Cause keywords and Effect keywords, you should use the placement of the keyword in the sentence to determine both evidence and conclusion. The most common patterns are as follows, though you can substitute just about any other Evidence keyword for "because" or Conclusion keyword for "therefore."

[Conclusion] **because** [evidence].

Because [evidence], [conclusion].

[Evidence]. **Therefore**, [conclusion].

MCAT EXPERTISE

Having trouble figuring out what part of the argument a Logic keyword is indicating? Try this simple substitution test: If you can replace the word or phrase with *because* or *because of*, then whatever follows is a piece of evidence. If, instead, *therefore* would preserve the meaning, the subsequent claim is a conclusion.

Counterpoint and Target

Counterarguments are logical structures that function like arguments but in the opposite direction: instead of supplying reasons to believe or accept a claim, they provide reasons to doubt or reject one. Like arguments, they consist of two parts: **counterpoints** are reasons for you to doubt a claim, while **targets** are the claims that the author wants you to doubt. Counterpoints are effectively the opposite of evidence, which is why another term for them is simply "counterevidence."

So how are counterarguments like arguments? First, they are also unidirectional: a counterpoint gives you a reason to doubt its target, but not vice-versa. Second, they are also relative: the same claim could be a counterpoint in one counterargument and a target in a different counterargument.

In fact, the same claim in the same passage could be featured in both arguments and counterarguments, especially when an author looks at multiple perspectives on an issue. For example, if an author offers pro and con arguments for a political proposal, that proposal serves both as a conclusion supported by the evidence in the pro argument and as a target challenged by the counterpoints in the con argument.

Consider the claim from before that "Chronic sleep deprivation impairs immune function." Before, we saw it used both as a conclusion supported by scientific studies and as a piece of evidence for an argument concluding that overworked medical residents get sicker. It could also serve as a *counterpoint* in the following counterargument.

> **Target:** There's no harm in premedical students skipping sleep for a few weeks to cram for exams.
>
> **Counterpoint:** Chronic sleep deprivation impairs immune function.

Perhaps not surprisingly, this claim could also be the *target* in a counterargument, such as the following:

> **Target:** Chronic sleep deprivation impairs immune function.
>
> **Counterpoint:** A new study reveals that premeds are actually impervious to the effects of sleep deprivation.

Sadly, this is a completely fictitious counterpoint, but it demonstrates how one and the same claim can play multiple (counter)argumentative roles. In fact, if you put these two counterarguments together, you can construct a positive argument. That new counterpoint, if it were true, would indirectly serve as evidence for the original target: a premed would not experience any harm from skipping sleep for a few weeks if they were immune to the effects of sleep deprivation. In other words, a counterpoint to a counterpoint effectively functions like evidence:

> **Evidence/Counterpoint to Original Counterpoint:** A new study reveals that premeds are actually impervious to the effects of sleep deprivation.
>
> **Conclusion/Original Target:** There's no harm in premedical students skipping sleep for a few weeks to cram for exams.

With that basic groundwork laid, let's see how keywords can help. **Counterpoint keywords** appear before counterevidence or reasons to doubt a claim, while **Target keywords** appear before the claims the author (or other perspectives discussed in the passage) wants you to doubt. Counterpoint keywords include *challenged by*, *undermined by*, *called into question by*, *objects that*, and *counters that*. Target keywords include *challenges*, *undermines*, *calls into question*, *objects to*, *critiques*, *criticizes*, *argues against*, *rejects*, and *doubts*. In addition, be aware that sometimes a counterpoint is introduced using a Contrast keyword like *however* or *despite*, especially when the author presents an argument in favor before introducing the counterargument.

Now that the variations of Logic keywords have been explained, let's return to the traffic light analogy. Most Logic keywords are red lights. The exception is Evidence keywords, which are green lights. Evidence keywords are more common than the other Logic keyword variations because any given conclusion can and often does have multiple pieces of evidence supporting it. A consequence of this is that any singular piece of evidence is less likely to show up in a CARS question than the conclusion it supports, making Evidence keywords inherently lower yield.

On the other hand, Conclusion keywords, as well as Counterpoint and Target keywords, are red lights. Not only should you slow down to make sure you can identify which evidence supports which conclusion (or which counterpoint challenges which target), but you should be sure to include conclusions and counterarguments in your distillation of the passage. See Chapter 5 for more on how to distill passages.

BRIDGE

Most Logic keywords are red lights because arguments and counterarguments are very high yield for CARS, appearing in questions on a variety of frequently tested skills, especially Evaluate Reasoning (see Chapter 14), Make Deduction (see Chapter 15), and Strengthen/Weaken Argument (see Chapter 19).

Examples of Logic Keywords

Table 3.2 presents a selection of Logic keywords of each of the four types.

Evidence Keywords	Conclusion Keywords
because (of)	therefore
since	thus
if	then
why	so
the reason is	argues (for/that)
on account of	concludes
is justified by	implies
after all	suggests
for example	can be inferred
for instance	**Target Keywords**
as evident in/as evidenced by	challenges
assuming	undermines
Counterpoint Keywords	calls into question
challenged by	objects to
undermined by	critiques/criticizes
called into question by	argues against
objects that	rejects
counters that	doubts

Table 3.2 Common Logic Keywords

3.3 Author Keywords

Author keywords reveal opinions in the passage, usually the passage author's. Opinions are commonly tested on the MCAT, which is why all Author keywords are treated as yellow lights in the traffic light metaphor. You should slow down when you encounter them and try to appreciate the often-subtle opinions that authors express in CARS.

In contrast to Connection and Logic keywords, which often include lesser-noticed parts of speech, Author keywords consist of the parts of speech everyone commonly thinks of: nouns, verbs, adjectives, and adverbs. What makes Author keywords distinctive is the choice of these words and the emotional resonance that the author's word choice carries.

One helpful model for understanding Author keywords can be borrowed from chemistry. This simplified picture won't account for every subtlety that CARS authors might demonstrate, but it at least gives you a starting framework for understanding how opinions can vary in CARS passages.

In chemistry, atoms and molecules possess a fundamental property called electrostatic charge, which is assigned an integer value. As you probably recall from reviewing chemistry for the MCAT, neutral atoms have a charge of 0, while ions have charges like +3 or –1.

BRIDGE

Author opinions are tested in a variety of ways in CARS. Two prominent ways are the Recognize Opinion and Anticipate Response skills.

Recognize Opinion questions are surface-level (Foundations of Comprehension), asking you to state what the author thinks or feels about a specific subject. These questions can often be answered by paying attention to the Author keywords used in the passage. See Chapter 9 for more on this skill.

With the Anticipate Response skill, you're bringing in some new info (Reasoning Beyond the Text). Many of these questions ask you to put yourself inside the author's head and give their opinion on a topic they didn't even discuss in the passage. Often you can answer these by paying attention to the Author keywords they use when describing analogous topics. See Chapter 17 for more on Anticipate Response.

In CARS, Author keywords have a **word charge**, a representation of the strength and direction of an opinion. Word charges aren't assigned numerical values because they're not that precise, but they do make up a simple spectrum of possible opinions.

In terms of direction, an opinion can be positive, neutral, or negative. Strength is a continuous quality, but for the sake of simplicity, you can divide it into three categories. For example, an opinion could be slightly positive or extremely positive or something in the middle, just "positive." Figure 3.2 presents the range of possibilities for word charge on this simplified model.

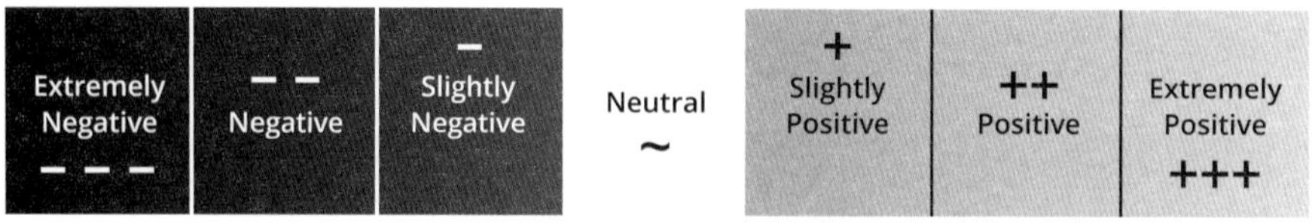

Figure 3.2 Word Charge

So how do you determine the word charge of any Author keyword? Just like electrostatic charge, word charge has both a direction and a strength or magnitude. Some Author keywords reveal the direction: Positive or Negative. Other Author keywords indicate the strength: Amplifiers indicate a stronger feeling, while Limiters indicate a weaker one. Let's look at each of these dimensions separately before we put the pieces back together.

Positive and Negative

Positive keywords indicate approval of the person writing, while **Negative keywords** indicate disapproval in some way.

Positive keywords include nouns such as *victory*, *asset*, and *competence*; verbs such as *excel*, *succeed*, and *know*; adjectives such as *compelling*, *impressive*, and *elegant*; and adverbs such as *skillfully*, *reasonably*, and *fortunately*.

Negative keywords include nouns such as *disaster*, *farce*, and *limitation*; verbs such as *miss*, *fail*, and *confuse*; adjectives such as *problematic*, *so-called*, and *deceptive*; and adverbs such as *questionably*, *merely*, and *purportedly*.

KEY CONCEPT

Keep in mind that "Author keywords" is just a term for words that carry emotional polarity, either positive or negative. Because of that, even though answer choices weren't written by the author of the passage, they can also contain Author keywords and have their own distinctive word charge.

Amplifying and Limiting

Amplifying keywords, or **Amplifiers**, are words that indicate a stronger or more extreme opinion, while **Limiting keywords**, or **Limiters**, are words that indicate a weaker or more qualified opinion.

Amplifiers are often adjectives or adverbs that accompany a Positive or Negative keyword, such as *very*, *really*, *quite*, *primarily*, *especially*, *obviously*, *foremost*, and *always*. Other Amplifiers include verbs like *need*, *must*, *should*, and *ought*, and phrases such as *in fact*, *above all*, and *it is clear that*. Sometimes Amplifying keywords will appear without Positive or Negative ones, which typically indicates that the author thinks something is important, without revealing whether it's important in a good or bad way.

Limiters are words that tone down the strength of an expressed opinion or qualify it in some way. They can be adjectives or adverbs attached to Positive or Negative keywords, such as *somewhat*, *moderately*, or *largely*, as well as phrases like *to some extent*, *in a manner of speaking*, or *in some sense*. Limiters may put limits on time, place, or frequency, such as *here*, *at times*, *in some cases*, and *in this instance*. Finally, Limiters include some verbs, particularly those that deal with possibility like *can*, *could*, *may*, *might*, and *is possible*. Sometimes authors will use limiters without Positive or Negative keywords when trying to distance themselves from a particular viewpoint or idea, like when they say something *is believed to be true* instead of just saying that it *is true*.

Determining Word Charge

On the word charge model, Positive and Negative keywords reveal the direction or "sign." If one of these keywords appears alone, without any other Author keywords, you can generally assume a word charge of simply "positive" or "negative." Some of these keywords, however, can be a little stronger or weaker. For example, describing a work of art as a *masterpiece* or a scientist as a *genius* would be "extremely positive" for most authors. Conversely, words like *adequate* and *satisfactory* have a word charge of "slightly positive" in most contexts.

Amplifiers and Limiters change the calculation a bit. When you see one of these keywords with either a Positive or a Negative, you'll need to take into account the entire "molecule" of Author keywords to determine the overall word charge. Fortunately, there's a simple rule you can use as a guideline: Amplifiers add *extremely* and Limiters add *slightly* to the word charge.

For example, "incredibly dangerous" has a word charge of extremely negative, because "incredibly" amplifies the negativity of "dangerous." Similarly, "somewhat optimistic" is slightly positive, because "somewhat" limits the positivity of "optimistic." Keep in mind that all the "atoms" of the Author keyword "molecule" may not be adjacent in the text, but they'll usually at least be confined to the same sentence.

One final complication with calculating word charge is the presence of words of negation like *not*. For example, "That idea is completely wrong" carries an overall word charge of extremely negative, with "completely" amplifying "wrong." However, "That idea is not completely wrong" isn't an extremely positive statement: it's not accurate to flip the direction from negative to positive. In most contexts, the full phrase "not completely wrong" indicates a slightly negative opinion about an idea: the author believes the idea isn't strictly true, which is negative, but that's offset in some way, perhaps by some countervailing evidence or by a deeper insight that the idea points to. So "not" commonly changes the strength of an opinion without impacting its direction.

There are a few exceptions to this rule. Phrases like *must not* and *should not* retain their strength but reverse their direction (*must* is extremely positive while *must not* is extremely negative). Similarly, the negation word *never* often acts as an Amplifier (resulting in an extreme opinion) in addition to reversing the direction of any Positive or Negative keyword.

Examples of Author Keywords

Table 3.3 lists examples of Author keywords in each of the four categories.

Positive Keywords	Negative Keywords	Amplifying Keywords	Limiting Keywords
breakthrough	oversight	must	can/could
virtue	miscommunication	need/necessary	may/might
benefit	shortcoming	always	possibly
validates	distorts	every	probably
masters	neglects	any	sometimes
clarifies	oversimplifies	should	on occasion
insightful	flawed	ought	often
sound	unsubstantiated	indeed	tends to
benevolent	dubious	very	here
effectively	superficially	especially	now
precisely	incorrectly	obviously	in this case
persuasively	vaguely	above all	in some sense

Table 3.3 Common Author Keywords

Conclusion

Keywords reveal some of the highest-yield material in CARS: the connections between ideas (Connection keywords), including argumentative relationships (Logic keywords), as well as the opinion of the author and any other perspectives (Author keywords). We covered a lot of subtypes of keywords in this chapter, but don't worry if you haven't yet mastered all of them. The most important to know are Continuity and Contrast, Evidence and Conclusion, and Positive and Negative.

The other subtypes are either less common or not as high yield, but they are helpful if you are aiming for a particularly high CARS score. You'll see some of these subtypes in later chapters when they're relevant to a specific skill. Feel free to return to this chapter if you ever need a refresher on these lower yield subtypes.

Now, moving on to Chapter 4 and the discussion of elaborative interrogation, you'll see the role that keywords play in the proven strategy of active reading.

Skill and Strategy Summary

Connection Keywords

- **Keywords** are words and short phrases that reveal important information such as passage structure and author intentions.
- The **traffic light system** assigns different color values to the keyword types to guide your reading:
  - **Green Light**: Keep reading at the same pace or pick up your speed.
  - **Yellow Light**: Slow down and reflect on what the keyword reveals before moving on.
  - **Red Light**: Slow down and identify the ideas that the keyword is connected to and how those ideas relate to each other; maybe outline or highlight what is revealed.

- **Connection keywords** reveal relationships between ideas in the passage, including how adjacent sentences in the passage connect.
  - **Continuity keywords** (green light) indicate more of the same, clarifying or elaborating upon ideas that have already been introduced. Examples: *furthermore, in other words, also.*
  - **Contrast keywords** (yellow light) signal a change in passage direction or another difference between ideas. Examples: *however, on the other hand, as opposed to.*
  - **Cause keywords** and **Effect keywords** (both yellow lights) indicate causal relationships in passages. Examples: *due to, caused by* (Cause); *resulting in, leading to* (Effect).

Logic Keywords

- In CARS, an **argument** consists of a **conclusion**, a claim made in the passage, and one or more pieces of **evidence**, reasons the passage provides for believing that claim to be true.
- A **counterargument** in CARS consists of a **target**, a claim made in the passage, and at least one **counterpoint**, a reason the passage provides for doubting that claim's truth.
- **Logic keywords** reveal the structure of arguments and counterarguments in the passage.
  - **Evidence keywords** (green light) precede reasons to believe a specific statement from the passage. Examples: *because, for example, after all.*
  - **Conclusion keywords** (red light) point to passage claims that are supported by other ideas in the passage. Examples: *therefore, then, argues for.*
  - **Counterpoint keywords** (red light) indicate reasons to doubt a specific statement from the passage. Examples: *undermined by, called into question by, objects that.*
  - **Target keywords** (red light) signal passage claims that are challenged by other ideas in the passage. Examples: *rejects, doubts, argues against.*

Author Keywords

- **Author keywords** (all yellow lights) signal how the author feels about subjects discussed in the passage, or sometimes how another point of view feels.
  - **Positive keywords** indicate author approval of something. Examples: *victory, excel, compelling.*
  - **Negative keywords** signal author disapproval of something. Examples: *disaster, miss, problematic.*
  - **Amplifying keywords**, or **Amplifiers**, show emphasis or a stronger feeling. Examples: *very, need, in fact.*
  - **Limiting keywords**, or **Limiters**, denote limitations or a weaker feeling. Examples: *moderately, at times, could.*
- Author opinions, as revealed by all types of Author keywords, range along a spectrum that can be simplified as follows: extremely positive, positive, slightly positive, neutral, slightly negative, negative, extremely negative.

CHAPTER 4

INTERROGATING PASSAGES

In This Chapter

Introduction 31

4.1 Passive vs. Active Reading 32

Active Reading: Worked Example 32

Why Active Reading? 34

Elaborative Interrogation 34

4.2 Chunking and Passage Architecture 35

Continuity Keywords: Chunk Glue 35

Contrast Keywords: Chunk Borders 35

Chunking: Worked Example 36

Expert Analysis 36

4.3 Chatting and Author Perspective 37

Chatting: Worked Example 38

Expert Analysis 39

Sample Question 40

Conclusion 40

Skill and Strategy Summary 41

LEARNING OBJECTIVES

After Chapter 4, you will be able to:

- Distinguish between passive and active reading
- Use keywords to break paragraphs down into meaningful chunks
- Ask the author questions to uncover high-yield passage information

Introduction

It's your second year of medical school, your first time on clinical rotations. A patient is admitted with a vague but serious complaint: shortness of breath. The supervising physician turns to you. "What do you want to ask her?" he says.

Your mind races. An untrained person might ask a general question like, "How are you feeling?" But you know that a vague question gets a vague answer. It probably won't help you figure out if the problem is her heart, her lungs, or something else entirely.

If you want a diagnosis, you'll need a more targeted approach. "Does it get worse when you lie down?" you ask. The patient nods. "Yes, I have to prop myself up with three pillows to sleep."

That single answer to that one strategic question changes everything. It's a classic sign that points you strongly toward a diagnosis of heart failure. An answer like that doesn't appear by passively observing the patient; you get it by knowing exactly what to ask.

The CARS section is not a matter of life and death, but otherwise a dense CARS passage is a lot like that patient. If you know what signs to look for and what questions to ask, you can home in on the important stuff, the high-yield information.

This chapter is dedicated to teaching you the art of interrogating CARS passages. We will equip you with the two core skills of an active reader: chunking and chatting. You will learn the technique of chunking to break down dense text and mentally map its underlying architecture. Then, you will learn the skill of chatting with the author, asking targeted questions to diagnose the author's underlying perspective and purpose in every chunk. But before examining these techniques, it's essential to understand the difference between reading passively and reading actively.

4.1 Passive vs. Active Reading

Many students, especially at the beginning of their prep, try to read CARS passages like they read textbooks. You scan the text quickly, latching onto the buzzwords (the major concepts and other content that you think might appear on the class exam) and ignoring everything else. This is passive reading, that is, processing textual information at a purely surface level. While it might work in some college classes, it's not enough if you want a good CARS score.

As we saw in the previous chapter on keywords, many easily overlooked words are actually pretty important for CARS. And unlike the academic jargon you find in a lot of CARS passages, keywords are often short every-day words (*so*, *but*, *and*, *like*, *since*, etc.) that any English language reader can recognize. Active readers pay attention to these keywords and the deeper truths they reveal about the passage.

To understand the difference between passive and active reading, recognize that any CARS passage can be appreciated on three levels. The surface level is **content**, or *what* the passage talks about. Beneath the surface is the **architecture**, the logical and conceptual structure of the passage, or *how* the passage is organized. At the deepest level is the author's **perspective**, the attitudes and intentions of the passage's architect, or *why* the passage was written. So **active reading** is simply the ability to read at all three levels, including the two deeper levels.

Passive readers stay at the surface, understanding what the words say, but not really grasping how the pieces of the passage fit together or appreciating why the author wrote it. Active readers, in contrast, go deeper, actively searching for insights about passage architecture and author perspective.

Active Reading: Worked Example

To see this in action, read through the following paragraph. Approach it the way you think a CARS passage should be read. Afterwards, compare how you read it to the analysis that follows to see what level you're starting off at. Remember that this is just a baseline: you can always improve from here, but it's good to know where your starting point is.

KEY CONCEPT

The three levels of active reading:

- Content: *What*
- Architecture: *How*
- Perspective: *Why*

> The artistic movement of Minimalism is often understood as a simple quest for aesthetic purity, wherein the artist strips away all non-essential forms to present an object's most fundamental nature. This interpretation, however, reduces the movement to merely a formal exercise in reduction. A more compelling analysis suggests that Minimalist works are not self-contained objects at all, but rather theatrical stages designed to generate a profound and often unsettling awareness of the viewer's own body within the gallery space.

Level 1: Content

At a surface level, this paragraph talks about an artistic movement called Minimalism. It explains what Minimalism is, with descriptions like "strips away all non-essential forms" and "formal exercise in reduction." It also mentions what viewers experience when seeing this art in galleries, an "unsettling awareness" of their own bodies.

Level 2: Architecture

Going a bit deeper, notice the use of the Contrast keyword "however" in the second sentence. This is a signal that there are actually two definitions of Minimalism being provided here. The beginning of the passage describes Minimalism as art that focuses on "aesthetic purity" and "an object's most fundamental nature." So the first one is a definition focused on the object that the artist produces.

The end of the passage offers a different description, one that says "Minimalist works are not self-contained objects at all." This second definition pivots from object to subject, that is, to the audience viewing the art: Minimalist works of art are "theatrical stages designed to generate a profound and often unsettling awareness of the viewer's own body." In other words, Minimalism (according to the second view) is distinctive because of the effects it has on people.

Level 3: Perspective

Moving beneath the architecture to the author's perspective, Author keywords (see Chapter 3) reveal how the passage architect feels about these two opposing views. The Limiting keyword "is often understood as" provides a clear signal that the author is distancing themself from the first definition. It's a recurring pattern in CARS passages for an author to introduce a "traditional" or "accepted" or "commonly understood" view, purely for the sake of tearing it down or replacing it with a newer view.

The author's preference for the new view over the old view is confirmed by two other Author keywords. First, the Negative keyword "merely" in the second sentence shows that the author is critical of the first view: it reduces Minimalism to "merely a formal exercise," which doesn't sound terribly artistic or creative. The second clue is the Positive keyword "more compelling" in the last sentence, which plainly reveals that the author thinks the second view is better.

Recognizing the author's preferences based on Author keywords can then let you answer the key question: Why did the author write this paragraph? Why would an author introduce two definitions of Minimalism, if they only really like one of them? The most likely reason someone would write such a passage is to change people's minds about Minimalism: to switch them from having one view about it (the commonly accepted view) to another (the author's preferred view).

So the active reader appreciates not only that the passage is defining what Minimalism is (the content), but that there are two opposing definitions (the architecture), and that the author wants to advocate for the second over the first (the perspective).

MCAT EXPERTISE

Just because most CARS questions test the deeper levels of reading doesn't mean that surface-level reading for content is unimportant. Indeed, with the difficult text characteristic of CARS passages, just figuring out what the author is saying can be a real challenge. Content is the main focus in Foundations of Comprehension (30% of CARS questions), but it also plays a supporting role in questions that probe into deeper levels. Rather than ignoring the content level, the active reader stays mindful of all three levels, prepared to answer questions of any depth.

Why Active Reading?

Why does this matter? Well, like anything in CARS prep, the reason it ultimately matters is that reading actively will earn you more points. Consider the following question that could accompany the preceding passage.

The author's primary purpose is to:

A. define Minimalism as art composed of aesthetically pure objects.
B. criticize Minimalism as an overly reductionistic approach to art.
C. contrast two subtly different views of what Minimalism really means.
D. argue for the superiority of a subject-centered interpretation of Minimalism.

A passive reader is more likely to answer **(A)** or **(B)**, depending on whether they pay more attention to the first or second sentence of the passage, but both are distortions of what the author actually says. The author doesn't present just one definition, but two, and actually prefers the second one, which rules out **(A)**. And although the author does criticize the first interpretation of Minimalism as too reductionistic, they don't criticize the movement entirely. Instead, they offer an alternative understanding of what it is, which eliminates **(B)**.

Someone who reads a little more deeply might notice the contrasting views and fall for trap answer **(C)**. While there definitely is a contrast, the author doesn't suggest that the views are only "subtly different." In fact, the views seem to focus on completely different aspects of the artistic experience—one emphasizes the artwork and the other emphasizes the audience. The contrast is important to the author, sure, but it's introduced in service to a larger purpose.

The active reader will recognize this larger purpose, as it's articulated in **(D)**, and get the point that passive readers would miss. Although the passage never uses the word "subject-centered," you can recognize that "viewer," which the passage does use, has a similar meaning as "subject": to be "subjected" to something is to observe or experience it. So a "subject-centered interpretation" is one that depends on the audience or viewer, just as the author describes Minimalism in the last sentence.

Elaborative Interrogation

Now that you've seen a glimpse of what active reading looks like, let's break it down into its specific components. Active reading uses an approach called **elaborative interrogation**, often just referred to as "interrogation," which is just a fancy term for having a conversation with the author. In fact, what makes "active reading" active is the fact that you're transforming the passage from a boring monologue into an interactive dialogue—and doing so by using the same two skills you use in everyday in-person conversations.

Imagine you're meeting up with a talkative friend who's excited to tell you about some topic they're really enthusiastic about. How do you make the interaction with them more interesting than just listening to them lecture you on their new obsession? Well, typically, you'll need to do two things.

First, you'll need to look for pauses in their speech, or places where it seems like they've finished talking about something or are about to start on a new train of thought. In other words, you'll look for the right moments for you to participate in the conversation.

Second, you'll need to come up with what you say. With a friend whom you're encouraging (or at least humoring), you'll probably want to ask them questions. Maybe you'll ask them to explain something they said but you didn't understand fully, or you'll ask them how they feel about a specific idea they mentioned.

The same considerations apply in CARS to interrogation, or having a conversation with the author. First, you need to look for the natural pauses in the author's stream of text. The spaces between paragraphs are usually breaks of this kind, but you can also subdivide paragraphs further into meaningful segments called chunks. So the first interrogation skill is what we call "chunking," which we'll discuss in section 4.2.

Second, you need to know what to ask. We call this skill "chatting," because it's really about picking the author's brain, asking them the same kinds of questions that you'd ask an obsessed and talkative friend. We'll return to chatting in section 4.3.

4.2 Chunking and Passage Architecture

Chunking is the skill of breaking down a passage and its paragraphs into smaller pieces, or **chunks**, each of which serves a distinctive function. It's your number one tool for uncovering the architecture of the passage, its logical and conceptual structure.

You've actually already seen an example of chunking in action. With the Minimalism passage in the preceding section, you might recall that we identified two distinct parts of the paragraph: the first part presented an older definition of Minimalism, while the second part offered a newer definition. This recognition of the distinctive functions of each chunk was essential for avoiding the trap answers that came with the sample question.

A single clue let us divide that passage into these two distinct chunks: it was the word "however," a Contrast keyword as discussed in Chapter 3. Indeed, the reason we devoted an entire chapter to keywords is that they're incredibly useful for getting at the deeper levels of meaning in a passage.
Keywords help you identify chunks in two central ways.

Continuity Keywords: Chunk Glue

First, there are Continuity keywords such as *this*, *furthermore*, and *that is*. Recall from Chapter 3 that these words typically indicate that we're seeing more of the same. If you read a sentence in a passage that introduces some idea, and then the next one begins with "in other words," you can be confident that the passage will continue to discuss the same idea, not something new.

In this way, Continuity keywords can serve as the "glue" that holds the different sentences in a chunk together. Every clause or sentence that starts with one of these is almost certainly a continuation of the same chunk from before.

Contrast Keywords: Chunk Borders

Another major way that keywords help with chunking is through Contrast keywords, which can mark the end of a chunk or the beginning of a new one. Words or phrases such as *while*, *instead*, and *on the other hand* are signals that the author is going to talk about something new. These shifts in direction are central features of the passage's architecture, ones likely to appear in questions.

Contrast keywords are often the "borders" between chunks. However, there are many possible contrasts beyond shifts in passage direction. In other words, not all Contrast keywords mark the beginning or end of a new chunk.

With practice, you'll learn how to differentiate a minor point of contrast from a chunk border. A good starting guideline is that most chunk boundaries will occur between sentences, rather than appearing in the middle of a sentence.

MCAT EXPERTISE

Continuity and Contrast keywords aren't the only types of keywords that can reveal information about chunks. Evidence keywords work a lot like Continuity keywords, so you can often treat them like chunk glue. Conclusion keywords, on the other hand, are more likely to serve as chunk borders. For example, a sentence in the middle of a paragraph that begins with the Conclusion keyword *therefore* will often indicate the start of a new chunk that talks about the conclusion of an argument, with any earlier chunks in the paragraph most likely being evidence for that conclusion. See Chapter 3 for more on these two types of Logic keywords.

Chunking: Worked Example

Let's now apply the skill of chunking to a longer passage. Read through the following text and try to divide it into chunks. Pay close attention to any keywords that might signal the "glue" that holds ideas together or the "borders" that separate them. Afterwards, compare your reading and chunking to our expert analysis.

> The concept of "high culture" has traditionally been used to describe artistic works thought to possess timeless value and intellectual complexity, such as classical music, opera, and literature. These are the works often seen as the foundation of a formal education, appreciated by a sophisticated elite. In contrast, "popular culture" has been characterized as the realm of the commercial and the ephemeral: pop music, television shows, and genre fiction created for mass consumption and immediate appeal. Yet this entire dichotomy, with its tidy separation, is intellectually problematic and fails to account for the complexities of how culture is actually created and consumed.
>
> The line between these two categories has never been blurrier. For example, art museums today regularly feature exhibits on street art and fashion design, while symphony orchestras perform live scores for popular films. Moreover, university literature departments, once the domain of the literary canon, now offer courses on graphic novels and science fiction. These examples demonstrate that cultural products once dismissed as "lowbrow" are increasingly gaining institutional legitimacy.
>
> Ultimately, an argument for the superiority of high culture is not based on any objective quality of the art itself. Aesthetic judgments are notoriously subjective and shift dramatically from one generation to the next; what is considered profound art in one era is often dismissed as sentimental kitsch in another. Rather, the very act of defining certain cultural products as "highbrow" often functions as a form of social gatekeeping. The distinction between high and popular culture is thus a tool used by educated and economic elites to signal their social status and to create a sense of cultural superiority that separates them from the masses.

Expert Analysis

Paragraph 1

I immediately notice "high culture" in quotation marks, revealing the topic of this opening chunk. The second sentence begins with the Continuity keyword *These*, gluing the first two sentences together in a single chunk.

In contrast is plainly a Contrast keyword, and I can tell we're in a new chunk with sentence 3 because that's followed by another phrase in quotes, "popular culture," which must be the new topic for this second chunk.

The last sentence starts with *Yet*, another Contrast keyword, giving us a third chunk. What's unique about this chunk is that it rejects the distinction between high culture and pop culture as "problematic."

So altogether we have three chunks: one that describes high culture, one that describes popular culture, and one that says high and pop culture aren't really different.

Paragraph 2

The opening sentence here seems to repeat a similar idea as paragraph 1's third chunk, saying that the division between the two types of culture is "blurrier" than it has ever been. I see Evidence and Continuity keywords throughout the rest of this paragraph that indicate additional support for this idea: *For example*, *Moreover*, *These examples*. Yes, this is all one chunk full of examples that support the idea that high and low culture can't be separated anymore.

Paragraph 3

In the final paragraph, the topic shifts to the idea that high culture is superior, which the author initially says is "not . . . objective." The next sentence doesn't have any clear keyword clues, so I'll have to be a little more thoughtful. I see the author says that judgments about art ("Aesthetic judgments") "are notoriously subjective," which suggests we're continuing in the same direction. Then there's a semicolon, which suggests even more in the same chunk. So this is all one chunk echoing the idea that high culture isn't objectively superior.

Finally, we get to a new chunk with *Rather* at the beginning of sentence 3. Here, the author introduces the idea of "social gatekeeping," suggesting that high or "highbrow" culture exists for this purpose. The last sentence contains a thus, which is sometimes a Conclusion keyword, but here it's actually functioning more like a Continuity keyword, similar to *this* or *these* in that it's referring back to something mentioned in the preceding sentence. So this last sentence continues the chunk by explaining what social gatekeeping is: status-signaling and elitism.

So paragraph 3 has two chunks: the first denies the objectivity of high culture's superiority, and the second asserts that labeling something as "high culture" is just showing off.

4.3 Chatting and Author Perspective

Chunking is just the first piece of interrogation: it gives you a sense of the basic architecture of the passage by highlighting shifts in its narrative. By chatting with the author, you can dig even deeper into the passage's structure, further enhancing your understanding of its logical and conceptual relationships. On top of that, you can gain insight into the author's perspective, the deepest level of active reading.

Chatting is asking the author targeted questions that you answer with the passage. Your ultimate objective is to reveal information that the test will ask about but which you'd miss with a passive reading of the passage. In other words, you want to reveal information about the passage's architecture and the author's perspective, as discussed in the opening section on active reading.

The wording of these chat questions can vary from person to person; fortunately, there are multiple correct ways to reveal the deeper passage insights that will earn you points. As you gain more experience with the CARS section, you may just be able to ask, "What's important here?" or "What's likely to show up in a question about this chunk?" After enough practice, you'll learn what tends to get tested in various kinds of passages.

If you're new to CARS or less comfortable with academic writing, you can approach it like the conversation with a friend that we described earlier. If your friend makes a bold statement, you'd probably ask them, "Why do you believe that?" Or if your friend suddenly went off on an unexpected tangent, you'd probably ask them, "Why are you telling me this?" or "How does this connect to what you were saying before?" or "Where are you going with this?" All of these can be powerful questions to chat with the author about in a passage interrogation.

- *Why do you believe that?* Uncovering the specific evidence for passage conclusions is high yield on CARS.
- *Why are you telling me this?* Many CARS questions ask about the author's intentions and the functions that different parts of the passage are supposed to serve.
- *How does this connect to what you were saying before?* More challenging CARS questions will require you to make connections across different paragraphs in the passage, so it's helpful to understand how the parts of the passage relate to each other.

- *Where are you going with this?* Thinking ahead to future paragraphs is another way of making connections across paragraphs. Some CARS questions ask you to anticipate what the author would do in new situations, so anticipating future paragraphs is good practice.

The answers to these and other chat questions are often revealed by keywords. Connection and Logic keywords, in addition to revealing information about chunking, can also reveal other architectural information, such as what is evidence and what is the conclusion in an argument (*why do you believe that?*). Similarly, Author keywords can reveal author opinions and beliefs, which are vital clues for uncovering the author's intentions and underlying motivations (*why are you telling me this?*).

If you find yourself with an especially tough chunk that makes it difficult to answer any of those four suggested chat questions, it's okay to fall back on a simpler question, even something like *What are you talking about?* Just getting a sense of the content of a chunk is better than nothing.

With practice, you may find yourself preemptively responding to your chats before you can even formulate a proper question. You'll just see an Author keyword and instantly recognize what it suggests about what the author likes and is trying to accomplish. Until that time, you should aim to pause whenever you encounter a new chunk and create one chat question for the chunk you just finished reading. The exact wording of the question doesn't matter as long as you are aiming to uncover the high-yield information in that chunk.

BRIDGE

These same questions can be useful when approaching passages in the three science sections of the MCAT. Though you'll also need a solid grasp of content for the sciences, critical reading and critical thinking are tested in every section.

MCAT EXPERTISE

Posing chat questions and answering them will slow down your reading at first, but that's just part of the learning process. After you internalize the habit of asking and answering these questions, you'll start to do it as you read, instead of having to force yourself to stop and do it after each chunk. So while you're still in training, don't pay too much attention to the clock!

Chatting: Worked Example

Let's see this in action with the sample passage that we've already chunked. For your convenience, the borders between chunks in paragraphs have been underlined. Try to pose a chat question for each chunk and respond to it by uncovering keywords or other clues in the text. Then compare your analysis to the expert approach that follows.

> The concept of "high culture" has traditionally been used to describe artistic works thought to possess timeless value and intellectual complexity, such as classical music, opera, and literature. These are the works often seen as the foundation of a formal education, appreciated by a sophisticated elite. <u>In contrast</u>, "popular culture" has been characterized as the realm of the commercial and the ephemeral: pop music, television shows, and genre fiction created for mass consumption and immediate appeal. <u>Yet</u> this entire dichotomy, with its tidy separation, is intellectually problematic and fails to account for the complexities of how culture is actually created and consumed.
>
> The line between these two categories has never been blurrier. For example, art museums today regularly feature exhibits on street art and fashion design, while symphony orchestras perform live scores for popular films. Moreover, university literature departments, once the domain of the literary canon, now offer courses on graphic novels and science fiction. These examples demonstrate that cultural products once dismissed as "lowbrow" are increasingly gaining institutional legitimacy.
>
> Ultimately, an argument for the superiority of high culture is not based on any objective quality of the art itself. Aesthetic judgments are notoriously subjective and shift dramatically from one generation to

the next; what is considered profound art in one era is often dismissed as sentimental kitsch in another. Rather, the very act of defining certain cultural products as "highbrow" often functions as a form of social gatekeeping. The distinction between high and popular culture is thus a tool used by educated and economic elites to signal their social status and to create a sense of cultural superiority that separates them from the masses.

Expert Analysis

Paragraph 1

Chunk 1 (defines high culture)

- **Chat:** Why do you define "high culture"?
- **Response:** The author says that the term "has traditionally been used to describe" the definition provided. That's a Limiting keyword, indicating that the author is describing a viewpoint held by others. In addition, *traditionally* is itself often used as a Contrast keyword to differentiate an older point of view from a newer one. So this definition is almost certainly introduced just so it can be challenged later.

Chunk 2 (defines pop culture)

- **Chat:** How does your discussion of pop culture connect to the previous discussion of high culture?
- **Response:** The author uses the Contrast keyword *In contrast* to establish a conceptual dichotomy, or division. The two are presented as direct opposites: high culture is "timeless" and complex, while pop culture is "commercial" and "ephemeral."

Chunk 3 (rejects dichotomy)

- **Chat:** How do you feel about this distinction between high culture and pop culture?
- **Response:** By using the Negative keyword "intellectually problematic," the author directly reveals their disapproval of the distinction. This helps to explain the purpose not only of this chunk, but of the two preceding ones. The author ultimately wants to argue against the dichotomy, using chunk 3 to communicate that thesis. The previous chunks introduced the two sides of the dichotomy only for the sake of letting the author tear them down.

Paragraph 2

Chunk 1 (examples of blurriness)

- **Chat:** How does this new paragraph connect to what you said before?
- **Response:** This paragraph provides direct evidence for the claim that the dichotomy between the two types of culture is "intellectually problematic." The Evidence keyword *For example* and the Continuity keyword *Moreover* introduce two examples that support the idea that the line between high and pop culture is extremely blurry now.

Paragraph 3

Chunk 1 (high culture not objective)

- **Chat:** Why do you believe that high culture is not objectively superior?

- **Response:** The author says that artistic judgments are "notoriously subjective" and "shift dramatically." This actually reinforces the point made in the previous paragraph that it's harder to tell the difference between high culture and pop culture these days.

Chunk 2 (high culture as social gatekeeping)

- **Chat:** Why introduce the concept of "social gatekeeping" at the very end of the passage?
- **Response:** The author treats social gatekeeping, which they describe as signaling elite "social status" and creating "a sense of cultural superiority," as an explanation for why the category of "high culture" even exists. Rather than reflecting any reality of the cultural artifacts themselves, the people who describe the art they like as "high culture" are just snobs, in the author's view.

Sample Question

Before concluding this chapter, let's see how chunking and chatting can help you to earn points on Test Day. Consider the following Reasoning Beyond the Text question:

> Based on the passage, how would the author most likely view a critically acclaimed, award-winning television series that is also a massive commercial success?
>
> **A.** As an artifact that challenges the conventional boundaries between high and popular culture
> **B.** As an example of popular culture, because its primary medium is commercial television
> **C.** As an example of high culture, because its critical acclaim establishes its artistic value
> **D.** As a rare exception that proves the rule about the general separation between the two categories

A question like this might seem challenging because it brings in completely new information and asks how the author would view it. But chatting with the author gives you a glimpse inside their mind and lets you anticipate how they would respond to a range of new scenarios.

The expert analysis above showed that the author presented the two definitions of high culture and pop culture not because they endorsed those definitions but ultimately to attack them. A passive reader might find **(B)** or **(C)** convincing by only paying attention to the first two chunks of paragraph 1. Either definition could apply since the new information is deliberately ambiguous. For some passive readers, **(D)** might even seem convincing if they recognize the ambiguity.

But understanding the importance of the end of paragraph 1, the active reader would choose correct answer **(A)**. The example in the question stem is similar to the examples provided in paragraph 2 of hybrids between high culture and pop culture, and all of those were used to support the author's rejection of the distinction between the two categories. So even though this seems like new information, it's directly connected to the passage. Active reading makes it easier to find these connections.

Conclusion

Some students find the idea of elaborative interrogation intimidating, but we hope that seeing it in action has reduced the intimidation factor. Remember that you're just trying to treat the author like they're a friend telling you about their latest hyperfocus, stopping them whenever they shift the subject (chunking) and asking them questions (chatting) such as "Why are you talking about this?" and "How does that connect to what you just said?" While the author won't be able to answer your questions directly, the keywords they've chosen will help you find the answers to a lot of them.

Chapter 3 on keywords and this chapter on interrogation collectively tackle Step 3 in the PCRD method, Read. The upcoming Chapter 5 will cover the final step of the Kaplan Method for CARS Passages, Distill, offering details on the two tools at your disposal to help you retain information from the passage: outlining and highlighting.

Skill and Strategy Summary

Passive vs. Active Reading

- **Passive reading** refers to a surface-level type of reading, which focuses only on what the passage says (the content).
- **Active reading**, also known as **elaborative interrogation**, instead engages with texts on three levels:
  - **Content** (*what*): the topics discussed in each paragraph
  - **Architecture** (*how*): the logical and conceptual structure of the passage
  - **Perspective** (*why*): the author's attitudes, intentions, and purpose
- Active reading/interrogation is recommended for CARS because most questions ask about more than the content.
- Interrogation consists of two activities: chunking and chatting.

Chunking and Passage Architecture

- **Chunking** is breaking down paragraphs into smaller, meaningful segments called chunks.
  - A **chunk** is unified by having each of its parts contribute to the same function.
- Keywords (see Chapter 3) are important clues for identifying paragraph chunks.
  - Continuity keywords (and Evidence keywords) serve as **chunk glue**: sentences that contain these typically continue the same chunk.
  - Contrast keywords (and Conclusion keywords) serve as **chunk borders**: sentences that contain these might mark the end of a chunk or the start of a new one.

Chatting and Author Perspective

- **Chatting** is asking the author targeted questions that you answer using keywords and other clues in the passage.
- For each chunk of the passage, chat until you can answer one of the following questions, or any other chat question that helps you uncover high-yield information:
  - *Why do you believe that?* Answer this with Evidence keywords that indicate the supporting reasons behind passage claims.
  - *Why are you telling me this?* Author keywords reveal opinions that can help determine the author's intent.
  - *How does this connect to what you were saying before?* Continuity and Contrast keywords demonstrate relationships between adjacent sentences; for more distant connections, look for repeated topics or terminology.

- *Where are you going with this?* Keywords in a paragraph's final sentence can give hints about what to expect next; for example, a Contrast keyword might signal a new direction for the upcoming paragraph.
- *What are you talking about?* If keywords are sparse or the text is otherwise difficult, try to at least understand the topics being discussed in the chunk.

CHAPTER 5

TEST DAY TOOLS: OUTLINING AND HIGHLIGHTING

In This Chapter

Introduction **43**
5.1 Outlining **44**
How to Outline 44
What to Outline 45
Outlining: Worked Example 1 46
Outlining: Worked Example 2 47
Outlining Under Pressure 49
5.2 Highlighting **50**
How to Highlight 50
What to Highlight 51
Highlighting: Worked Example 1 52
Highlighting: Worked Example 2 53
Highlighting Under Pressure 55
5.3 Choosing Your Tool **55**
When Should You Highlight? 55
When Should You Outline? 56
Can You Specialize? 56
Do You Have to Choose One? 56
5.4 Practice Passage **57**
Expert Analysis 58
Full Passage Outline 62
Full Passage Highlights 63
Practice Question 64
Conclusion **64**
Skill and Strategy Summary **64**

LEARNING OBJECTIVES

After Chapter 5, you will be able to:

- Use your notes to outline the purpose of each paragraph in a passage
- Use the highlighter tool in the MCAT interface to flag important passage information
- Choose the tool that better helps you to distill the most important info in the passage
- Practice interrogating a passage and distilling it through outlining or highlighting

Introduction

You've spent the better part of an hour with Mrs. Santiago's chart, and you've got a decent handle on the basics. You know she's a 76-year-old woman with a history of COPD and congestive heart failure who came in last night with shortness of breath. You've reviewed her labs, her recent medications, and the overnight nursing notes. The information is in your head, but it's a jumble of facts and figures. Now comes the hard part: how to present it all to the attending physician in a way that sounds coherent and confident.

You glance at the clock. Rounds start in fifteen minutes. You have two options for how to prepare your presentation.

On one hand, you could grab a notepad and sketch out a quick outline. You'd create a clear structure, maybe organizing your thoughts by problem—a section for her pulmonary issues, another for her cardiac problems. This would help you build a logical narrative, explaining how her elevated BNP points to a heart failure exacerbation, which could possibly be the main reason for her breathing trouble. The outline would be your script, ensuring you don't get lost or flustered. But is there time?

On the other hand, you could simply take a highlighter to a printout of the existing chart. You could mark the most important data points—the low oxygen saturation, the new cough, the recent medication change. This would be much faster, and it would keep you anchored to the data. But it could also be messy. When the attending starts firing questions, you might find yourself frantically flipping through pages, trying to connect the highlighted dots on the fly.

This is the strategic choice every medical student faces when confronted with a dense, complex "passage" like Mrs. Santiago's chart. There isn't one right way to distill the information, but you must choose a way.

If you haven't yet read Chapter 3 on keywords and Chapter 4 on interrogation, we strongly recommend you do so before continuing with this chapter. Chapter 5 builds on the reading strategy developed in the last two chapters, exploring two powerful tools for the final step of the Preview-Choose-Read-Distill (PCRD) method: outlining and highlighting. We'll break down how each one works, what it works best for, and how your choice of tool can turn an overwhelming passage into an opportunity for more points on the CARS section.

5.1 Outlining

On Test Day, you'll receive a laminated booklet and wet-erase marker (or some kind of equivalent tool) for taking notes. While you won't need to write out math calculations like you will in the Chem/Phys section, you can still put your notes to valuable use during the CARS section. The best way to use this tool is **outlining**, building a paragraph-by-paragraph schematic of the passage.

How to Outline

Use your note space wisely. Make sure you leave enough space in your notes for up to nine outlines, one for each passage in the section. Within each outline, leave room to allow a separate line for each paragraph, plus an extra line at the bottom for the passage goal. Adjust the size of your handwriting, if necessary, to fit.

Label everything clearly. At the top of your outline, include the passage number and its range of questions (for example, "Pass. 1: Q1–6"). Label each line of your outline by paragraph number ("P1", "P2", "P3", etc.). Label the bottom line of your outline "Goal" to capture the author's overall purpose for writing the passage. Figure 5.1 illustrates how you might set up an outline for a 5-paragraph passage.

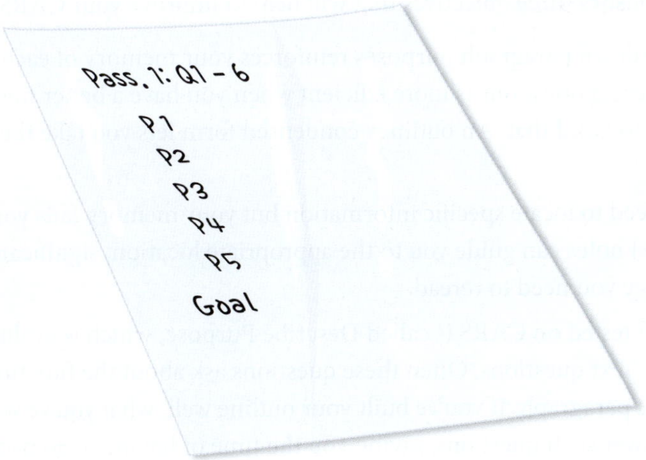

Figure 5.1 Preparing Your Outline

Read the whole paragraph before distilling it. Authors can do a lot in a paragraph, shifting in directions that aren't obvious at the start. Wait until you've read the entire paragraph and completed your interrogation of it before writing anything down for its label.

Write only as much as you need to. Your outline is ultimately a memory tool. If you only need a few words to remember what's important for a paragraph, just write down those few words. On the other hand, if you eventually find yourself puzzling over the labels in your outlines, often unsure of what you meant, then write a bit more. Use abbreviations, symbols, emojis, or any other shorthand that works for you to communicate ideas quickly.

Don't forget the overall goal. Leave a space at the bottom to write down your statement of the author's goal. Answer any one of the following questions: Why did the author write the passage? What was the author trying to accomplish with the passage? What effect was the author trying to have on their intended audience? Try to start with a verb, such as *argue*, *criticize*, or *explain*.

What to Outline

There are a lot of ways that you could build a paragraph-level outline of the passage, but you probably would prefer to do it the way that's going to earn you the highest CARS score. That's why we recommend a **functional** outline, that is, an outline that spells out the author's main purpose for including each paragraph, or the role that each paragraph plays in the passage.

As discussed in the preceding chapter on reading by elaborative interrogation, the reason to actively read passages by interrogating them is to uncover deeper levels of meaning that are commonly featured in CARS questions. Specifically, CARS questions love to ask about **passage architecture**, or the logical and conceptual connections between ideas in the text, and about **author perspective**, or the purposes and opinions of the passage's writer.

A functional outline is one that focuses on the deepest level of reading, author perspective, by describing the author's purpose for each paragraph. Interrogation equips you to recognize these purposes: after you become practiced with this approach to reading, you'll find that outlining is just writing down the results of your interrogation. You'll finish interrogating the whole paragraph first, and then you'll write down your description of its purpose in your outline.

This approach to outlining accomplishes three objectives that will help to improve your CARS score:

- **Memory reinforcer:** Writing down paragraph purposes reinforces your memory of each paragraph and the passage as a whole. Answering questions is more efficient when you have a better mental map of the passage, and an outline helps to build that. An outline's condensed form lets you take the whole passage in at a glance.
- **Navigation aid:** When you need to locate specific information but your memory fails you, your outline can help. Your paragraph-level notes can guide you to the appropriate location, significantly narrowing down how much of the passage you need to reread.
- **Question answerer:** One skill tested on CARS is called Describe Purpose, which is evaluated in about 30% of Reasoning Within the Text questions. Often these questions ask about the function of a paragraph or of some element within the paragraph. If you've built your outline well, what you've written in your notes might be enough to answer such questions, saving you the time of having to go back to the passage.

Outlining: Worked Example 1

Let's look at some examples. We'll start with just a single paragraph in isolation, before considering how interactions between multiple paragraphs can affect your outline. Try to actively read and outline the following paragraph yourself and then compare your approach to the expert analysis that comes after.

> The early twentieth-century "discovery" of N-rays by French physicist Prosper-René Blondlot serves as a formidable cautionary tale in the history of science. After claiming to have identified a new form of radiation, Blondlot and his colleagues published numerous papers describing its properties, all based on perceiving minute changes in the brightness of a spark in a darkened room. Despite the fact that visiting scientists could never replicate the results, Blondlot's laboratory continued to produce data, a testament to the powerful influence of confirmation bias. The entire field was ultimately debunked as a case of mass self-deception, illustrating that even trained scientists can see what they expect to see, rather than what is actually there.

MCAT EXPERTISE

It's easy to see how a functional outline can help if a question asks for the overall purpose of a paragraph, because that's exactly what you write down in your outline. But even when a Describe Purpose question asks for the function of something more specific, you can use your outline to help. For example, if you've determined that paragraph 3 of a passage provides evidence for the author's thesis, then you can be pretty confident that the second example provided in paragraph 3 is included to support the thesis in some way. See Chapter 13 for more on the Describe Purpose skill.

Content Outline

As discussed in Chapter 4, a passive read of the paragraph would just stick to the surface level, focusing on the content that the paragraph talks about. Someone reading at this level would focus on details like "N-rays" and the physicist Blondlot. This type of reading will tend to miss the deeper purpose of the paragraph and will usually lead to a content-based outline like the following:

P1. Blondlot's false discovery of N-rays

Functional Outline

The active reader, also discussed in Chapter 4, knows to interrogate the passage and dig deeper. Active readers would ask why the author is discussing this example from history ("Why are you telling me this?"), looking for clues in the author's choice of keywords (see Chapter 3). "Formidable cautionary tale" is an Author keyword, suggesting a highly negative opinion of the "discovery," which makes sense since it's not a real discovery.

Other strong language in the paragraph reveals more: "powerful influence of confirmation bias" uses an Amplifying keyword "powerful" to stress that the author thinks something is important. Crucially, "influence of" is a phrase that serves as a Cause keyword: the author is asserting a connection between confirmation bias and the "discovery" of N-rays, specifically that confirmation bias caused this false discovery.

So with active reading, you'll see that the author didn't write this paragraph just for the sake of discussing a weird scenario from history. That's what the content outline seems to suggest, but that's a misreading. Instead, it's about providing an example of how powerful confirmation bias can be and the types of scientific fiascos it can cause. An active reader would create a functional outline such as this one:

P1. shows power of confirmation bias, example: N-rays

To be clear, we wouldn't expect you to produce that exact label word-for-word. This is just one expert opinion on what to label for that paragraph. Any label that makes the crucial connection between confirmation bias and N-rays would suffice. The important part is that you're expressing something about those deeper levels of reading that CARS questions love to ask about.

MCAT EXPERTISE

On Test Day, feel free to use abbreviations in your outline. In our sample outline here, you could abbreviate "confirmation bias" as CB or "example" as *ex*. For the sake of clarity, we'll keep abbreviations to a minimum in all our sample outlines, but we encourage you to use whatever shorthand works best for you.

Outlining: Worked Example 2

The value of actively reading for author purpose (and reflecting that in your outline) becomes more obvious as you start to consider how things get more complex when multiple paragraphs interact. As before, practice the active reading approach described in Chapter 4 and try to build a functional outline of the following two-paragraph mini-passage. Then compare your analysis to what the experts say.

> The Efficient Market Hypothesis (EMH) posits that asset prices in a market fully reflect all available information. A direct implication of the EMH is that it is impossible for any investor to consistently "beat the market," as stocks are always trading at their fair value, making it fruitless to search for undervalued assets. This elegant theory, which assumes rational actors and instantaneous information flow, however, struggles to account for numerous real-world phenomena, perhaps none more glaring than the dot-com bubble of the late 1990s.
>
> During that period, hundreds of internet-based companies achieved astronomically high stock valuations despite having minimal revenue, no profits, and in some cases, no finished products. A frenzy of speculative buying, fueled by media hype rather than financial fundamentals, drove the share prices of companies like Pets.com and Webvan to unsustainable heights. When the bubble inevitably burst in 2000–2001, these same companies became worthless virtually overnight, erasing trillions of dollars in market value and demonstrating a clear-cut case of market-wide irrationality.

Content Outline

A passive read would focus only on the main topics of each paragraph, producing an outline like this:

P1. Efficient Market Hypothesis

P2. dot-com bubble

Functional Outline

The active reader will notice a lot more. They'll see the Contrast keyword "however" in the last sentence of P1, indicating a new chunk of information. Most of P1 is devoted to explaining what EMH is, but "however" indicates something new. In this last short chunk, the author is introducing a criticism of EMH, one that we won't actually see until P2.

We also get a better sense of the author's opinion in this second chunk of P1: EMH "struggles" to account for "glaring" examples in the real world. These Negative keywords indicate the author is skeptical of the theory, despite recognizing that it is "elegant" in the first chunk.

A more practiced CARS student would go a little further and recognize that "struggles to account for" is not just negative in its word charge, but it's a Counterpoint keyword, introduced in Chapter 3. Whatever follows this keyword ("numerous real-world phenomena ...") is a counterpoint that challenges the truth of whatever comes before it ("This elegant theory ..."), also known as the target. So the target here is the EMH.

Putting those pieces together, you can deduce that EMH is only introduced for the sake of being criticized later. You could outline that as follows:

> P1. introduces EMH to set up criticism

Before reading it, you can anticipate that the next paragraph is going to give some details on this "glaring" counterexample.

And that's precisely what we see in P2. Even though this paragraph doesn't mention the EMH at all, the active reader goes into the paragraph anticipating that it's going to give a criticism of that theory based on a real-world example.

The active reader confirms this expectation by noticing the Conclusion keyword "demonstrating" in the last sentence of P2. The phrase "clear-cut case" is an Amplifier, signaling the importance of this conclusion for the author. These keywords tell the reader that this part of the paragraph is more important than the details that precede it.

What's this important conclusion then? The author says that the dot-com bubble was ultimately evidence of "market-wide irrationality." That does sound incompatible because the EMH "assumes rational actors," according to P1. In other words, the EMH says that people are going to be reasonable, but the dot-com bubble showed they often aren't.

The active reader would outline something like the following for P2:

> P1. introduces EMH to set up criticism
>
> P2. challenges EMH with irrational dot-com bubble

A content outline gives you a disconnected list of topics: a theory and a stock market event. A functional outline tells you the story of the passage: the author defines a theory and then details a counterexample to undermine it. This active, functional approach will pay off in points when you get to all those questions on passage architecture and author perspective.

Overall Goal

While it would have been redundant with the one-paragraph worked example, now that we have a multi-paragraph passage, we can reflect on all the paragraphs as a whole. Whenever you build an outline on Test Day, you should be sure to take some time at the end to reflect on how the author's various purposes fit together. Why did the author even write the passage?

If the author's overall goal for the passage isn't clear to you after reading it, examine your completed outline and look for common threads. In our functional outline for the EMH passage, we see in P1 that the author is trying to "set up criticism" of the Efficient Market Hypothesis, while P2 "challenges EMH." The words "criticism" and "challenge" mean more or less the same thing, so the author's overall purpose must be to criticize the EMH.

Here's our completed functional outline for the passage:

P1. introduces EMH to set up criticism

P2. challenges EMH with irrational dot-com bubble

Goal: criticizes EMH

Whenever you encounter a CARS question about the author's overall goal for writing the passage, you already have a prediction right in your outline. These questions aren't the most common, but they are a variation of the Describe Purpose skill that you can expect to see perhaps a couple of times on Test Day (see Chapter 13).

You might also be surprised by how many wrong answers you can eliminate in a wide variety of questions just by knowing the author's goal. For example, if the author's purpose is to advocate for an environmentally friendly energy policy, any answer choice that suggests the author is critical of that policy would be wrong, as would any choice that had the author endorsing environmentally unfriendly actions, like burning coal and drilling for oil. This super-charging of the process of elimination is why the overall goal is perhaps the single highest-yield piece of information in a typical CARS passage.

Outlining Under Pressure

Functional outlining is a skill. It takes practice to look past what a paragraph says and identify why the author put it there. On Test Day, you may encounter a passage so dense, abstract, or confusing that you struggle to identify a clear purpose for one or more paragraphs, or even for the passage as a whole. Alternatively, you may just be low on time and need to work through a passage more quickly than usual.

In these moments, it is perfectly okay to fall back on a content-based outline.

Don't panic or waste precious time trying to force a functional analysis that isn't coming to you. Simply writing down the main topic of a challenging paragraph accomplishes two of our three primary objectives of outlining. It will still help you to remember the passage more easily, and it will still give you a navigational tool to locate information more quickly. It won't be as helpful for directly answering questions, but that's a small price to pay for maintaining your momentum and confidence.

MCAT EXPERTISE

Though not as high yield as the purpose, the main idea of a paragraph or the overall thesis of the passage can earn you points on Test Day too. The Summarize Text skill, discussed in Chapter 11, tests your ability to boil down a paragraph—or the entire passage—to its key points.

This is just an introduction to outlining, a skill you will ultimately master by practicing it. To see how outlining works with a full-length CARS passage, check out section 5.4 below. Before turning to that, let's look at the other strategic option for the Distill step of the PCRD method: highlighting.

5.2 Highlighting

The MCAT interface contains a highlighting function, which allows you to leave lasting highlights on text selections from passages and questions. Using the tool, including switching between the yellow and blue color options, is less streamlined than you might hope, but it is still usable. In fact, it becomes quite useful with Kaplan's **highlighting** strategy, which captures important passage information at every level.

How to Highlight

Less is more. Ever buy a used textbook with so much highlighting that the words that weren't highlighted stood out more than the ones that were? You highlight to draw attention to specific ideas, but the more terms you highlight, the less any one of them can stand out. Set yourself a limit on how much you can highlight in a paragraph. We generally recommend that CARS test-takers make one or two highlights per paragraph, allowing for three if it's an especially long or dense paragraph. Feel free to adjust these limits if you find something else works better for you in practice.

Read the whole paragraph before distilling it. You may remember this rule from outlining; it also applies to highlighting. If you just impulsively highlight things that seem important as you read, you'll almost certainly highlight too much. Wait until you've interrogated the entire paragraph, identifying all its distinct chunks of meaning, before you decide which highlights to make.

Learn the shortcuts. The highlighting tool on the MCAT can be clunky. If you used it without taking any shortcuts, here's what you would need to do for every single highlight you make:

Click and drag to select some text in a passage or question.
Click on the colored box next to Highlight above the passage.
Select the yellow, blue, or white box (white removes existing highlights).
Click on the Highlight button to highlight the selected text in the selected color.

Under timed conditions with nine passages, each consisting of several paragraphs, each of which you'll mark up with 1–3 highlights, the seconds spent on this cumbersome process would add up to minutes, probably costing you points on CARS.

Fortunately, there's a better, faster way: double-click + Alt-H. When you double-click on a word in a passage or question, it selects that whole word automatically, without you having to click and drag the precise text. Then, pressing the Alt and H keys on the keyboard simultaneously will highlight the text for you. Every highlight takes only a fraction of a second with this process. If you want to highlight two or three consecutive words, you can just repeat the process—highlighting more than three words in a row is generally not recommended.

Don't change colors or remove highlights. If the MCAT interface made changing highlight colors or removing highlights a seamless process, then this wouldn't be one of our basic recommendations. Unfortunately, there just isn't enough value in adding a second highlight color, so most students should stick

MCAT EXPERTISE

You might be surprised at how effective highlighting only one word in a longer phrase can be. It usually performs the exact same function of drawing your attention to that important phrase, provided you don't have too many other highlights in the surrounding paragraph. But if you're committed to highlighting several words at once, we strongly recommend a quick and dirty click-and-drag over a precise one. Your highlight is 100% as effective if it includes three extra letters you didn't intend or misses the first letter of the first word. Taking the extra time to be exact just isn't worth the points it could cost you, especially if it would mean using the cumbersome process to remove highlights.

with the default yellow. A second color wouldn't change the fact that there are only so many points of interest that can be effectively marked in a paragraph. The same goes for removing highlights: if you accidentally highlight something you didn't intend to, just try to ignore it. It's rarely worth the extra time required to switch from yellow to remove highlighting and then back to yellow.

Writing down the goal still helps. While it's often impossible to highlight a passage in a way that effectively communicates the author's overall purpose, it is still useful to identify this when you distill by highlighting. Since you won't be using your notes for anything else, consider writing down a brief summary of the overall goal you identified at the conclusion of your interrogation of the whole passage. This is an optional part of the highlighting strategy, but we recommend it because the overall passage goal is the highest yield piece of information in CARS.

What to Highlight

A typical CARS paragraph contains around 100 words, but if you follow the Kaplan strategy, you can only highlight two or three of them at the most. How do you decide? Like any other strategy decision on the MCAT, you're looking for the method that's going to get you the highest score on the exam. With outlining, we saw that the most important thing to focus on was the author's purpose, but with highlighting we don't always have the ability to represent that directly. That's why we recommend a **hybrid** approach to highlighting, one that spans the different levels of CARS reading.

Chapter 4 discusses three levels at which you can read a CARS passage (or really any text): content, architecture, and perspective, or the *what*, *how*, and *why*. Our highlighting strategy is hybrid because it includes all three of these elements.

Content

In the discussion of the outlining strategy, we aimed to move beyond content-based outlines to functional outlines based on author purposes. With highlighting, you can only work with what the author said directly, so you can't afford to be so picky.

After you read a paragraph, think about what new content this paragraph introduced, and identify a term or two in the paragraph that best represents this new content. Your best candidates will usually be proper names, "ism"s and other ideologies or theories, and other nouns that get used repeatedly. Nouns attached to Author keywords that suggest strong feelings are also viable for highlighting. Highlight the first appearances of the most important nouns to give yourself a visual map of where different content is introduced in the passage.

Architecture

The first half of interrogation is chunking paragraphs into meaningful segments, an important part of passage architecture. Rather than representing these chunks with what you choose to highlight, you represent them in space by *where* you highlight.

For example, imagine you read a paragraph that shifts focus halfway, creating two chunks of roughly equal length. You should aim to highlight one term in the upper half that best captures what content is unique to that chunk, and another term in the lower half, doing the same there.

Perspective

MCAT CARS rarely features passages that state their purposes plainly and in few words. But there are clues in the passage that can help, typically Author keywords (introduced in Chapter 3). These won't usually tell you the author's purposes directly, but they will uncover attitudes that can be used to deduce motivation.

When a chunk of the passage doesn't introduce a new topic but instead focuses on the author's response to a topic that was introduced earlier or on their feelings about that topic, find an Author keyword that best represents the author's reaction and choose that as your highlight for that chunk. If a passage features multiple author opinions, don't try to highlight them all, but focus on the ones that seem the strongest or the most important to the author.

A finished set of highlights will typically feature one highlight per chunk of the passage, with a few chunks having two highlights. These highlights will usually focus mainly on content, but in more opinionated passages, there will likely also be some Author keywords that indicate perspective. The spatial arrangement of these highlights will reveal the architecture of the passage and make navigating it easier.

We mentioned in section 5.1 that outlining has three aims: memory reinforcer, navigation aid, and question answerer. Highlights will rarely be enough by themselves to give you an answer, but they will help to reinforce your memory of the passage. On top of that, they are a superior navigation aid because they coexist with the text of the passage: you don't have to dart your eyes back and forth between the passage and your notes, as when navigating with an outline.

Highlighting: Worked Example 1

Both Distill tools, outlining and highlighting, are viable options for any passage. To demonstrate that, let's return to the same examples we saw in the Outlining section above and show you one way to approach them with highlighting. As with the sample outlines we shared above, where you didn't need to use identical phrasing in your own paragraph labels, you don't need to make the exact same highlights as our CARS experts to build an effective distillation of the passage.

Let's start with an unmarked version of the one-paragraph passage from earlier. Assuming you finished section 5.1, you've already interrogated this one and even seen our expert analysis. Reread it if you need to and then highlight one to three terms. Afterwards, compare your highlighting choices to the ones made by our experts.

> The early twentieth-century "discovery" of N-rays by French physicist Prosper-René Blondlot serves as a formidable cautionary tale in the history of science. After claiming to have identified a new form of radiation, Blondlot and his colleagues published numerous papers describing its properties, all based on perceiving minute changes in the brightness of a spark in a darkened room. Despite the fact that visiting scientists could never replicate the results, Blondlot's laboratory continued to produce data, a testament to the powerful influence of confirmation bias. The entire field was ultimately debunked as a case of mass self-deception, illustrating that even trained scientists can see what they expect to see, rather than what is actually there.

Hybrid Highlights

Earlier, we determined that the author's purpose for this paragraph was to demonstrate the power of confirmation bias, using the example of Blondlot's false discovery of N-rays. It would be tricky to capture that purpose in short highlights, but you can at least highlight where the major ideas in that purpose are introduced. Thus, the CARS expert will definitely highlight "confirmation bias," to show where this piece of content is introduced in the next-to-last sentence.

For the other major idea from the purpose, Blondlot's "discovery" of N-rays, you can make a case for highlighting either "N-rays" or "Blondlot" in the first sentence. Some CARS experts elect to highlight neither, because they appear in the first sentence in capital letters, which already makes them stand out.

So we've got one or two highlights primarily about content, but can we communicate anything more directly about perspective? Well, let's go back to the expert interrogation of the paragraph from before. The CARS expert quickly recognized the author's feelings about the subject by noticing the Author keyword "formidable cautionary tale." This perfectly encapsulates the role that the story of Blondlot's laboratory plays for the author; it's a tale of caution about the "powerful influence of confirmation bias." Now "formidable" is just an Amplifier, a keyword that indicates a stronger author feeling, so you don't need to highlight that. But "cautionary tale" is a great clue about the author's purpose worth highlighting.

Putting this all together, here's one expert way to highlight the paragraph:

> The early twentieth-century "discovery" of N-rays by French physicist Prosper-René Blondlot serves as a formidable cautionary tale in the history of science. After claiming to have identified a new form of radiation, Blondlot and his colleagues published numerous papers describing its properties, all based on perceiving minute changes in the brightness of a spark in a darkened room. Despite the fact that visiting scientists could never replicate the results, Blondlot's laboratory continued to produce data, a testament to the powerful influence of confirmation bias. The entire field was ultimately debunked as a case of mass self-deception, illustrating that even trained scientists can see what they expect to see, rather than what is actually there.

As noted, you might also opt to highlight either "N-rays" or the first appearance of "Blondlot," but the expert opted against it here since they stand out in the first line of the paragraph.

Highlighting: Worked Example 2

Now let's highlight the multi-paragraph example. As before, we'll give you the passage blank to let you choose your own highlights. Then, we'll provide the expert analysis with highlights chosen based on the interrogation from earlier in this chapter.

> The Efficient Market Hypothesis (EMH) posits that asset prices in a market fully reflect all available information. A direct implication of the EMH is that it is impossible for any investor to consistently "beat the market," as stocks are always trading at their fair value, making it fruitless to search for undervalued assets. This elegant theory, which assumes rational actors and instantaneous information flow, however, struggles to account for numerous real-world phenomena, perhaps none more glaring than the dot-com bubble of the late 1990s.
>
> During that period, hundreds of internet-based companies achieved astronomically high stock valuations despite having minimal revenue, no profits, and in some cases, no finished products. A frenzy of speculative buying, fueled by media hype rather than financial fundamentals, drove the share prices of companies like Pets.com and Webvan to unsustainable heights. When the bubble inevitably burst in 2000–2001, these same companies became worthless virtually overnight, erasing trillions of dollars in market value and demonstrating a clear-cut case of market-wide irrationality.

Hybrid Highlights

Beginning with paragraph 1, earlier we identified two chunks during interrogation. The first one explained what the EMH was, while the second introduced a criticism that isn't fully explained until P2. So, to make this architecture more easily visible, the expert would opt to highlight at least one term in the first chunk and at least one in the second.

For the first chunk, "EMH" is a good choice for content highlighting, though it is also something that stands out in all caps in the first line of the paragraph. However, unlike with the previous sample, we don't really have a good alternative with this passage. Nothing quite sums up what the EMH is in three words or fewer. Perhaps the simplest statement of it is "stocks are always trading at their fair value," so you could highlight "fair value," but that could misleadingly suggest a positive author appraisal of the theory if you're not careful. So the expert opts to highlight "EMH" for lack of a better alternative.

In the second chunk, "dot-com bubble" is your best option for highlighting content. This not only captures a major idea in the second chunk of P1, but also the subject of all P2. Paragraph 2 never uses the term "dot-com bubble," so having it highlighted right before the paragraph is better than nothing.

Those are two content highlights, but can we capture anything about perspective? Before we saw that the overall purpose of the passage was to criticize the EMH. What words from the passage let us recognize this? It was the Counterpoint keyword "struggles to account for." That's actually four words, so it's sufficient to highlight "struggles," which by itself suggests a point of conflict between EMH and the dot-com bubble, as we were hoping to communicate.

Now, let's turn to paragraph 2. During our interrogation, we noticed that P2 supplied details about the dot-com bubble, and that there was an important conclusion, signaled by a combination of Amplifying and Conclusion keywords, "demonstrating a clear-cut case." So the expert will aim to highlight something about this important conclusion, for sure, and potentially also something about the details if there are any good one-to-three-word summaries in the passage text.

For the conclusion, we noted before that the dot-com bubble provided an example of "market-wide irrationality," which shouldn't exist according to the EMH, so the CARS expert would highlight that phrase or just "irrationality." In terms of characterizing the details, there are a few candidates: "astronomically high stock," "frenzy," "unsustainable heights." Any of these would work fine, but the best option is probably "bubble inevitably burst" at the start of the third sentence, because it conveys the key detail that the dot-com bubble came to a dramatic end.

Putting those pieces together, here is one way that a CARS expert would highlight these two paragraphs:

> The Efficient Market Hypothesis (EMH) posits that asset prices in a market fully reflect all available information. A direct implication of the EMH is that it is impossible for any investor to consistently "beat the market," as stocks are always trading at their fair value, making it fruitless to search for undervalued assets. This elegant theory, which assumes rational actors and instantaneous information flow, however, struggles to account for numerous real-world phenomena, perhaps none more glaring than the dot-com bubble of the late 1990s.
>
> During that period, hundreds of internet-based companies achieved astronomically high stock valuations despite having minimal revenue, no profits, and in some cases, no finished products. A frenzy of speculative buying, fueled by media hype rather than financial fundamentals, drove the share prices of companies like Pets.com and Webvan to unsustainable heights. When the bubble inevitably burst in 2000–2001, these same companies became worthless virtually overnight, erasing trillions of dollars in market value and demonstrating a clear-cut case of market-wide irrationality.

Highlighting Under Pressure

Say you finally make it to the last CARS passage on Test Day and glance at the clock to see there are only five minutes left! What's your best strategic option?

Unless you've gotten really quick at interrogation, you're likely not going to have time to ask yourself questions like "Why did the author write that?" and "Where is this passage going?" Instead, you have to find a way to read more quickly. One option is to skim the passage and build a quick content outline, as discussed in the "Outlining Under Pressure" section earlier. But there's another possibility that can work if you're worried you won't have time to jot down notes.

Start by reading more quickly than you ordinarily would, leaning more heavily on keywords as guideposts. Once you have an idea of what the author is discussing in one part of the passage, it's okay to skip over sentences until you reach a keyword signaling something important, usually a Contrast keyword. When sentences start with Continuity (or Evidence) keywords, skip over them entirely because you don't have time to read more of the same.

When skimming the passage in this manner, you'll just highlight important-looking words as they appear. By the time you get to Test Day, you'll have practiced enough CARS to have a better sense of what these should be, so just trust your gut. In addition to major nouns, Author keywords that suggest particularly strong author opinions are another solid choice. It's permissible when the clock is running out to highlight more than three things, but keep in mind that every additional highlight makes it that little bit harder to find what you want when researching a question.

This whole process should take only a couple of minutes because you need to save time to work on the questions. You'll heavily triage the questions, primarily looking for surface questions that you can quickly research with your highlights and wildly guessing on everything else. This same triaging approach can also work if you opt for the quick version of outlining instead.

5.3 Choosing Your Tool

So far, we've discussed two options for distilling the passage: outlining lets you distill in your own words, while highlighting is distillation in the author's original words. How do you know which to use on any particular CARS passage?

Rest assured that both are viable options, so there's no wrong answer. We encourage you to experiment with both tools, at least early in your CARS prep, to get a feel for how they work with different kinds of passages. We offer a few general guidelines to get you started, but we want to emphasize that you may find things work out differently for you with practice, and that's okay. See Chapter 7 for more on developing a plan for CARS practice.

When Should You Highlight?

Many students identify two distinct use cases for highlighting. First, passages that are more straightforward, with an author who expresses themself directly and concisely, are often easier to find short highlights for. If you don't have to guess at what the author is talking about, highlighting can be significantly more efficient than jotting down an outline.

The other case is in high-pressure situations. If there's very little time left or if a passage is so difficult that you can barely make sense of it, highlighting is better because it's a bit faster. In some cases, you may even want to use the approach to highlighting described earlier in the "Highlighting Under Pressure" section.

When Should You Outline?

Provided you're not pressed for time and not completely confused by what you're reading, outlining is a safe bet for most passages. You decide what to write in your paragraph labels, so you're not constrained to use only the words contained in the passage.

Outlining can be an especially good choice with an author who is wordy or indirect. If the author talks around ideas instead of giving them simple names, it can be almost impossible to find good highlights. It's better with such passages to cut to the chase and put short paraphrases in an outline.

Can You Specialize?

Perhaps you're notorious for marking up your science textbooks with a rainbow of highlights, or maybe you love creating outlines as part of writing assignments. Either way, it's okay to choose one tool and use it for everything. You can become a specialist in highlighting or outlining.

Just be aware that if you choose one tool because you're accustomed to using it elsewhere, you're almost certainly not going to use it the same way here. Follow the guidelines in section 5.1 for outlining or section 5.2 for highlighting, and practice with them until using the Kaplan strategy becomes a habit. Try to reflect on how our strategy differs from your past approach so you can better catch yourself if you start to fall back into old habits that aren't optimized for the MCAT.

Do You Have to Choose One?

You don't strictly have to choose one tool. Using both at the same time is not recommended because it's almost impossible not to be redundant, which wastes time that would be better spent on answering questions. On the other hand, using neither is a viable option in some cases.

While not recommended for most students, some test-takers find success on the CARS section by only reading actively (interrogating) without an outline or highlights. If you're already someone who's highly comfortable with academic writing in the humanities and social sciences, and you have a strong enough memory to retain most of what you've read, using the tools might actually slow you down.

Think of using these tools like you would using a calculator. Many students aren't great at mental math or don't enjoy doing it, and so they generally get the fastest results by using a calculator when they have to do math. Other students, after mastering the multiplication tables and getting enough math practice, actually find they save time with mental arithmetic, enabling them to reach an answer quicker than the time it takes to type in the digits. The same applies to highlighting and outlining; they save time for most students, but not necessarily all.

It's also perfectly acceptable to start practicing with these tools and then stop using them once you've gotten in the habit of active reading. Remember what's important here: maximizing your CARS score (and your medical school prospects). Active reading is inherently valuable for the CARS section because it reveals high-yield information on passage architecture and author perspective. That's why every student who wants to succeed on CARS should interrogate passages.

Highlighting and outlining, in contrast, are worthwhile only because they help students to become better active readers (and to remember the insights from their interrogation). So if you learn to read actively without them (and if you don't need a memory aid to locate details for CARS questions), it's okay to stop using the tools.

Regardless of what you choose, make sure you leave yourself plenty of time to practice with the approach that you plan to use on Test Day. It's okay to change things up during your prep, but you can only build accuracy and efficiency with your approach by practicing it. So let's start practicing now!

5.4 Practice Passage

We'll skip Steps 1 and 2 (Preview and Choose) of the Kaplan Method for CARS Passages and go straight to Read and Distill. Interrogate the following passage and distill it with your choice of either outlining or highlighting. An expert interrogation will follow, along with sample expert outlines and highlight selections, for you to compare against.

The archetype of the Russian anti-hero, when summoned in the popular imagination, often coalesces into a singular, gloomy figure: a man alienated from society, tormented by metaphysical questions in a cramped St. Petersburg apartment. While this Dostoevskian image is not without merit, viewing it as the definitive statement on the subject flattens a dynamic literary evolution into a monolithic cliché. In reality, the celebrated Russian anti-hero undergoes a profound transformation across the nineteenth century, beginning as the passive "superfluous man" and evolving into the ideologically committed nihilist. This literary trajectory directly reflects a nation's tumultuous journey toward modernity.

The genesis of this archetype is the "superfluous man" (*lishniy chelovek*), a figure born of the early nineteenth-century Russian nobility. Crystallized in Pushkin's Eugene Onegin, the superfluous man is defined by a deep-seated ennui. Endowed with intelligence and a Western education, he is paralyzed by his own privilege, perceiving the vacuity of his social milieu—the endless balls, the insipid gossip, the rigid codes of honor—but finds himself unable to commit to any genuine passion. His alienation is not a product of rebellion but of profound listlessness. Onegin's casual cruelty, culminating in a pointless duel, stems not from malice but from a bored adherence to a social script he inwardly scorns, leaving him a ghost at the feast of his own life.

A decisive break from this paradigm emerges mid-century with Ivan Turgenev's character Bazarov in *Fathers and Sons*: the nihilist. Unlike the superfluous man, Bazarov's alienation is not a passive affliction but a programmatic creed. A member of the *raznochintsy*, or classless intelligentsia, his rejection of the old order is active and absolute. He dismisses art, romance, and tradition in the name of a strict materialism and faith in science. Where Onegin was bored by the societal structure, Bazarov wishes to demolish it, famously asserting that "a good chemist is twenty times more useful than any poet." This shift represents a crucial move from an alienation of feeling to an alienation of ideology.

This ideological fervor finds its most tortured culmination in the works of Fyodor Dostoevsky. Here, the anti-hero internalizes the radical ideas of the era and pushes them to terrifying conclusions. While Raskolnikov in *Crime and Punishment* tests an ideology through violent action, the narrator of *Notes from Underground* represents a more disturbing endpoint. He is a spiteful, hyper-conscious intellectual who has retreated from a world governed by a rationalism he despises. His inaction is not Onegin's bored listlessness but a deliberate philosophical rebellion, championing the caprice of free will against the deterministic certainty of "two plus two equals four." The ideological project collapses inward into a state of paralyzed, self-devouring spite, creating an anti-hero whose alienation is total.

The arc from Onegin to the Underground Man is a mirror held up to Russian history. The superfluous man was the product of a static, autocratic state that offered its educated elite no outlet for their political energies. The nihilist, by contrast, was the child of a society in flux, born from the Great Reforms of the 1860s and the rise of radical movements that sought to violently remake Russia. The literary journey from aristocratic ennui to ideological rebellion and, finally, to psychological implosion charts the very course of the nineteenth-century Russian intellectual's search for meaning in a world where old certainties were crumbling and the shape of the future was not yet clear.

Expert Analysis

Paragraph 1

The opening sentence introduces the topic of this passage, "the Russian anti-hero." There, the author suggests that "in the popular imagination" this "archetype" is "a singular, gloomy figure." CARS authors love to discuss "traditional," "accepted," and "popular" views, but usually so they can be critical or so they can offer some new alternative, often both.

That's what I'm seeing here, as confirmed by the Contrast keyword "While" in the next sentence. The author introduced this view on Russian literature but is then immediately critical of it. With that Contrast keyword, I could interpret this as a new chunk, but it certainly seems like the author introduced that view from the first sentence just to criticize it. I conclude that these two sentences have that unified purpose, so it's just simpler to treat them as a single meaningful chunk.

Another Contrast keyword, "In reality," starts the next sentence, so I'm almost certainly into a new chunk now. I'm expecting to see the author's alternative view, which of course the author would regard as reflecting "reality." Looking for more keywords, I see that the author claims a "profound transformation" occurred with the anti-hero, a Positive keyword that contrasts with the Negative keywords in the preceding sentence that described the popular view ("flattens a dynamic literary evolution into a monolithic cliché").

I also notice that "beginning as" and "evolving into" serve as Contrast keywords, marking steps of this transformation that the author introduced. A sentence like this in the opening paragraph is often a preview of what the passage will discuss. The terms that follow these keywords ("superfluous man" and "nihilist") are likely to reappear in the passage, as the author goes into more detail about this evolution.

The last sentence begins with the Continuity keyword "This," suggesting more detail about the transformation. Here, the author says that it is connected to "a nation's tumultuous journey toward modernity." What could this mean? Given that this paragraph focuses on the "Russian anti-hero" and mentions "transformation across the nineteenth century," the author is probably just describing Russian history in the 1800s. So the author is suggesting the change in literature expresses an actual change in Russian life.

Reflecting on the whole paragraph, I see that the author introduces a view to criticize it in the first chunk and then presents their preferred viewpoint in the second chunk, which they say better reflects reality and Russian history. If I could have a chat with the author, I'd want to ask "Where are you going with this?" but I already have a pretty good idea based on the keywords I saw. The author will most likely go into depth on the only remotely positive idea discussed in the whole paragraph, the "profound transformation" of the Russian anti-hero. Maybe they'll say more about how Russian history also changed, based on the very last sentence of P1.

The purpose of this paragraph seems to be to introduce an idea (the anti-hero changed) that the author will defend against the alternative view (the anti-hero didn't change). Here's how I'd outline this, though I could add a verb like "claims" or "contends" to the beginning if I wanted to remind myself more forcefully of that purpose:

> P1. Russian anti-hero evolved, not "singular"

I wouldn't quite be able to capture all of that with highlights. Brief highlights will let me stress what the author's preferred view is, but there's not a good way to concisely capture the idea that there's an alternative the author is opposing. Here's what I'd highlight if I used that tool instead:

> The archetype of the Russian anti-hero, when summoned in the popular imagination, often coalesces into a singular, gloomy figure: a man alienated from society, tormented by metaphysical questions in

a cramped St. Petersburg apartment. While this Dostoevskian image is not without merit, viewing it as the definitive statement on the subject flattens a dynamic literary evolution into a monolithic cliché. In reality, the celebrated Russian anti-hero undergoes a profound transformation across the nineteenth century, beginning as the passive "superfluous man" and evolving into the ideologically committed nihilist. This literary trajectory directly reflects a nation's tumultuous journey toward modernity.

Paragraph 2

Moving on to a new paragraph, I'm not surprised to meet the "superfluous man" again. This was the "beginning" of the transformation according to P1, so it makes sense the author would start here. Before reading any further, I anticipate that the rest of this paragraph will supply details about this figure, probably mentioning specific characters from Russian literature. I expect this because I've read enough literature passages to know that they typically back up their arguments with quotes and paraphrases from famous literary works.

And that's what I find in P2. The author introduces an example of one character from the works of Pushkin, a figure named Onegin. The remainder of this paragraph describes this character. What's important here among the details? There are two possibilities: something that is called out as important by keywords, or something that gets repeated over and over.

As it happens, I find both in this paragraph, and they point to the same idea. The Amplifying keyword "is defined by" tells us that we're seeing an important characteristic of this "superfluous man." Specifically, this man experiences "a deep-seated ennui." That means intense boredom, but even if I didn't know that, the same idea is repeated throughout this paragraph: "vacuity," "insipid," "listlessness," "pointless," and "bored adherence." So that's the most important idea here: the superfluous man, the first version of this Russian anti-hero, is just really, really bored.

Here's what I'd outline for paragraph 2 to remind me how the author begins the story of the anti-hero's transformation:

> P2. 1st anti-hero: superfluous man (Onegin) = bored

Here's what I'd highlight to capture most of that:

> The genesis of this archetype is the "superfluous man" (*lishniy chelovek*), a figure born of the early nineteenth-century Russian nobility. Crystallized in Pushkin's Eugene Onegin, the superfluous man is defined by a deep-seated ennui. Endowed with intelligence and a Western education, he is paralyzed by his own privilege, perceiving the vacuity of his social milieu—the endless balls, the insipid gossip, the rigid codes of honor—but finds himself unable to commit to any genuine passion. His alienation is not a product of rebellion but of profound listlessness. Onegin's casual cruelty, culminating in a pointless duel, stems not from malice but from a bored adherence to a social script he inwardly scorns, leaving him a ghost at the feast of his own life.

Regardless of which tool I chose to use, I'd include the character Onegin in case he's mentioned in questions. I'm imagining there are going to be more Russian names appearing in this passage, and they can be hard to keep straight since I don't know that language.

Paragraph 3

Paragraph 3 begins with "a decisive break," suggesting that we've reached a turning point in the story of the anti-hero's evolution. This break comes both with an example, a character named Bazarov, but also with a name we already saw in P1: "the nihilist." Because CARS authors often follow patterns, we can expect this paragraph to look a lot like the previous one. P3 will probably give us some details about the "nihilist" using Bazarov as an example, just as P2 detailed the "superfluous man" with Onegin.

The last paragraph was a single chunk, and I anticipate this one will be as well, but I'll look out for Contrast keywords since sometimes they mark new chunks. The second sentence starts with a Contrast keyword, "Unlike," and features another Contrast construction: "not … but." Is this a new chunk?

Digging a little deeper, this actually seems to have the same purpose as the opening sentence of explaining who the nihilist anti-hero is. The contrast is actually one drawn between the nihilist and the superfluous man, and it's drawn to better define the nihilist, so this is not a new chunk. Unfortunately, it's not immediately clear what the author means by "programmatic creed," so while that contrast might have been helpful for the author's original audience, I'll need to look for other clues to explain the nihilist.

In the next sentence, I see some Amplifying keywords that signal importance: "his rejection of the old order is active and absolute." Then, in the next-to-last sentence, there's another contrast between the example of the superfluous man and the nihilist: "Where Onegin was bored by the societal structure, Bazarov wishes to demolish it." So the nihilist is not acting out of "a deep-seated ennui," but from an intentional effort to destroy society.

The last sentence begins with the Continuity keyword "This" and seems to supply another way of talking about the move from superfluous man to nihilist. I'm not sure what "alienation of feeling" and "alienation of ideology" are supposed to mean, but I do know that the first must describe the superfluous man and the second must describe the nihilist.

So we have the next step in the transformation: the destructive nihilist. Here's how I would outline that:

> P3. 2nd anti-hero: nihilist (Bazarov) = destructive

And here's what I'd highlight:

> A decisive break from this paradigm emerges mid-century with Ivan Turgenev's character Bazarov in *Fathers and Sons*: the nihilist. Unlike the superfluous man, Bazarov's alienation is not a passive affliction but a programmatic creed. A member of the *raznochintsy*, or classless intelligentsia, his rejection of the old order is active and absolute. He dismisses art, romance, and tradition in the name of a strict materialism and faith in science. Where Onegin was bored by the societal structure, Bazarov wishes to demolish it, famously asserting that "a good chemist is twenty times more useful than any poet." This shift represents a crucial move from an alienation of feeling to an alienation of ideology.

Paragraph 4

P4 begins with the Continuity keyword "This," so I'll start by trying to figure out the specific reference. The phrase "ideological fervor" sounds similar to "alienation of ideology" in the last sentence of P3, which I know was associated with the second anti-hero, the nihilist. So, this opening sentence is talking about the nihilist's "most tortured culmination." This mix of Negative and Amplifying keywords suggests an important idea: the final endpoint of the nihilist anti-hero is in Dostoevsky's works.

If this paragraph is anything like the previous two, I'll see an example of one of Dostoevsky's characters and some descriptions that will help to explain who this ultimate nihilist is. As I continue, I indeed find more explanation of this last form of the Russian anti-hero. The Continuity keyword "Here" signals a first piece of explanation, with Negative keywords like "radical ideas" and "terrifying conclusions" indicating strong author feelings.

The third sentence starts with a Contrast keyword, but I recall that paragraph 3 had such a sentence without starting a new chunk. What's the contrast here? First, we have "Raskolnikov in *Crime and Punishment*," who must be one of Dostoevsky's characters. Then, we have "the narrator of *Notes from Underground*," but who is that? This book was not mentioned earlier, so the context suggests it must be another of Dostoevsky's works, one in which the narrator is a distinctive character. The latter "represents a more disturbing endpoint," which suggests that the anti-hero continued to evolve from one work of Dostoevsky's to another.

The next sentence starts with "He," which must refer to the last character mentioned, the narrator of *Notes from Underground*. In the remaining sentences of the paragraph, there are more Author keywords that paint an extreme portrait of this narrator anti-hero: "spiteful," "despises," "collapses," "paralyzed, self-devouring spite," "alienation is total." These characteristics give the overall impression that this is an amplified form of the destructive nihilist anti-hero from the previous paragraph.

The author mentions two examples here, but only elaborates on one of them, so I'll include only that one in my outline. Here's what I'd outline for this paragraph to remind me how the author is bringing the transformation story to a close:

> P4. final anti-hero (Underground narrator): extreme nihilist

And here's what I'd highlight instead:

> This ideological fervor finds its most tortured culmination in the works of Fyodor Dostoevsky. Here, the anti-hero internalizes the radical ideas of the era and pushes them to terrifying conclusions. While Raskolnikov in *Crime and Punishment* tests an ideology through violent action, the narrator of *Notes from Underground* represents a more disturbing endpoint. He is a spiteful, hyper-conscious intellectual who has retreated from a world governed by a rationalism he despises. His inaction is not Onegin's bored listlessness but a deliberate philosophical rebellion, championing the caprice of free will against the deterministic certainty of "two plus two equals four." The ideological project collapses inward into a state of paralyzed, self-devouring spite, creating an anti-hero whose alienation is total.

Paragraph 5

As I begin the final paragraph, I wonder what is left to say after introducing the final version of the Russian anti-hero. Each of the last three paragraphs provided descriptions of specific characters along this transformational path. Now what?

The opening sentence jogs my memory about an earlier line from the passage, at the end of P1. The author noted that "This literary trajectory directly reflects a nation's tumultuous journey toward modernity." Before, I thought that might be a fancy way of describing Russian history, and the first sentence of P5 confirms that. I infer that "the Underground Man" must be another name for the narrator of *Notes from Underground,* since Onegin was the beginning of the "arc" of evolution, and this narrator was the end. So this last paragraph will likely explain how Russia's people changed from being more like Onegin to being more like the Underground Man.

The next two sentences begin "The superfluous man" and "The nihilist," exactly as expected. The first comes from "a static, autocratic state" and its unfulfilled elite, while the second comes from "a society in flux" that led to "the rise of radical movements that sought to violently remake Russia." Here, I might chat with the author: "How does this connect to what I read earlier?" Well, the superfluous man was bored in the same way the autocratic state's elite sound, while the nihilist was characterized by destruction and radical ideology, like the movements described here. The final sentence is lengthy, but it just seems to echo what I've already read.

The author explains how Russian history parallels its literature in this last paragraph, so I could start my label with a verb like "shows" as a way to stress that purpose. However, in the interest of being a little more concise, this is what I would outline:

P5. anti-hero change reflects Russian history

As usual, I won't be able to capture all of that if I decided to highlight instead. However, every other paragraph addresses the idea that the anti-hero changes, so I can instead focus on what's new in P5. So here's what I'd highlight:

The arc from Onegin to the Underground Man is a mirror held up to Russian history. The superfluous man was the product of a static, autocratic state that offered its educated elite no outlet for their political energies. The nihilist, by contrast, was the child of a society in flux, born from the Great Reforms of the 1860s and the rise of radical movements that sought to violently remake Russia. The literary journey from aristocratic ennui to ideological rebellion and, finally, to psychological implosion charts the very course of the nineteenth-century Russian intellectual's search for meaning in a world where old certainties were crumbling and the shape of the future was not yet clear.

Overall Goal

As I reflect on the passage as a whole, looking at either my assembled highlights or my complete outline (I naturally wouldn't do both on Test Day), I can see a definite structure emerge. The author started P1 by talking about a static view of the Russian anti-hero, but only to reject that view and focus on the anti-hero's evolution. Paragraphs 2–4 illustrated the steps of that evolution, while P5 tied it to Russian history in the 19th century.

So the passage's overall purpose is to argue, contrary to the view that the anti-hero never changed, that the 19th-century Russian anti-hero evolved in response to Russian historical events. I'd write something like the following in my notes:

Goal: argues anti-hero changed with Russian history

Full Passage Outline

P1. Russian anti-hero evolved, not "singular"

P2. 1st anti-hero: superfluous man (Onegin) = bored

P3. 2nd anti-hero: nihilist (Bazarov) = destructive

P4. final anti-hero (Underground narrator): extreme nihilist

P5. anti-hero change reflects Russian history

Goal: argues anti-hero changed with Russian history

Full Passage Highlights

The archetype of the Russian anti-hero, when summoned in the popular imagination, often coalesces into a singular, gloomy figure: a man alienated from society, tormented by metaphysical questions in a cramped St. Petersburg apartment. While this Dostoevskian image is not without merit, viewing it as the definitive statement on the subject flattens a dynamic literary evolution into a monolithic cliché. In reality, the celebrated Russian anti-hero undergoes a profound transformation across the nineteenth century, beginning as the passive "superfluous man" and evolving into the ideologically committed nihilist. This literary trajectory directly reflects a nation's tumultuous journey toward modernity.

The genesis of this archetype is the "superfluous man" (*lishniy chelovek*), a figure born of the early nineteenth-century Russian nobility. Crystallized in Pushkin's Eugene Onegin, the superfluous man is defined by a deep-seated ennui. Endowed with intelligence and a Western education, he is paralyzed by his own privilege, perceiving the vacuity of his social milieu—the endless balls, the insipid gossip, the rigid codes of honor—but finds himself unable to commit to any genuine passion. His alienation is not a product of rebellion but of profound listlessness. Onegin's casual cruelty, culminating in a pointless duel, stems not from malice but from a bored adherence to a social script he inwardly scorns, leaving him a ghost at the feast of his own life.

A decisive break from this paradigm emerges mid-century with Ivan Turgenev's character Bazarov in *Fathers and Sons*: the nihilist. Unlike the superfluous man, Bazarov's alienation is not a passive affliction but a programmatic creed. A member of the *raznochintsy*, or classless intelligentsia, his rejection of the old order is active and absolute. He dismisses art, romance, and tradition in the name of a strict materialism and faith in science. Where Onegin was bored by the societal structure, Bazarov wishes to demolish it, famously asserting that "a good chemist is twenty times more useful than any poet." This shift represents a crucial move from an alienation of feeling to an alienation of ideology.

This ideological fervor finds its most tortured culmination in the works of Fyodor Dostoevsky. Here, the anti-hero internalizes the radical ideas of the era and pushes them to terrifying conclusions. While Raskolnikov in *Crime and Punishment* tests an ideology through violent action, the narrator of *Notes from Underground* represents a more disturbing endpoint. He is a spiteful, hyper-conscious intellectual who has retreated from a world governed by a rationalism he despises. His inaction is not Onegin's bored listlessness but a deliberate philosophical rebellion, championing the caprice of free will against the deterministic certainty of "two plus two equals four." The ideological project collapses inward into a state of paralyzed, self-devouring spite, creating an anti-hero whose alienation is total.

The arc from Onegin to the Underground Man is a mirror held up to Russian history. The superfluous man was the product of a static, autocratic state that offered its educated elite no outlet for their political energies. The nihilist, by contrast, was the child of a society in flux, born from the Great Reforms of the 1860s and the rise of radical movements that sought to violently remake Russia. The literary journey from aristocratic ennui to ideological rebellion and, finally, to psychological implosion charts the very course of the nineteenth-century Russian intellectual's search for meaning in a world where old certainties were crumbling and the shape of the future was not yet clear.

Practice Question

Just to remind you why these strategies pay off, let's tackle a CARS question. Try it yourself, using the expert's (or your own) outline or highlights as needed to find the answer. Then compare to the expert analysis to check your accuracy and efficiency.

Which character described in the passage would the author be most likely to associate with "psychological implosion" (paragraph 5)?

A. Bazarov

B. Onegin

C. Raskolnikov

D. The narrator of Notes from Underground

Expert Analysis

In paragraph 5, I find "psychological implosion" in the very last sentence. There, the author seems to retrace the evolution of the anti-hero, so I can map each term to a specific character: "aristocratic ennui" is the superfluous man Onegin, "ideological rebellion" is the nihilist Bazarov, and "psychological implosion" describes the extreme nihilist.

Looking at my highlighting or outline, I'd see that this extreme nihilist is described in paragraph 4, where the author actually mentions two characters, Raskolnikov and that narrator who is called "the Underground Man" in P5. The author says at the beginning of P5 that the second character was the end of the "arc" that began with Onegin, so it stands to reason that "psychological implosion" probably describes the narrator. This is confirmed by some of the language I see in P4 describing the narrator, whose "ideological project collapses inward into a state of paralyzed, self-devouring spite." **(D)** must be correct.

Conclusion

We have now covered every aspect of the Kaplan Method for CARS Passages. You've seen how to Preview and Choose when to complete passages, as well as how to Read them actively through interrogation, and how to Distill their most important information by building an outline or making highlights.

The next chapter is all about our other major CARS method, the Kaplan Method for CARS Questions. We'll examine every step of this method with examples, empowering you to tackle any question on Test Day like a CARS expert.

Skill and Strategy Summary

Outlining

- **Outlining** is building a schematic of each paragraph of the passage, using the instruments provided on Test Day for taking notes.
  - Leave enough space in your notes to outline every passage.
  - Label the passage number (and its questions) and leave space for each paragraph and the goal.
  - Read the full paragraph before writing a label for that paragraph.
  - Be concise and use abbreviations.
  - Label the author's overall goal after finishing the passage.

- A **functional outline**, the most effective for CARS, is one that maps the role each paragraph plays in the passage or, in other words, the author's purpose for each paragraph.
  - Building a functional outline reinforces your memory of the passage, creates a map to locate specific details for CARS questions, and helps you answer some questions without needing to reread.
- A **content outline**, which just labels the topics or main ideas of paragraphs instead of the purposes, is a good fallback option when under the pressure of a difficult passage or reduced time.

Highlighting

- **Highlighting** is marking up select terms in each paragraph of the passage, using the MCAT interface's built-in functionality.
  - Highlight one to three terms per paragraph.
  - Read the full paragraph before choosing your highlights.
  - Use double-click + Alt-H to highlight efficiently.
  - Stick with yellow and don't remove mistaken highlights.
  - Optional: Write down the author's goal in your notes.
- Highlighting is typically a better navigation tool than an outline, making it easier to find specific details, but it is less effective at helping you to answer questions without rereading.
- **Hybrid highlights** capture high-yield information on all three levels of active reading, making this the best approach for CARS.
  - Content: Highlight proper names, theories, or whatever is the most important topic in the chunk.
  - Architecture: Space out your highlighting, only one or two per chunk.
  - Perspective: Highlight the Author keywords that best communicate author motivation.
- Under the pressure of low time or a tough passage, you can bend the rules of highlighting: just trust your gut and highlight whatever seems important as you go, ignoring the limit of three.
  - This approach is your best option if you need to complete a full passage in five minutes or less on Test Day.

Choosing Your Tool

- Highlighting and outlining are both viable tools: the best choice depends on the passage and your preferences.
  - Highlighting is often better for straightforward passages or high-pressure situations.
  - Outlining can work with any passage but is especially useful with wordy or indirect authors.
  - Ultimately, let your practice guide you and use the tool that grants you the most success with similar passages.
- You can specialize in one tool, using it for every passage, but make sure you use it in the way that's optimized for CARS, as described in this chapter.
- Interrogation only (no outline or highlights) is an acceptable strategy for some students.
  - Best for students who are comfortable with academic writing and with active reading, either through prior experience or through extensive CARS prep
  - Best for students who don't need memory aids to maintain a detailed recollection of the whole passage
  - Should only be used on Test Day after extensive practice without tools

CHAPTER 6

QUESTION STRATEGY, TYPES, AND SKILLS

In This Chapter

Introduction 68

6.1 The Kaplan Method for CARS Questions . 68

Step 1: Type the Question................. 69

Step 2: Rephrase the Stem 72

Step 3: Investigate Potential Solutions 73

Step 4: Match Your Prediction to an Answer Choice................................ 74

6.2 Question Types and Skills 75

Foundations of Comprehension Skills 76

Reasoning Within the Text Skills 77

Reasoning Beyond the Text Skills.......... 77

Question Skill Summary.................. 78

6.3 Wrong Answer Pathologies 79

Faulty Use of Detail...................... 79

Out of Scope............................ 80

Opposite............................... 80

Distortion.............................. 80

Healthy Answer Choices.................. 80

6.4 Practice Question Set 81

6.5 Answers and Explanations 84

Conclusion.......................... 90

Skill and Strategy Summary 90

LEARNING OBJECTIVES

After Chapter 6, you will be able to:

- Distinguish the steps of Kaplan's TRIM method
- Identify CARS questions by their AAMC question type
- Recognize the set of skills tested by each AAMC question type
- Rephrase questions into actionable tasks
- Make answer predictions based on your distillation or passage research
- Diagnose common traps in wrong answer choices

Introduction

A patient is rushed into the emergency department, the paramedics calling out the classic signs: the left side of his face is drooping, his speech is slurred, and he can't lift his left arm. Your attending physician turns to you.

"Symptoms started 30 minutes ago. The clock is ticking."

Your mind starts to race, but you center yourself and focus. These are traditional symptoms of a stroke. You know there is a narrow window of only a few hours to administer a powerful clot-busting drug that can reverse an ischemic (clot-based) stroke's devastating effects. You also know that this same drug, given to a patient whose stroke is caused by a brain bleed instead of a clot, could be fatal. An untrained person might order a dozen different scans and labs, a "shotgun approach" hoping to find an answer somewhere in the data. But there's no time for that. Every minute of delay means more brain tissue is lost forever.

So what do you do? Based on the patient's history and classic presentation, you form a clear, testable prediction: if this isn't an ischemic stroke, there will be evidence of a brain bleed. You order the single quickest test to find out: a non-contrast CT scan of the head. When it comes back negative, you give the patient the clot-busting drug. Another life saved.

This high-stakes medical reasoning—forming predictions to find fast answers—is the same skill you'll use to conquer CARS questions. Faced with a question and four answer choices, too many students laboriously evaluate each option, trying to build a case for or against each one from scratch. This is the inefficient shotgun approach. The expert test-taker, however, uses the passage to form a prediction of the answer *before* ever reading the choices, transforming the task from a slow deliberation into a quick, confident search for a match.

This chapter introduces the Kaplan Method for CARS Questions, a four-step strategy that, with practice, will turn you into that expert. You'll learn to approach questions with a clear prediction in mind, allowing you to efficiently identify the correct answer. We will also preview the different skills that CARS questions test and analyze the most common wrong answer traps, equipping you with a complete strategic toolkit for conquering questions on Test Day.

6.1 The Kaplan Method for CARS Questions

In Chapter 2, we introduced the **Kaplan Method for CARS Passages**, or **PCRD**, a systematic approach for reading passages actively and uncovering high-yield information like passage architecture and author perspective. The active reading approach that works best for CARS can be challenging to master, so Chapters 3–5 provided greater detail on the primary components of this strategy: keywords, elaborative interrogation, and the tools of outlining and highlighting. Before continuing with this chapter, we strongly recommend you read through each of those chapters at least once.

To turn the heightened understanding of the passage provided by PCRD into points, you need an equally reliable strategy for the questions. The **Kaplan Method for CARS Questions** is exactly that, a structured plan of attack for any CARS question.

We use the abbreviation **TRIM** to represent its four steps: **T**ype, **R**ephrase, **I**nvestigate, and **M**atch. Figure 6.1 spells out each of the steps fully, and we'll explain each one in more detail below. At the end of the chapter, you'll have an opportunity to try this method out with a practice passage and question set.

The Kaplan Method for CARS Questions

TYPE the question

Read the question stem and glance at the choices to identify the AAMC question type and difficulty and decide whether to do it *now* or *later*

REPHRASE the stem

Simplify the phrasing of the question stem to determine the specific tasks required to answer it

INVESTIGATE potential solutions

Use your distillation and the passage, if necessary, to predict what you can about the answer

MATCH your prediction to an answer choice

Look for an answer choice that is synonymous with your prediction or eliminate choices that conflict with it

Figure 6.1 The Kaplan Method for CARS Questions

Step 1: Type the Question

Chapter 2 explained how the first two steps of PCRD, Preview and Choose, amounted to a decision about how to **triage** the passage. Much like the physician triaging patients to better save lives, the MCAT student triages passages to better save points. A hard passage is worth the same number of points as an easy one (provided they have an equal number of questions), so it's better to do the easy ones first. The same principle applies to questions as well.

The ultimate aim of the **Type** step is to make a triage decision: attack the question *now* or *later*. Within a passage's question set, "later" means after completing all the "now" questions for that passage, but *before* moving on to any other passages. There's a powerful benefit to this strategy. Your understanding of a passage deepens significantly not just after the initial read, but also during the process of answering its questions. By tackling the more straightforward "now" questions first, you build a more robust mental map of the text. When you return to the "later" questions, you can leverage this enhanced understanding to answer them more quickly and accurately. This approach ensures you tackle the most difficult questions when your familiarity with the passage is at its peak, giving you the best chance of getting them correct.

Just like with passages, a question triage decision should be made quickly: we recommend 10 seconds or fewer. If the question stem is only a couple of lines, read the entire thing. If it's longer, skim it until you get a sense of what the question is asking for. Glance down at the answer choices, *but don't read them.* Your only goal is to get a sense of how long they are, and potentially some other characteristics when the question stem is ambiguous, like whether the choices contain ideas the passage didn't talk about.

To make triaging in 10 seconds possible, you should decide based on just two pieces of information: the AAMC question type and the apparent difficulty. The **AAMC question type** uses the official CARS typology released by the Association of American Medical Colleges, the maker of the MCAT. According to the AAMC, 30% of CARS questions test the Foundations of Comprehension, 30% test Reasoning Within the Text, and 40% test Reasoning Beyond the Text. The **apparent difficulty** is a judgment you make about how hard or time-consuming the question would be to answer, which may override any triaging decision based on type alone.

Foundations of Comprehension

Foundations of Comprehension (FOC) questions tend to ask about the **content** of the passage, either in its details or general trends, without delving much into the deeper levels of meaning described in Chapter 4. Because of this tendency to focus on the shallowest level, we call them **surface questions**.

Surface questions may ask about specific ideas that the author discussed, or particular claims that the author made. They may ask about big picture themes of individual paragraphs or the passage as a whole. They may ask you to identify how the author feels about certain ideas or what precisely the author believes. Or they may simply ask you to explain what the author meant by using a particular word or phrase.

Just because these questions stick to content does not mean they are necessarily easy; some are certainly more challenging than others. But the default triage recommendation for surface questions is *now*. Most of the time, these questions will ask either about broad themes that you likely picked up on during active reading or about specific details isolated within a single paragraph. The challenge of these questions can be finding the particular detail you need, but at least you won't need to connect ideas across distant paragraphs, which is more likely to happen with the other two question types.

Because the default is *now*, you only need to watch out for signs that a surface question is particularly challenging. For example, a question that asks for one specific thing the author says is not as hard as a question that asks for the one idea among the answer choices that the author *doesn't* say.

Other factors that could increase the difficulty of a surface question and change your triage decision include a particularly long stem or answer choices, an absence of paragraph references (when you don't already know where to look), or a vague question that lacks context clues, making it difficult to form a prediction of the answer. Chapters 8–11 discuss other variations in these questions that could affect difficulty. Those chapters also include many sample questions if you're looking for some concrete examples of FOC.

BRIDGE

Chapter 4 explains how active reading appreciates passages on *three* levels:

- Content: *what* the paragraphs say
- Architecture: *how* the passage is organized
- Perspective: *why* the author wrote it

These are directly relevant for understanding the differences between AAMC question types.

KEY CONCEPT

Questions that use negations like "NOT" or "LEAST," as well as those that use Roman numerals containing multiple details, are collectively known as **scattered** questions. They often need to be approached with a more time-consuming process of elimination, requiring you to find three or four specific details in the passage instead of just one. Thus, they are often best to save for *later*, even when they're FOC.

Reasoning Within the Text

Reasoning Within the Text (RWT) questions focus on passage **architecture** and author **perspective**, the two deeper levels of meaning revealed by active reading. In other words, these questions ask about conceptual interconnections, logical arguments, and author intentions. Content, of course, plays a role in these questions, but their challenge comes from their depth. Consequently, we refer to these as **deep questions**.

Deep questions may ask you how two passage ideas are related, how the author supports their thesis, or where the central argument contains a flaw. They may ask you why the author wrote the passage or why they included a particular detail. They may even ask you to derive conclusions that were never stated in the passage by connecting ideas from far-flung paragraphs or by following through a chain of reasoning that the author starts but never finishes.

There is no default triaging recommendation for this type, so trust your gut-level appraisal of the difficulty. If your interrogation of the passage went well, a question asking for the purpose of a particular paragraph could be one that you pull directly from your distillation without having to reread, so it's definitely one that you'd want to do *now*. On the other hand, a vague question with few context clues and long answer choices could involve some pretty intense reasoning and a lot of searching through the text, so it's best saved for *later*. Chapters 13–15 discuss other variations in these questions that could impact difficulty and provide many examples.

Ultimately, after you read an RWT stem, ask yourself, "Do I already have a sense of what the answer might be or an idea of how to find it quickly?" Yes means *now*; no means *later*. If you're not sure, try it *now*, especially if you have a tendency to triage a lot of questions for *later*. Too much triaging can actually be counterproductive: at some point, you have to attack the questions to earn their points.

Reasoning Beyond the Text

Reasoning Beyond the Text (RBT) questions are distinctive not because of the level of meaning they target (though they do tend to focus more on architecture and perspective) but because of their inclusion of information that never appears in the passage. This characteristic is the reason we refer to them as **new info questions**.

New info questions may ask you to determine how a novel hypothesis affects passage arguments or to identify a new fact that would impact the passage in a specific way. They may ask you to supply examples of concepts the author discussed or to identify seemingly unrelated ideas with hidden similarities to the passage. They may ask you to predict how the author would respond in a new situation or how they might answer an objection they didn't consider. Or they may ask you to extend the logic of the passage into new realms, anticipating outcomes the author didn't address or offering plausible explanations of concepts the author left unexplained.

Keep in mind that the new info in these questions is never completely unconnected to the passage. Indeed, one main aspect of the challenge of RBT questions is that you need to find the point or points of connection between the passage and what's new in the question. These connection points aren't always obvious, especially for students who are relatively new to CARS. For that reason, the default triage recommendation for these questions is to save them for *later*.

That said, RBT questions are the most common, making up 40% of the questions on Test Day, so you need to look for opportunities to do the relatively easier ones *now* whenever you can. For example, a question asking for a new example of an idea the author introduced might have one- or two-word answers, so jump at these and others that have shorter stems and choices. If you immediately know where to look in the passage for the point of connection, do that question *now* as well. Chapters 17–20 discuss more variations that can affect RBT difficulty and include example questions.

Identifying the Specific Skill

Kaplan has conducted an extensive analysis of AAMC CARS questions, subdividing each AAMC type into three or four specific critical thinking skills. Section 6.2 below provides an overview of these 11 skills, while Units 2–4 later in the book go into greater depth on each. It's often (though not always) possible to identify the specific skill as part of the Type step, by reading the question stem and glancing at the answer choices. You can use this information to assist with your triage decision, based on which skills you're more comfortable with.

Just don't forget to adjust for difficulty. Even if one skill is your top strength, a scattered question on that skill would still probably be better saved for *later.* Similarly, a skill that you struggle with may be worth attempting *now* if it's being tested in a short question with a clear context clue and a numbered paragraph reference.

Step 2: Rephrase the Stem

Once it's time to attack the question, your next objective is to make a plan for answering it. The most efficient way to do that is to take the question stem and **Rephrase** it into a concrete task. With tougher questions, you may need to specify two or more tasks.

Start by reading the stem fully. You may have already read it once during the Type step, but now you're reading it with a very practical aim in mind: deciding how to answer it. It's okay to glance at the answer choices again to refresh your memory about their length and other characteristics, because that can be very relevant for a rephrase. Just don't read them word-for-word at this stage because three of them are wrong answers. If you latch onto the interpretation offered by a wrong answer, it may completely distort your approach to the question.

When you rephrase, you're not just trying to put the question into synonymous language. You're trying to devise an action plan that you can follow to earn the point. For example, if the question stem said:

> The author characterizes the films of Alfred Hitchcock (paragraph 2) as:

You can rephrase the question into a concrete task like:

- Go to paragraph 2, see what the author says about Hitchcock's films, including Author keywords, and summarize the author's feelings.

The more specific you can be, especially about where to go in the passage to find the relevant info, the less time the Investigate step will take. A vague question with few context clues makes this difficult, but see if you notice any patterns when glancing again at the answer choices.

To see how the answer choices can have an impact on rephrasing, consider the following question stem with only one useful clue, "masterpiece":

> Which of the following would the author most likely describe as a masterpiece?

If the answer choices were all titles of paintings that you remember seeing in paragraph 2, such as *Starry Night*, then you might rephrase your task as follows:

- Go to paragraph 2 and see which paintings mentioned there are singled out as special, for instance, with Positive and/or Amplifying keywords.
- The one with the most positive description is the answer.

If the answer choices were instead lengthy descriptions like "A peaceful still life composed with crisp lines and precise brush strokes," but you don't remember seeing anything quite like that in the passage, then your rephrase will look very different. In a situation like this, you'll have some additional tasks to accomplish.

In this case, you'll want to rely on your distillation of the passage, your outline or selection of highlights, as discussed in Chapter 5. If you built an outline during the Distill step of PCRD, your rephrase of the masterpiece question with the long descriptions for answer choices might be something like this:

- Search my outline for paragraphs that reference masterpieces, standards for good art, or anything similar.
- Go to the passage, starting with the paragraphs that seemed helpful in my outline, until I find positive descriptions of art.
- Use the most positive description I can find to generate a prediction of the answer.

As this example shows, a rephrase can be one relatively straightforward task, or a series of steps, all depending on the exact character of the question when considering the stem and answer choices as a whole.

Your rephrase also depends on how much you've retained of the passage. For example, the version of the masterpiece question that used paintings from the passage as choices would have an extra step or two if you forgot those paintings were mentioned in paragraph 2. By the same token, if you happened to remember that the author detailed several criteria for good paintings in paragraph 3, then your rephrase of the other version of that question might have fewer steps.

Step 3: Investigate Potential Solutions

The **Investigate** step begins with your plan from the Rephrase step and usually ends when you have a **prediction** in your own words of the correct answer. It may also involve a pivot or two if your initial rephrase of the question wasn't quite the right plan.

Start by trying to complete the task or tasks from your rephrase. If all goes as planned, you'll find that after completing these steps you have a good sense of the right answer. While occasionally you can formulate a prediction just relying upon your distillation, more often than not you will have to go back to the text and reread at least a sentence or two. The more solidly your prediction is grounded in specific sentences from the passage, the more likely it is to be accurate and useful.

REAL WORLD

It might be helpful to remember that the AAMC could theoretically be called upon to defend any CARS answer choice as correct or incorrect in a court of law. Medical school admissions is a serious business, and the MCAT needs to be fair. As with *much* in the legal realm, the precise wording of texts makes all the difference. Thus, the AAMC ensures that every choice is indisputably justified as correct or incorrect with backing from one or more lines of the passage. Kaplan's practice materials emulate this standard to best prepare you for the exam.

Know When to Pivot

Sometimes the best-laid plans fall through. Imagine you were attacking a question like this one:

> The author most likely believes that the *Lord of the Rings* trilogy is:

You remember the trilogy was introduced in paragraph 1, so you rephrase the question as:

- Go to paragraph 1 and see what the author says about the trilogy, including Author keywords that reveal how they feel about it.

But you go to paragraph 1 and there are no strong claims about the trilogy and no Author keywords at all, just a vague introduction that sets up a more detailed (and opinionated) account of the three books in the paragraphs that follow. So, going to one place and finding a specific description of the author's feelings is not a viable plan. What do you do instead?

It's time for a new plan. The most challenging thing about this part can be staying calm and remaining strategic in how you adapt. If you panicked and just started rereading paragraphs 2 to 4 to see what the author said about each book, you'd end up wasting a lot of time. Instead, rely on the tools we introduced earlier, including the highlighting and outlining tools from the Distill step.

Let's say you highlighted the passage and, following the advice from Chapter 5, you highlighted the title of the book that is the main content focus of each of those paragraphs, along with an Author keyword that summarizes the general feelings expressed in that paragraph. Now, you can simply glance at your highlights to see how the author feels about each book. So you pivot to a new plan:

- Look for trends in my highlights of the paragraphs about each book. Reread the sentences containing the highlights if necessary to reach a prediction.

Perhaps you highlighted "adequate start" in the paragraph on *The Fellowship of the Ring*, "strong narrative" in the paragraph on *The Two Towers*, and "captivating conclusion" in the paragraph on the trilogy's final book, *The Return of the King*. Based on just noticing that trend in your highlights, you could predict that the author thought the trilogy improved as it went on. No rereading would even be necessary.

When Prediction Isn't Possible

Sometimes, even after pivoting, reaching a specific conclusion about the answer isn't possible. On some questions, you might at best be able to set expectations that you can use to evaluate the question. For example, you can detail one or more conditions that the correct answer would need to satisfy or a set of disqualifiers that would immediately rule out an answer.

If no prediction or only a limited prediction is possible, then you're likely going to need to use the **process of elimination**. When you have to eliminate answers, your Investigate step changes focus from the question stem to the answer choices. Stop if you can find textual support directly confirming one answer, but until then search your distillation and the passage for information to eliminate wrong choices.

If it's not too far along in the question set and you haven't triaged too much for *later* yet, it's okay to put a question you can't predict on pause. As you investigate other questions, you may come across information that will make it easier to rule out wrong options or recognize the correct answer in the triaged question when you return to it.

MCAT EXPERTISE

It can be very useful to write down your rephrase and prediction during initial untimed practice, since it will help you remember to do these steps consistently until they become second nature. It also makes it much easier to review your work and improve your approach. The process of rephrasing and predicting will take time at first, but it leads to big gains as you become more comfortable with the strategy. As you advance in your studies and approach Test Day, you'll find yourself implementing these steps more quickly and habitually, without the need to write either of them down.

Step 4: Match Your Prediction to an Answer Choice

The **Match** step is where the TRIM method pays off: it's time to get those points that you've earned through your sound strategic approach. The extra effort of forming a prediction pays dividends when you save time finding the correct answer.

Keep in mind that you're looking for an idea-for-idea match, not a word-for-word match. Synonyms are okay, so be flexible about wording while watching out for the little words that can have a big impact on meaning like "not" or "all." Perhaps not surprisingly, a lot of these words are keywords, as introduced in Chapter 3. If after paying close attention to the wording of the choice, you recognize it has the same meaning as your prediction, then select it, get the point, and move on.

Sometimes the correct answer will be more general than the specific prediction you've made. For example, you might predict that the purpose of paragraph 4 is to defend Abraham Maslow's hierarchy of needs, but the correct answer might read "provide support for a psychological theory." Similarly, it could go in the other direction with the correct answer being more specific than you expect, especially when you're only able to make a vague prediction. As long as your prediction is still fully consistent with the answer choice, whether it's more general or more specific, it still counts as a match.

Why bother with this prediction matching approach? Consider possible alternatives. Some advise using the process of elimination as a default. But the AAMC is good at making wrong answers look like correct answers. By reading all of the answer choices and looking for the "best" one, you are much more likely to be swayed by these tempting traps. Making a prediction and matching it avoids this trap by letting you focus on what the right answer *must* look like instead of trying to bend a wrong answer to convince yourself it's right.

Also, let's just do the math. There are roughly an equal number of A, B, C, and D correct answers on the test. So if you stop reading answers after you've found a match for your prediction, as Kaplan recommends, you'll read an average of two or three answer choices for each question. With an elimination-first strategy, you always read all four choices, so it's usually slower.

A particularly misguided version of the elimination strategy advises reading answer choices in pairs, comparing them to each other and eliminating the worse one each time. But that means you not only have to read every single answer choice, but that you're also rereading some of them, potentially multiple times. That's far less efficient than the Kaplan prediction-first approach.

Don't waste your time trying to compare every answer choice. As suggested earlier in this chapter, the test maker backs up each answer choice as right or wrong primarily by comparison to the text of the passage. When you have to use the process of elimination, aim to take each choice individually and rule it out only because of something in the passage (or your distillation) that justifies it.

If the process of elimination itself fails, and you're only able to eliminate some answer choices, then you'll have to make an **educated guess**. Every choice you can confidently eliminate increases your chances of a successful guess, but every additional second spent investigating the remaining options takes away time from other questions. At a certain point, you have to balance accuracy and speed and just trust your gut.

A **wild guess** is generally not recommended unless you're totally stumped or almost completely out of time. Still, it is much better than leaving a question blank. There is no wrong answer penalty on the MCAT, so a wild guess has a 25% chance of earning you a point of pre-scaled score (which just might increase your scaled 118–132 CARS section score), while an unanswered question automatically earns zero.

MCAT EXPERTISE

There are limited exceptions to the rule against comparing answer choices, such as when you can't find a clear match for your prediction. But you'll likely never need to compare everything. First rule out whatever choices you can with the process of elimination, and then only compare those that remain.

BRIDGE

These guidelines about matching predictions, process of elimination, educated guessing, and wild guessing apply to the science sections of the MCAT as well. The only difference is that you'll sometimes need to draw on outside science knowledge to find a match or eliminate wrong options.

6.2 Question Types and Skills

The AAMC question types, Foundations of Comprehension, Reasoning Within the Text, and Reasoning Beyond the Text, were discussed extensively in the previous section. We also mentioned in that section that we further subdivide each AAMC type into distinctive critical thinking skills. Now we'll explain more about those skills.

Question skills refer to the specific critical thinking skills that are tested in CARS questions. You should use skills primarily as diagnostic tools: they prominently feature in much of the feedback that Kaplan provides with our CARS practice materials. After completing some CARS practice, you can examine your results and look for opportunity areas, skills that you seem to be struggling with and have room to improve.

As noted above, skills can optionally be identified as part of the Type step of the TRIM method, for students who want to make more precise triage decisions based on their personal strengths and weaknesses. This is not recommended for students who are beginning their CARS prep, because there is already a lot of information to juggle in the CARS section.

Regardless of whether you're using skills to diagnose your strengths and weaknesses or as a direct part of your strategy, they are helpful categories. Students who are looking for a high CARS score should identify which skills they've already mastered and then seek to build the remainder to mastery as well. For students who would be satisfied with a respectable, above-average score, skills are still useful categories to identify high-yield areas of opportunity for targeted improvement. If you're in this category, you don't need to master every skill or even be able to recognize them all; you should just be aware of your weak points, so you can devote more practice time there.

While all 11 skills are discussed below, don't feel the need to try to memorize all this information, especially if you are early in your prep. This section is intended primarily as a reference to help you make better use of the skill chapters in Units 2–4.

MCAT EXPERTISE

What do you do after you've identified a skill as an area of opportunity? Try to incorporate some occasional targeted practice into your CARS routine. See Chapter 7 for more on establishing a practice routine and improving your skills. The targeted practice materials provided in this book include the Skillbuilders at the end of every skill chapter as well as Chapters 12, 16, and 21, which contain practice passages with only FOC, only RWT, or only RBT questions, respectively.

Foundations of Comprehension Skills

Kaplan has identified four component skills that make up Foundations of Comprehension, discussed below. Approximate frequencies here and for the other skills are based on our analysis of AAMC's official CARS practice materials.

MCAT EXPERTISE

Just remembering 11 different skills can be a challenge, let alone learning how to recognize each one, so don't force it. Instead, start with the simpler three-part division of surface, deep, or new info questions. That's all you need (along with difficulty) to make a triage decision and set initial expectations for answering the question.

Interpret Meaning

> Use context to determine what a word/phrase from the passage is intended to communicate.

CARS authors sometimes use language in weird ways. This skill is all about taking a particular part of the passage and unpacking what it means. About 20% of FOC questions target this skill. It's discussed in greater detail in Chapter 8.

Recognize Opinion

> Identify what the author or someone else feels about a passage idea based on word choice or other context clues.

Opinions in CARS passages can sometimes be subtle, depending only on one or a few choice words (these are Author keywords, discussed in Chapter 3). This skill, which also accounts for about 20% of FOC, is about identifying some of the subtleties of opinion in the passage. Chapter 9 provides a full treatment of this skill.

Paraphrase Detail

Recognize a specific piece of information that is stated or strongly implied at one location in the passage.

This is the most commonly tested FOC skill, accounting for about 40%, or roughly twice as frequent as the other skills. These questions just ask for specific pieces of information, but be warned that they can sometimes be difficult to distinguish from the more complex Make Deduction, a RWT skill. What is distinctive about Paraphrase Detail is that it only requires one specific part of the passage to yield an answer. See Chapter 10 for more on this skill.

Summarize Text

Articulate the main idea of the passage or of a part of it.

Rather than asking about specific details, this skill will require you to generalize across an entire paragraph or the whole passage, supplying the major takeaway or theme. This skill is tested in about 20% of FOC questions and is covered in Chapter 11.

Reasoning Within the Text Skills

For Reasoning Within the Text, there are only three key skills.

Describe Purpose

Identify why the author wrote the passage or a part of it.

This skill targets the deepest level of reading, author perspective, as discussed in Chapter 4. Rather than identifying the content of part of the passage, you instead identify its function, the role that the author intends for it to play in the passage. This skill is tested in about 30% of RWT questions. Chapter 13 focuses on this skill.

Evaluate Reasoning

Characterize logical connections between ideas in the passage.

This skill targets passage architecture, the other deep level of meaning discussed in Chapter 4. It requires you to unpack specific types of conceptual connections between ideas in the passage, especially logical arguments. It's a little more frequent than the other RWT skills, accounting for about 40%. See Chapter 14 for a lot more on this skill.

Make Deduction

Infer a claim that follows from multiple parts of the passage, such as an assumption in an argument.

The last 30% of RWT questions also focus on passage architecture, requiring you to make conceptual connections across the passage to uncover deep conclusions. These questions can appear deceptively simple but are some of the most time-consuming on the test to answer. Chapter 15 provides a thorough overview of the Make Deduction skill.

Reasoning Beyond the Text Skills

Reasoning Beyond the Text tests four distinctive critical thinking skills.

Anticipate Response

Identify what the author or someone else would feel/say/do about a new situation based on its similarities to passage ideas.

With this skill, you need to put yourself inside the author's head and imagine things from their point of view. These questions contain information that wasn't in the passage, but you'll have to supply the author's response, usually on the basis of passage ideas that are similar to the new information. This skill accounts for 15% of RBT and is covered in Chapter 17.

Predict Outcome/Explanation

Apply causal reasoning or another connection from the passage to a new situation.

The key to this question skill is understanding causal relationships and other similar kinds of connections in passages. Most often, you'll be given some kind of new situation and either need to find its probable outcome or offer a likely explanation of how it could happen, using causal or other conceptual relationships from the passage. This skill is also tested in 15% of RBT questions. See Chapter 18 for more details.

Strengthen/Weaken Argument

Characterize the logical relationship between a new claim and arguments from the passage.

This is the single highest yield skill on the CARS section, making up a full 50% of RBT. In other words, about one-fifth of all CARS questions test this skill in some way, so you can usually expect to see at least one with most passages. This skill tests your understanding of the logic of arguments and how they change in response to new evidence. Chapter 19 covers everything you need to know about this important skill.

Imagine Example/Analogy

Identify new examples of categories defined in the passage or analogies of passage concepts.

Sometimes CARS authors provide unique definitions of concepts in passages, establishing their own set of standards for something to qualify as an example of that concept. They may do this directly with a formal definition or a list of criteria, or more indirectly, for instance by providing their own set of examples of the concept. With this skill, you have to identify new examples, applying the criteria that the author directly or indirectly established. Analogies are similar to examples, but require a little more abstraction. This skill is tested in about 20% of RBT and discussed in Chapter 20.

Question Skill Summary

Figure 6.2 breaks down all CARS skills by AAMC question type, including approximate frequencies. Note that percentages included for skills are relative to the question type (FOC, RWT, or RBT), not to all CARS questions.

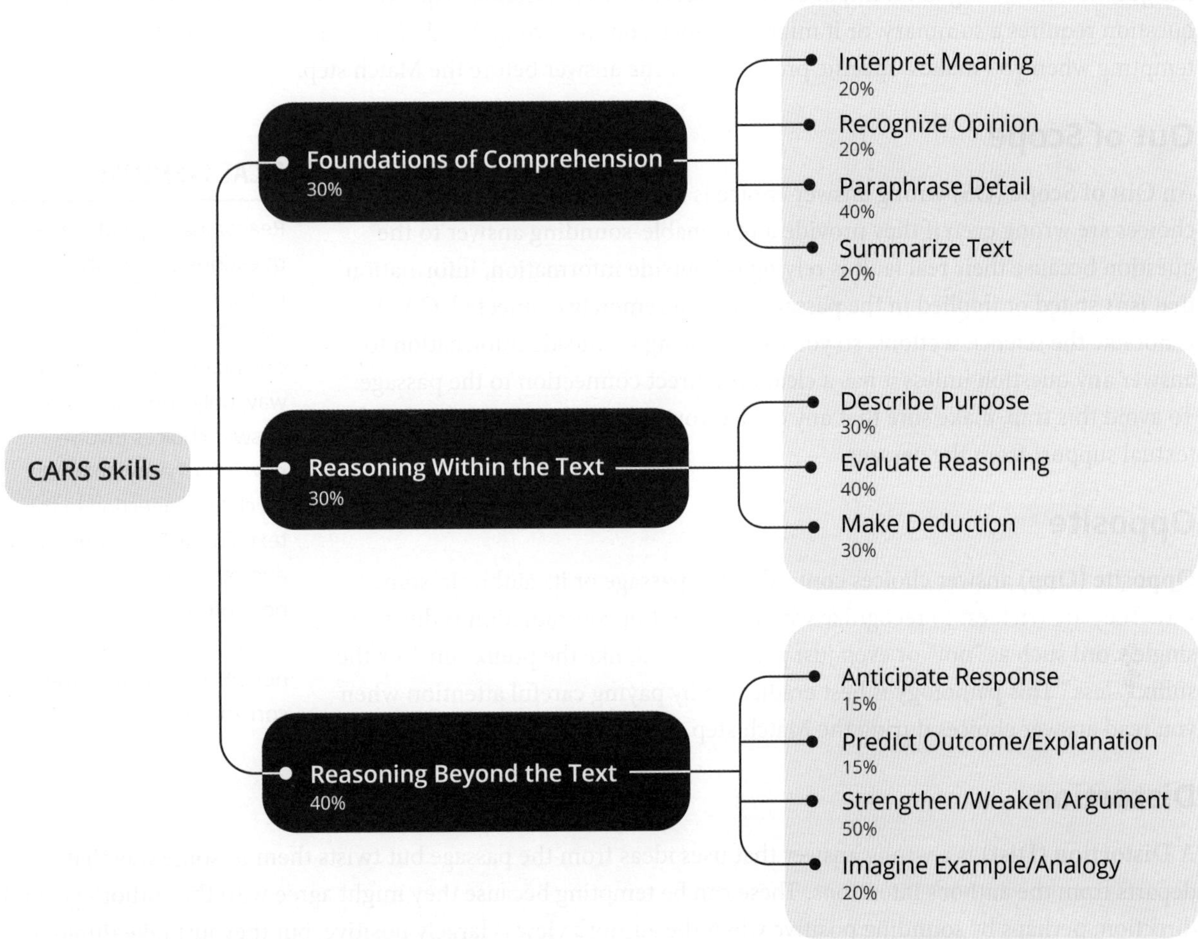

Figure 6.2 CARS Question Types and Skills

6.3 Wrong Answer Pathologies

We've already stressed in this chapter that wrong answers to CARS questions are always incorrect for a justifiable reason. At a basic level, that reason is always going to be some version of a disconnect between the answer choice and the passage the author wrote. There are recurring patterns to these misconnections, the most common of which Kaplan calls **wrong answer pathologies**. These pathologies are symptoms of unhealthy answer choices, yearning to be eliminated. For examples of all pathologies, see the analysis of the practice questions in section 6.4 below.

Don't expect every incorrect answer choice to have exactly one pathology. Some answer choices suffer from multiple pathologies, while others have different problems that aren't covered by this list. Still, being aware of these four common wrong answer traps will reduce the chances that you fall into any of them.

Faulty Use of Detail

Faulty Use of Detail (FUD) wrong answers contain details from the passage (words or ideas) but simply fail to answer the question asked. A FUD may be true and accurately reflect what the passage says, but it is irrelevant to what

MCAT EXPERTISE

Some question skills have wrong answer traps that are unique to them, such as the dictionary definition trap for Interpret Meaning questions (see Chapter 8). If a question skill has a unique trap, it is covered in the discussion of applying the Match step to that skill.

the question is looking for. It might be too general when a question requires a detail or too specific when a question requires a summary, or it might just focus on the wrong details. This trap is much less likely to be tempting when you make a specific prediction of the answer before the Match step.

Out of Scope

An **Out of Scope (OS)** wrong answer choice is like the flipside to a FUD. OS choices are wrong even if they provide a reasonable-sounding answer to the question because their real fault is relying on outside information, information that isn't stated or implied in the passage or even remotely connected. CARS is not like the science sections, so you cannot bring in outside information to answer any question unless it has a clear and direct connection to the passage. To avoid this trap, make sure that any choice you judge to be correct has solid textual support from the passage.

MCAT EXPERTISE

Reasoning Beyond the Text questions always bring in new information in some way. OS applies to those questions in a more limited way, only applicable when answer choices involve new information that has no clear connection to the text. For RBT questions, any answer choice containing new information that connects to the passage is not OS and could be the correct answer.

Opposite

Opposite (Opp) answer choices contradict the passage or its author in some way. They are trickiest to recognize when the point of contradiction is due to a single word such as "not" or even just part of a word, like the prefix "un-" or the suffix "-less." This pathology is best eradicated by paying careful attention when you read answer choices during the Match step.

Distortion

A **Distortion (Dist)** is a wrong answer that uses ideas from the passage but twists them in some way that departs from the author's intentions. These can be tempting because they might agree with the author's general direction, perhaps by sounding positive when the author's view is largely positive, but they just take things a little too far. Strong opinions and radical proposals are relatively uncommon in CARS passages, so a Dist is usually an extreme answer choice. Watch out for language like "all," "every," "only," or "never." In rarer cases, a Dist answer choice might misrepresent a relationship described in the passage, such as by portraying a correlation as cause and effect. Dist are best handled in the same way as Opp wrong answers: consider how every word in the answer choice impacts its meaning, paying special attention to the role played by keywords (see Chapter 3).

MCAT EXPERTISE

With scattered questions that contain words like "not," "least," or "except," the correct answer is going to look like an Opp would in a normal question. If you find yourself confused by the need to resolve double- or triple-negatives, it might help to remember that you're always looking for the one choice that is different from the other three. If three choices are consistent with the passage in a scattered question, you know you're looking for the one that will be opposite to the passage.

Healthy Answer Choices

While there aren't simple patterns that let you automatically recognize a correct answer, reflecting on where the pathologies go wrong can give you a better idea of what to expect when searching for a match to your prediction. Correct answers often possess the following characteristics:

- **Relevant.** Unlike a FUD, a correct answer needs to answer the question posed.
- **In Scope.** Unlike an OS, it needs to stay within the established scope of the passage.

- **Passage Agreement.** A correct answer should stick closely to what the author actually says in the passage, neither twisting it nor contradicting it, like a Dist or an Opp.
- **Measured.** Because most CARS authors aren't extreme, a correct answer is more likely to be a mild or limited statement than a strong or unqualified one.

Some exceptions to these trends are noted in the discussion of the pathologies above.

6.4 Practice Question Set

Now is your chance to practice the TRIM method. We'll return to the practice passage from Chapter 5, now with a full question set! The passage is reproduced below for your convenience.

If you recently completed Chapter 5 and the passage is still fresh in your mind, you can move straight on to the questions. Otherwise, you should Read *and Distill* the passage as you normally would and then attempt the questions that follow. Use the TRIM method on each question and don't hesitate to triage some questions for *later*, coming back to them after you've made a full pass through the questions. Full explanations, including a TRIM walkthrough for each question, can be found in Section 6.5.

> The archetype of the Russian anti-hero, when summoned in the popular imagination, often coalesces into a singular, gloomy figure: a man alienated from society, tormented by metaphysical questions in a cramped St. Petersburg apartment. While this Dostoevskian image is not without merit, viewing it as the definitive statement on the subject flattens a dynamic literary evolution into a monolithic cliché. In reality, the celebrated Russian anti-hero undergoes a profound transformation across the nineteenth century, beginning as the passive "superfluous man" and evolving into the ideologically committed nihilist. This literary trajectory directly reflects a nation's tumultuous journey toward modernity.
>
> The genesis of this archetype is the "superfluous man" (*lishniy chelovek*), a figure born of the early nineteenth-century Russian nobility. Crystallized in Pushkin's Eugene Onegin, the superfluous man is defined by a deep-seated ennui. Endowed with intelligence and a Western education, he is paralyzed by his own privilege, perceiving the vacuity of his social milieu—the endless balls, the insipid gossip, the rigid codes of honor—but finds himself unable to commit to any genuine passion. His alienation is not a product of rebellion but of profound listlessness. Onegin's casual cruelty, culminating in a pointless duel, stems not from malice but from a bored adherence to a social script he inwardly scorns, leaving him a ghost at the feast of his own life.
>
> A decisive break from this paradigm emerges mid-century with Ivan Turgenev's character Bazarov in *Fathers and Sons:* the nihilist. Unlike the superfluous man, Bazarov's alienation is not a passive affliction but a programmatic creed. A member of the *raznochintsy*, or classless intelligentsia, his rejection of the old order is active and absolute. He dismisses art, romance, and tradition in the name of a strict materi-

MCAT EXPERTISE

Any passage written by an author who takes extreme positions could also have some correct answers that appear extreme. When dealing with radical views in a passage, a Dist would actually be an answer choice with too weak of an opinion.

Also be aware that some RBT questions use the words "if true" or other similar language that asks you to assume the truth of each choice. Strengthen/Weaken Argument (see Chapter 19) is one skill in which this tends to occur. In such questions, a choice that is more extreme than anything in the passage might have the greatest strengthening or weakening impact, making it correct and not a Dist wrong answer.

BRIDGE

For a full expert analysis of the passage, including advice on how to interrogate it, along with recommendations for outlining and highlighting, return to Chapter 5.

alism and faith in science. Where Onegin was bored by the societal structure, Bazarov wishes to demolish it, famously asserting that "a good chemist is twenty times more useful than any poet." This shift represents a crucial move from an alienation of feeling to an alienation of ideology.

This ideological fervor finds its most tortured culmination in the works of Fyodor Dostoevsky. Here, the anti-hero internalizes the radical ideas of the era and pushes them to terrifying conclusions. While Raskolnikov in *Crime and Punishment* tests an ideology through violent action, the narrator of *Notes from Underground* represents a more disturbing endpoint. He is a spiteful, hyper-conscious intellectual who has retreated from a world governed by a rationalism he despises. His inaction is not Onegin's bored listlessness but a deliberate philosophical rebellion, championing the caprice of free will against the deterministic certainty of "two plus two equals four." The ideological project collapses inward into a state of paralyzed, self-devouring spite, creating an anti-hero whose alienation is total.

The arc from Onegin to the Underground Man is a mirror held up to Russian history. The superfluous man was the product of a static, autocratic state that offered its educated elite no outlet for their political energies. The nihilist, by contrast, was the child of a society in flux, born from the Great Reforms of the 1860s and the rise of radical movements that sought to violently remake Russia. The literary journey from aristocratic ennui to ideological rebellion and, finally, to psychological implosion charts the very course of the nineteenth-century Russian intellectual's search for meaning in a world where old certainties were crumbling and the shape of the future was not yet clear.

1. Which of the following discoveries, if true, would most WEAKEN the author's central argument?

- **A.** Archival evidence shows that the character of the nihilist Bazarov was based on a real person who lived decades before the Great Reforms of the 1860s.
- **B.** The private letters of many Russian authors in the 19th century reveal that they were personally preoccupied with their own feelings of alienation.
- **C.** Turgenev's novel *Fathers and Sons* was initially banned by state censors, who feared it would inspire radical movements.
- **D.** Literary critics in the 20th century consistently praised Dostoevsky's characters for their profound psychological realism.

2. As it relates to the first paragraph, the final paragraph:

- **A.** contradicts the initial claim that the popular image of the anti-hero is a cliché.
- **B.** introduces an entirely new argument about the role of the intellectual in society.
- **C.** questions the validity of the historical evidence used to support the thesis.
- **D.** provides a causal explanation for the literary transformation introduced there.

3. The author most likely includes Bazarov's assertion that "a good chemist is twenty times more useful than any poet" (paragraph 3) in order to:

- **A.** suggest that the author endorses the nihilist's worldview.
- **B.** provide a concrete example of the nihilist's rejection of traditional cultural values.
- **C.** contrast the practical education of the *raznochintsy* with the scientific education of the nobility.
- **D.** argue that Russian society had become overly focused on scientific progress at the expense of literature.

4. The central thesis of the passage is that the 19th-century Russian anti-hero:

- **A.** remains one of the most compelling and tormented figures in world literature.
- **B.** was primarily a product of the classless intelligentsia known as the *raznochintsy*.
- **C.** developed through several distinct stages that correspond to Russian political history.
- **D.** culminated in the works of Dostoevsky, whose characters are the most psychologically complex.

5. How would the author of the passage most likely react to a modern critic's claim that "the anti-hero is a constant in literature that represents a fundamental aspect of the human condition"?
   - **A.** The author would agree because of the passage's acknowledgment of the enduring power of the "Dostoevskian image."
   - **B.** The author would agree because all the figures described in the passage share a fundamental sense of alienation from society.
   - **C.** The author would disagree because the passage contends that the anti-hero archetype is dynamic and historically contingent.
   - **D.** The author would disagree because the modern critic fails to consider that only Russian literature produced true anti-heroes.

6. In describing Bazarov's alienation as a "programmatic creed" (paragraph 3), the author most likely means that it was:
   - **A.** directly copied from a popular religious text.
   - **B.** based on a consciously adopted set of principles.
   - **C.** a spontaneous emotional reaction to his social status.
   - **D.** a public performance intended to gain political power.

7. According to the logic of the final paragraph, a 19th-century Russian novel featuring an educated nobleman who, though frustrated, successfully channels his energies into a political reform movement would likely be explained by the passage author as a product of:
   - **A.** a static, autocratic state that paradoxically inspired action.
   - **B.** the rise of radical movements that sought revolution over reformation in Russia.
   - **C.** the novelist's ignorance of the true nature of aristocratic ennui and listlessness.
   - **D.** a historical period that offered the elite meaningful avenues for political engagement.

6.5 Answers and Explanations

Question 1 (A)

Type

The "if true" language in the question stem suggests that new information will appear in the answer choices, which are themselves on the long side. This is a new info (RBT) question, and it doesn't seem to be on the easier side, so most students would be better off triaging this question for *later*.

Rephrase

When coming back to attempt this, the prominent "WEAKEN" in the question stem makes it clear that this question is testing the Strengthen/Weaken Argument skill, specifically looking for a weakener. The tasks needed to answer this question might be characterized as follows:

- Find a statement of the central argument in your distillation or the passage.
- Look for weaknesses, assumptions, or requirements of this argument in your distillation or the passage.
- Make a prediction about what would weaken the central argument based on that info.
- If no match, investigate each choice for similarities in the text and eliminate those that don't produce the desired effect (weakening) or that otherwise conflict with the passage.

Investigate

The last two lines of paragraph 1 provide a good summary of the central argument: "In reality, the celebrated Russian anti-hero undergoes a profound transformation across the nineteenth century, beginning as the passive 'superfluous man' and evolving into the ideologically committed nihilist. This literary trajectory directly reflects a nation's tumultuous journey toward modernity." In other words, the author argues that the anti-hero changed in response to Russian history.

While there aren't obvious weaknesses or assumptions in the argument specified in the passage, the argument is ultimately about cause and effect. One requirement of cause-effect relationships involves the order of events: the cause has to precede the effect. So any choice which challenged this cause-effect connection would definitely weaken the central argument.

Though on the vague side, a solid prediction for this question would be: the correct answer will reorder the timing of events or otherwise challenge the cause-effect relationship between Russian history and the anti-hero's development.

Match

(A) matches the prediction because it does challenge the order of events described in the passage. According to paragraph 5, the nihilist anti-hero "was the child of a society in flux, born from the Great Reforms of the 1860s and the rise of radical movements that sought to violently remake Russia." This is relevant to paragraph 3, where the author writes, "A decisive break from this [superfluous man] paradigm emerges mid-century with Ivan Turgenev's character Bazarov in *Fathers and Sons:* the nihilist." However, **(A)** suggests that, rather than being "born from the Great Reforms of the 1860s," the nihilist Bazarov "was based on a real person who lived decades before." That directly challenges the cause-effect relationship in the author's central argument, making it correct.

Wrong Answers

(B) Every development of the anti-hero that appears in the passage is associated with some type of "alienation," so it would not be surprising if Russian novelists wrote letters about the topic. If anything this choice would strengthen the central argument, which makes it an Opposite.

(C) This choice is also an Opposite, producing a strengthening effect. Paragraph 5 associates the nihilist, connected in paragraph 2 to Turgenev's *Fathers and Sons*, with "the rise of radical movements," and this choice just reinforces that connection.

(D) The concept of "psychological realism" is not discussed in the passage, nor does the author make claims about how realistic Dostoevsky's characters are, so this choice has no impact on the passage. All the novels and events discussed in the passage are confined to the 19th century, so a statement about the 20th century is simply irrelevant.

Question 2 (D)

Type

This is a deep (RWT) question that asks about the logical relationship between two key paragraphs of the passage: the introduction and the conclusion. It requires an understanding of the passage's overall architecture. For a student who has successfully distilled the passage's structure, this should be a moderately difficult question to attack *now*; for others, it may be better to save for *later* in the question set.

Rephrase

This question tests the Evaluate Reasoning skill. The task is to define the specific function of the final paragraph as it connects to the argument presented in the first paragraph. A good plan would be to:

- Identify the primary purpose or main idea of the first paragraph.
- Identify the primary purpose or main idea of the last paragraph.
- Characterize the logical relationship between these two points.

Investigate

Use your distillation to identify the important ideas from the first and last paragraphs, or return to the passage if necessary. Paragraph 1 argues that the Russian anti-hero changed over time, concluding with the line "This literary trajectory directly reflects a nation's tumultuous journey toward modernity." The final paragraph, in contrast, describes how versions of the anti-hero arose in response to historical circumstances: "The superfluous man was the product of a static, autocratic state … The nihilist, by contrast, was the child of a society in flux …" Predict that the final paragraph is providing evidence to back up the claim the author makes at the end of paragraph 1.

Match

(D) matches the prediction. The evidence presented in the last paragraph comes in the form of a causal explanation of how the anti-hero changed.

Wrong Answers

(A) The last paragraph only provides details on 19th-century Russian history and does not address the point about the "popular imagination" from the first paragraph.

(B) Although the final paragraph mentions "the nineteenth-century Russian intellectual's search for meaning," this is actually in service to the argument introduced in the first paragraph about the anti-hero. The author connects the historical plight of the Russian intellectual to the development of specific literary characters discussed earlier in the passage. It is not "an entirely new argument."

(C) This is an Opposite. Rather than "question" the historical evidence, the final paragraph actually provides that evidence.

Question 3 (B)

Type

This question asks about the author's intentions with the phrase "in order to," indicating that it is a deep (RWT) question, testing you on the author's perspective. If your active reading of the passage was successful and you were able to identify the purposes of each paragraph, or at least of paragraph 3 in particular, then you should tackle the question *now*. Otherwise, save it for *later*.

Rephrase

This question tests the Describe Purpose skill, asking for the purpose of a specific element within paragraph 3. One efficient plan would be:

- Look at your distillation of paragraph 3 to determine that paragraph's purpose.
- Determine how the quoted text contributes to paragraph 3's purpose, rereading the surrounding context in the passage if necessary.
- State the quoted text's purpose in your own words as a prediction.

Investigate

A good distillation, whether an outline or highlighting, will show that the purpose of paragraph 3 is to explain the second stage in the evolution of the Russian anti-hero, the nihilist, as introduced in the novel *Fathers and Sons* and its character Bazarov. So it stands to reason that a quotation from this character should help to explain who the nihilist anti-hero really is. This by itself can serve as a prediction, but the sentence that precedes the quoted text can let you get more specific: "He [Bazarov] dismisses art, romance, and tradition in the same of a strict materialism and faith in science." By contrasting a chemist (connected to "science") with a poet (connected to "art"), the quotation from the novel provides textual support for the author's general description of the character and the archetype (the nihilist) that he represents. Predict that this quotation supports the author's description of the nihilist.

Match

While it is more specific than you might have predicted, **(B)** is a solid match. The passage said that the nihilist Bazarov "dismisses art, romance, and tradition," which sounds very similar to **(B)**'s "rejection of traditional cultural values." That line from the novel provides a "concrete example" of how this nihilistic attitude manifests in Russian literature.

Wrong Answers

(A) The author never endorses the nihilist's worldview or the worldview of any of the other anti-heroes described in the passage. In fact, the author later seems somewhat skeptical of this view by describing the extreme version of the nihilist that appears in Dostoevsky's works in negative terms: "The ideological project [of the nihilist] collapses inward into a state of paralyzed, self-devouring spite."

(C) According to paragraph 3, Bazarov prefers science over traditional culture and is a "member of the *raznochintsy*, or classless intelligentsia." In contrast, paragraph 2 described the Russian nobility as represented by the figure of Onegin, who is said to have a "Western education." Describing the nobility as having a "scientific education" is thus inconsistent with the passage, nor is there strong support for the idea that the *raznochintsy*'s education was especially "practical." This choice is a Distortion of how the two classes (and their respective educations) are described in the passage.

(D) The author never makes this argument. While the author doesn't endorse the nihilistic worldview, they never suggest anything in the passage that is specifically critical of science or the idea of scientific progress. The author is only unambiguously critical of the extreme form of nihilism found in Dostoevsky that rebels against "two plus two equals four," a view that suggests a rejection of mathematics (and probably science as well). Similarly, the detailed description of Russian society in the final paragraph never suggests too much focus on science or too little focus on literature.

Question 4 (C)

Type

The mention of "central thesis" in the stem indicates a question asking for the big picture, something the active reader will attempt to identify with every CARS passage. Rather than asking for the author's overall purpose, which would be a deep dive into the author's intentions, this is just asking for the main takeaway, making it a surface (FOC) question. Attempt this question *now*, when you first encounter it, especially since it gives you a clue that the thesis involves "the 19th-century Russian anti-hero."

Rephrase

This question tests the Summarize Text skill. Such questions can often be answered without having to do extensive rereading, or perhaps any rereading at all. Here's one way to rephrase it that works if you wrote down a goal for the passage in your notes (required for outlining and optional but recommended for highlighting):

- Look at the author's overall goal in my notes and use that to articulate the passage's thesis in my own words.

Investigate

In Chapter 5, we offered one possible statement of the author's overall goal, suggesting that the author "argues [that the] anti-hero changed with Russian history." The question stem already includes the mention of the Russian anti-hero, so you can simply predict that the correct answer will say it changed in some way in conjunction with Russian history.

Match

(C) is a perfect match. The "several distinct stages" are articulated in paragraphs 2, 3, and 4, with paragraph 5 showing how they "correspond to Russian political history." This choice adequately captures the full scope of the passage and its thesis.

Wrong Answers

(A) This choice may be tempting because "compelling and tormented" echoes some of the language in the opening sentence of the passage: "the Russian anti-hero, when summoned in the popular imagination, often coalesces into a singular, gloomy figure." But the author never goes so far as to say that the Russian anti-hero is "one of the most" compelling figures, or even to compare the anti-hero to other "figures in world literature." Moreover, the author immediately rejects the description in the opening sentence, calling it "a monolithic cliché."

(B) Although the *raznochintsy* is mentioned in paragraph 3, the author only connects them to the middle stage of the evolution of the anti-hero, the nihilist in its early form. Because two other stages of the anti-hero are described that are not directly connected to this class, it is inaccurate to say the anti-hero was "primarily a product" of the *raznochintsy*.

(D) The author makes it clear in paragraph 1 that their focus is not on talking about how Dostoevsky represents a culmination of the anti-hero, even though that statement has some truth to it: "While this Dostoevskian image is not without merit, viewing it as the definitive statement on the subject flattens a dynamic literary evolution into a monolithic cliché." Rather than just focusing on the final stage, like this answer choice suggests, the author is interested in discussing the entire evolution of the archetype, particularly as it relates to Russian history. This choice is a Faulty Use of Detail.

Question 5 (C)

Type

The quotation in the question stem is attributed to a "modern critic," indicating the introduction of new information. Most new info (RBT) questions should be saved for *later*, but the stem here is a manageable size and the new info is directly relevant to the overall thesis of the passage, which you probably just articulated to answer Q4. Most students are better off doing this question *now*.

Rephrase

This question tests the Anticipate Response skill, asking how "the author of the passage" would "react" to a new statement from a critic. One way to rephrase it into tasks is as follows:

- Find the point of connection between the situation presented by the new quotation and the point of view of the responder (the author).
- Predict how the author would act in light of this specific type of connection.

Investigate

You'll start to investigate this question by further unpacking the quotation in the stem. The modern critic is making a claim about the anti-hero, saying it is "a constant in literature" and that it "represents a fundamental aspect of the human condition." The theme here is that the anti-hero doesn't change. How does that connect to the passage? As we saw when working through question 4, the author's thesis is that the anti-hero changed in response to Russian history, which is a direct contradiction of the idea that the anti-hero is unchanging. So the point of connection is actually a contradiction, which means a negative response from the author. Predict that the author would reject this statement because it conflicts with the thesis of the passage.

Match

Based on the recommended prediction, either **(C)** or **(D)** must be correct because both acknowledge that the passage author "would disagree." (C) is in fact the match because it better summarizes the passage's thesis: "the passage contends that the anti-hero archetype is dynamic and historically contingent."

Wrong Answers

(A) This choice is an Opposite, directly contradicting what the author would say. Not only would the author disagree, but they specifically state that accepting the Dostoevskian image "as the definitive statement on the subject [of the anti-hero] flattens a dynamic literary evolution into a monolithic cliché." That is far from an "acknowledgement of the enduring power" of this image.

(B) This choice may be tempting because the author does *in fact* mention "alienation" as a recurring characteristic of the anti-hero appearing in each of paragraphs 2, 3, and 4. But while the author uses the same word throughout, they focus more on how this alienation changes from one stage to another, for example by talking about the transition from "an alienation of feeling to an alienation of ideology" in paragraph 3. Indeed, the emphasis on change appears consistently throughout this passage, so this choice is incorrect for suggesting that the author would agree with the quotation's vision of the anti-hero as a constant.

(D) While the passage author would definitely disagree with the modern critic's statement, this choice provides the wrong reason for that disagreement. The author never talks about anti-heroes outside the context of 19th-century Russia, so there is no basis for making a claim about the anti-hero more broadly, as this choice requires. There's not enough information in the passage to know whether the author believes that literature from other countries has produced worthwhile or "true" anti-heroes.

Question 6 (B)

Type

This is a surface (FOC) question that asks you to explain a short quotation from the passage, with the paragraph number given. On top of that, glancing at the answer choices reveals the shortest ones in the whole set. Definitely do this question, and others like it, *now*.

Rephrase

This is an Interpret Meaning question, so you'll want to find the quoted text and use the surrounding context to unpack its meaning. Here's a good rephrase:

- Locate "programmatic creed" in paragraph 3 and read the entire sentence that contains it, looking for keywords and other clues that might suggest a definition.
- Read sentences before or after if more clues are needed, until you can state a prediction of the quotation's meaning.

Investigate

Start your investigation with the sentence that contains the quote: "Unlike the superfluous man, Bazarov's alienation is not a passive affliction but a programmatic creed." This first sentence provides a contrast, letting us know that this alienation isn't passive, so it must be something that the nihilist Bazarov actively does. That's too vague to be a good prediction for this question, so read on for more clues. The next sentence states that "his rejection of the old order is active and absolute," which confirms that the contrast was intended to show that Bazarov is more active, while the sentence after that says something a little more substantive: "He dismisses art, romance, and tradition in the name of a strict materialism and faith in science." So we have Bazarov rejecting traditional values and embracing "materialism" and "science" instead. Predict that a "programmatic creed" means something that actively sets up different values to live by.

Match

The match here is **(B)**. The term "set of principles" corresponds closely to the values of "materialism" and "science" mentioned in the passage, while "consciously adopted" indeed suggests an active process that contrasts with a "passive affliction." This choice best explains the meaning of "programmatic creed" as the author uses it.

Wrong Answers

(A) This choice is Out of Scope because religion is not described in the passage. This choice plays on a dictionary definition of "creed," which can refer to a set of religious beliefs.

(C) Much like the "passive affliction" that the author directly contrasts with "programmatic creed," a "spontaneous emotional reaction" suggests something beyond the individual's control, rather than a deliberate action. This might better describe the character of Onegin from paragraph 2 than Bazarov from paragraph 3, so it is not a sound interpretation of "programmatic creed."

(D) While politics is discussed in other parts of the passage, particularly in the treatment of Russian political history in the final paragraph, it is not addressed in paragraph 3, where "programmatic creed" appears. This choice is Out of Scope because the passage says nothing that pertains to gaining political power or to public performances, either in the context of the quotation or elsewhere.

Question 7 (D)

Type

This lengthy question stem presents a scenario that is similar to ideas discussed in the passage but unique, making it a new info (RBT) question. There is a reference to a specific paragraph, but it's a vague one, so this one would be better for most students to attempt *later*. Since this is the last question in the set, you should go back to all the questions you already triaged for *later* and then return to this one last.

Rephrase

The skill tested here is Predict Outcome/Explanation. It asks you to extend a cause-effect relationship described in the passage to a new context. More exactly, the "product of" language at the end of the stem indicates that you're looking for a cause: a cause produces an effect, so it follows that an effect is a "product of" its cause. Understanding that the new situation is the effect and you're looking for the cause, you can rephrase as follows:

- Look at your distillation of the last paragraph and summarize the cause-effect logic there, rereading parts of paragraph 5 only if needed.
- Match the effect given in the new information to the effects described in the last paragraph.
- Predict what would have to be true of the cause of this new effect, based on how the corresponding causes are described in paragraph 5.

Investigate

In Chapter 5, we distilled the final paragraph to arrive at the idea that the development of the anti-hero in literature reflected Russian political history. In other words, historical events were causes of literary developments. The language in the last paragraph even parallels the language in this question stem: "The superfluous man was the product of a static, autocratic state that offered its educated elite no outlet for their political energies." This language is close to the new information in the question stem, but in fact contradicts it by mentioning "an educated nobleman who, though frustrated, successfully channels his energies into a political reform movement." Is such a figure described elsewhere in the last paragraph? No, but the nihilist is described as "the child of a society in flux, born from the Great Reforms of the 1860s and the rise of radical movements that sought to violently remake Russia." The common thread between these two is that the political situation produces certain types of people, and then these types of people feature as characters in novels. So, even though there's no exact correspondence between the new information and the passage, we can make a prediction that this kind of character must be the product of a society that contained actual people like the character. For this question, that would mean we're looking for a society in which nobles can freely engage in political activities.

Match

Though no such period is described in the passage, **(D)** is a match because it successfully extends the causal logic in paragraph 5. If there were *in fact* a period in 19th-century Russian history in which elites had "meaningful avenues for political engagement," then you would expect to see characters who had the same kind of experience. Thus, the cause of a literary character who could become a political reformer would have to be a society that allowed for political reform and similar activities, as suggested in **(D)**.

Wrong Answers

(A) While this exactly uses the language in the second sentence of the final paragraph, there is no reason given in the passage to suppose that such a state could "paradoxically inspire action." This departs too greatly from the discussion in the passage.

(B) This choice is an Opposite. While this choice describes the kind of society that produced the nihilist anti-hero, the character detailed in the question stem is explicitly connected to reformation rather than revolution, so it would be expected as the product of a society that didn't prioritize revolution.

(C) While this might provide a plausible explanation of how such a literary character could arise given the author's description of Russian history, it departs too far from the "logic of the final paragraph." In that last paragraph, the author never singles out specific characteristics of novelists that led them to create the characters they did, but instead simply focuses on how social circumstances produce certain kinds of people that then become characters in novels.

Conclusion

This chapter covered all aspects of question strategy: the Kaplan Method for CARS Questions (TRIM), the three AAMC question types with their 11 question skills, and the four common wrong answer pathologies. Using these tools on Test Day can improve your score by increasing your accuracy and efficiency in attacking questions. However, it's not enough to start using these strategies on the day of your MCAT: you need to practice regularly and review your practice to learn from your mistakes. The next chapter, the final one in Unit 1 on CARS strategy, covers these essential topics of practice and review.

Skill and Strategy Summary

The Kaplan Method for CARS Questions

- The **Kaplan Method for CARS Questions**, or **TRIM**, is a four-step process you can use to attack any question.
  - **Type the question**. Read the question stem and glance at the choices to identify the AAMC question type and difficulty and decide whether to do it *now* or *later*.
  - **Rephrase the stem**. Simplify the phrasing of the question stem to determine the specific tasks required to answer it.
  - **Investigate potential solutions**. Use your distillation and the passage, if necessary, to predict what you can about the answer.
  - **Match your prediction to an answer choice**. Look for an answer choice that is synonymous with your prediction or eliminate choices that conflict with it.
- You **triage** questions during the Type step, deciding whether to attempt them now or later. The main factor in this decision is the **AAMC question type**, but the **apparent difficulty** also plays a role.
  - **Foundations of Comprehension (FOC/surface questions)**: These questions focus on passage **content**. Complete these *now* unless especially difficult or time-consuming (for example, **scattered** variations that use a word like "not" or Roman numerals).
  - **Reasoning Within the Text (RWT/deep questions)**: These questions focus on passage **architecture** and author **perspective**. Choose *now* if your interrogation was successful regarding what the question asks, but save for *later* if you expect difficulties, such as the need to draw on info from multiple paragraphs.
  - **Reasoning Beyond the Text (RBT/new info questions)**: These questions always provide information not contained in the passage. Save for *later* unless they're short or you see a clear way to connect the new info to the passage.
- When you rephrase a question, you will set yourself one or more tasks to complete to arrive at an answer.
  - The number of tasks depends both on the exact wording of the question stem and on the format of the answer choices, as well as on how well you remember passage information that is relevant to the question.
  - Plan to use your distillation (highlights or outline) to help you locate relevant details when you don't know which paragraph to start with.
  - If your distillation doesn't provide an immediate answer, plan to look for specific lines in the passage that can justify a correct answer.

- At the end of the Investigate step, always try to make a specific **prediction** in your own words of the correct answer. Finding a match for your prediction is the quickest way to get the point.
    - If you are unable to predict, or if your prediction has no clear match, you'll need to use the **process of elimination**.
    - If you can't eliminate all three wrong answers, make an **educated guess** from among the remaining choices.
    - If you're low on time or unable to eliminate any choices with confidence, a **wild guess** is recommended because there's no penalty for wrong answers on the MCAT. Don't leave any question unanswered when time runs out.

Question Types and Skills

- Foundations of Comprehension is subdivided into four skills:
    - **Interpret Meaning**: Use context to determine what a word/phrase from the passage is intended to communicate.
    - **Recognize Opinion**: Identify what the author or someone else feels about a passage idea based on word choice or other context clues.
    - **Paraphrase Detail**: Recognize a specific piece of information that is stated or strongly implied at one location in the passage.
    - **Summarize Text**: Articulate the main idea of the passage or of a part of it.
- Reasoning Within the Text is subdivided into three skills:
    - **Describe Purpose**: Identify why the author wrote the passage or a part of it.
    - **Evaluate Reasoning**: Characterize logical connections between ideas in the passage.
    - **Make Deduction**: Infer a claim that follows from multiple parts of the passage, such as an assumption in an argument.
- Reasoning Beyond the Text is subdivided into four skills:
    - **Anticipate Response**: Identify what the author or someone else would feel/say/do about a new situation based on its similarities to passage ideas.
    - **Predict Outcome/Explanation**: Apply causal reasoning or another connection from the passage to a new situation.
    - **Strengthen/Weaken Argument**: Characterize the logical relationship between a new claim and arguments from the passage.
    - **Imagine Example/Analogy**: Identify new examples of categories defined in the passage or analogies of passage concepts.

Wrong Answer Pathologies

- **Wrong answer pathologies** are the four most common patterns in incorrect answers:
  - **Faulty Use of Detail (FUD)**: A choice that may accurately reflect the passage but doesn't answer the question
  - **Out of Scope (OS)**: A choice that answers the question but does so by using information that is neither stated nor implied in the passage and is unconnected to the ideas in the passage
  - **Opposite (Opp)**: A choice that contradicts the passage or author in some way, sometimes because of a single word or phrase
  - **Distortion (Dist)**: A choice that twists passage information beyond what the author says, often by being more extreme, sometimes because of a single word or phrase
- Not all wrong answers suffer from a single pathology. Some suffer from multiple issues, and others are incorrect for unique reasons.
- Correct answer choices tend to be relevant, in scope, measured, and in agreement with the passage and its author.

CHAPTER 7

PRACTICING AND REVIEWING CARS

In This Chapter

Introduction 93

7.1 Structuring Your CARS Prep 94

Phase 1 – Skillbuilding 94

Phase 2 – Diagnosis and Troubleshooting . . . 95

Phase 3 – Timing and Endurance 95

7.2 Effective Review of CARS. 98

Why I Missed It (WIMI) 98

How I'll Fix It (HIFI). 100

Thinking Like the Test Maker: Post-Phrasing. 102

Conclusion. 104

Skill and Strategy Summary 104

LEARNING OBJECTIVES

After Chapter 7, you will be able to:

- Structure your preparation for the CARS section in three phases
- Review CARS questions effectively using WIMI, HIFI, and post-phrasing

Introduction

Hours before scrubbing in, you review the day's case: a standard laparoscopic cholecystectomy. You skim the patient's chart, recognize the procedure, and feel a familiar comfort. You know the steps, at least in theory, the same way you might know the general topic of a book chapter you'd been assigned. You feel ready for what's coming up, or at least you think you do.

Later, in the OR, the gap between familiarity and true preparation became clear. During the closure, your attending stopped you. You reached for a cutting needle when the delicate tissue required a tapered one. It was a mistake born not of ignorance, but of a mind not fully engaged in the present step because it hadn't been rigorously prepared for the sequence. Now, in the quiet of the surgeon's lounge, the debrief begins.

"Talk me through it," your attending says, her tone analytical, not accusatory. You start with the easy out: "I just grabbed the wrong one. A silly mistake." She gently dismisses that. "There are no 'silly mistakes' in here, only flaws in a process that we need to fix. Let's do a root cause analysis. Was it a knowledge gap? Did you forget which suture to use? Or was it a cognitive lapse? Were you already thinking three steps ahead, rushing the immediate task?" The question forces you to look past the excuse. It wasn't a lack of knowledge. "A cognitive lapse," you admit. "I was worried about the time."

"Good," she replies. "That's a specific diagnosis." A vague problem like "being careless" gets a useless solution like "be more careful." A specific diagnosis, however, leads to a concrete, actionable step. You formulate one on the spot: "Before starting a closure, I will state the tissue layer and my intended suture out loud. It will force a cognitive pause."

The goal of that surgical debrief isn't to demand perfection—no one expects a physician, least of all an intern, to be flawless. The goal is to build a reliable process for improvement, because surgical skill is not a fixed talent, but one that is meticulously developed. This is the growth mindset required for CARS. *Your ability on this section is not a fixed trait you are born with.* Like the intern, you will make mistakes. The key is to treat them not as evidence of a permanent weakness, but as invaluable data. By reflecting on your errors and tracing them back to their root causes—whether in your preparation or your execution—you can systematically refine your approach and prove that this set of skills, like any other in medicine, can be learned.

In this chapter, we'll review strategies to help you improve by understanding both the test maker's patterns as well as your own behavioral patterns. We'll also discuss how your findings can be translated into concrete action steps by adjusting the way you practice CARS moving forward. True improvement comes from refining your entire process, from preparation to execution to review.

7.1 Structuring Your CARS Prep

The standard advice for CARS is "just practice," but we know from countless students who complete hundreds of CARS passages and questions that completion alone doesn't necessarily correspond to an increase in scores. Practicing without changing anything about your approach just reinforces a consistent score. While practice is a very important component, your path to CARS mastery must be more deliberate. We have organized this journey into a preparation path designed to build your abilities from the ground up. We also recognize that not everyone starts at the same place with CARS, so we also provide recommendations that depend on where you're scoring with a baseline practice exam.

Phase 1 – Skillbuilding

The points are in the questions, and as a Critical Analysis and Reasoning Skills section, developing the skills to tackle MCAT questions should be the top priority. As such, we recommend that you carefully review the three AAMC question types found in the CARS section, which are then broken down by skills in the following chapters of this book.

- Chapters 8–11 cover the Foundations of Comprehension Skills
- Chapters 13–15 cover the Reasoning Within the Text Skills
- Chapter 17–20 cover the Reasoning Beyond the Text Skills

Working on a skill is a type of procedural learning, and you learn best from doing rather than reading. More than just a description of these skills, each chapter contains a unique exercise called a Skillbuilder, which allows you to practice a specific skill that the AAMC wants you to master. This differs from a full CARS passage and question set in that it's a shorter passage with questions that focus on just one skill at a time, with additional Active Reading Check questions that aim to promote interrogation of each paragraph. Each set of chapters then has a cumulative exercise allowing you to practice all of the question skills within that type (Chapters 12, 16, and 21, respectively).

→ Action Step

If your initial score is 125 or below, we strongly recommend you begin with Phase 1: Skillbuilding. A score in this range typically indicates a need to build or reinforce the fundamental skills of how to actively read a passage, identify an author's main argument, and systematically analyze questions. Phase 1 is designed to construct this essential groundwork from the bottom up, ensuring you have a solid and reliable skillset.

If you are starting with a score above 125, you can proceed directly to Phase 2: Diagnosis and Troubleshooting. A score at this level suggests you already have a functional grasp of the skills. Your primary goal is to identify the specific, recurring patterns that are holding you back—whether it's timing, a particular passage topic (like philosophy), or a certain question skill. For you, the Skill-building chapters of this book should be used as a targeted "remediation" tool. For example, if your diagnostic review reveals a consistent weakness in Evaluate Reasoning questions, you can return to that specific chapter to strengthen that particular skill.

MCAT EXPERTISE

When you're first developing your strategy, it's best to do CARS passages and questions untimed. Trying to learn a new set of processes and managing the timer simultaneously is a recipe for frustration. Untimed practice allows you to isolate the variable of strategy. You can focus solely on executing your method correctly, step-by-step, until it becomes second nature.

Phase 2 - Diagnosis and Troubleshooting

With a solid foundation in the skills required for CARS, the next step in your CARS preparation is data mining. The value in practicing CARS is not only found in the experience you gain, but in the way practice serves as a source of data on how you think about CARS passages and questions. During Phase 2, you will learn to diagnose the thought patterns that lead you to incorrect answers and create action steps to troubleshoot for future passages and questions. Many students just read through the explanation, and like the intern in the introduction of this chapter, dismiss errors as "silly mistakes" without truly reflecting on why an error was made. Section 7.2 of this chapter is devoted to pattern analysis and generating action steps to help you learn how to effectively take advantage of the mistakes you're making. In this phase, we recommend regularly working through 1-2 CARS passages and their question sets at a time using Kaplan and AAMC question resources.

For all students, regardless of score, this phase may involve heading back to the Skillbuilders from Phase 1 if a particular question skill appears as a pattern in your errors. This iterative process is how you customize your review to what you need specifically.

Phase 3 - Timing and Endurance

This final phase is where it all comes together. Many students find that they run out of time in the CARS section, and for good reason: it's challenging working through so many dense passages and complex questions in a short period of time. Here, we recommend you gradually increase the number of CARS passages you complete in one sitting and start timed practice.

Timing

Proper management of the clock can make a significant difference to your score in any section, but the timing constraints in the CARS section differ from those of the other sections. Consider a few basic facts about the CARS section:

- There are 9 passages.
- There are 53 questions.
- It lasts 90 minutes.

It's a simple matter of arithmetic to see that 9 passages in 90 minutes allows you 10 minutes for each passage. Passages vary in difficulty, meaning that some will certainly take longer to read than others, but as a rule of thumb you should aim to complete the passage analysis in about 4–5 minutes, and around 1 minute per question. Because all of the points actually come from answering the questions, you must ensure that you allot enough time for them.

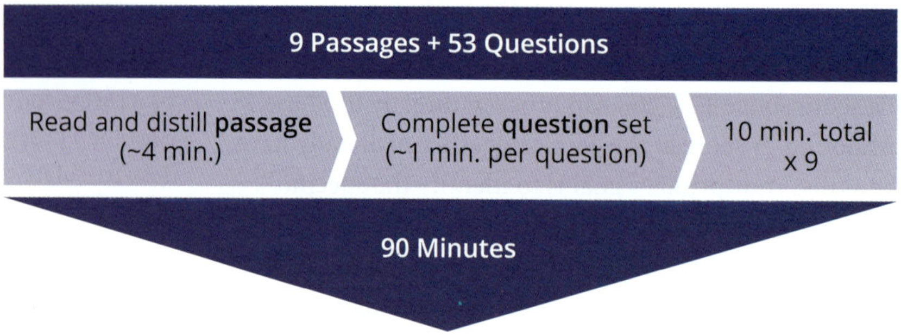

Figure 7.1 CARS Section Timing

Now, trying to ensure that each passage takes 4–5 minutes and each question a little less than one minute would actually be counterproductive: not only would you lose a substantial amount of time checking the clock, you'd likely heighten your anxiety each time you came across a question that takes a little extra time to get through. A better approach to managing your time is to check your timing only at a limited number of predetermined points during the section.

We recommend checking the clock after every other passage. Assuming that you take 10 minutes to read a passage and answer its questions, you should ideally be no more than 20 minutes further into the section each time you check the clock. Use the following guideposts:

2 passages complete: 70 minutes left

4 passages complete: 50 minutes left

6 passages complete: 30 minutes left

8 passages complete: 10 minutes left

If your timing appears to go off course, then during your review of the test, note which passages (and potentially your choice between the Distill tools of highlighting and outlining) seem to have caused this trouble. Could you have triaged these time-consuming passages or distilled them differently and answered more questions correctly in the limited time you had left?

Hitting these recommended time points does not leave you much of a cushion for going back to previous passages and questions, but this approach is by far the best way to maximize your score. Given that each CARS passage contains between 500 and 600 words, jumping between passages is far less realistic in CARS than in any of the science sections, where passages can be less than half that length. While it is recommended that you skip passages that you decide will be too time-consuming in your Preview step, we recommend that you answer all questions associated with a passage before moving on to the next one. In other words, once you decide to work on a passage, commit to finishing it.

→ Action Step

Consider utilizing a drill like this to work on pacing: First, time how long it takes for you to comfortably complete a CARS passage and question set. If you're already fairly close to 10 minutes, then congratulations, that's average test day timing! If not, then set yourself a time limit for subsequent CARS practice, starting by rounding down to the nearest 30 seconds from your latest timing, multiplied by the number of passages you're practicing at once. For example, if your timing starts at 14 minutes and 44 seconds, and you're practicing with two passages at a time, set a timer for two times 14 minutes and 30 seconds, or 29 minutes.

With each new practice session, reduce the time limit you set by 30 seconds for each CARS passage and question set, and continue doing so until you're at 10 minutes per passage. Extending the example from before and assuming you stayed with only two passages at a time, your next session's time limit would be reduced by twice 30 seconds or one minute, leaving you 28 minutes total, then 27 minutes the following session, and so on. You may find that you hit a point where the accuracy takes a hit due to the increased speed; at that point, consider heading back to some of the tips in Phase 2 to work on diagnosing what's taking the additional time.

MCAT EXPERTISE

If the seconds ticking down cause you too much anxiety, an alternative way of working on your timing is to use the timer on your phone or some other timepiece to "time up"—that is, to count upwards from zero to see how much time it's taking you to read the passage and to complete each question. Timers with "lap" functions can be especially useful because these can record how long each question takes. Generally, this method works best with only one or two passages at a time. Keep in mind, however, that an alternate timer cannot be used on Test Day!

Cognitive Endurance

Cognitive endurance is your brain's ability to maintain a high level of focus, concentration, and analytical thinking over a prolonged period. It's the mental resilience that allows you to resist fatigue, stay engaged, and perform consistently on demanding tasks. Just as a marathon runner trains their body to withstand 26.2 miles, you must train your brain to withstand 90 minutes of dense, academic reading. You may find that this is an issue for you if you notice that you do well with shorter sets of CARS practice but really struggle maintaining concentration for an entire section.

MCAT EXPERTISE

Some students see a boost in their CARS section score just from implementing regular practice of CARS passages, all from increasing their cognitive endurance!

Each passage demands that you build and hold a complex mental model of the author's argument. A momentary lapse in focus on a passage can cause you to miss the author's tone or a key transition, leading to multiple incorrect answers. Without strong cognitive endurance, your reading speed slows, your attention wanders, and you start making careless errors on questions you would have gotten right at the beginning of the test. In fact, the evidence of low cognitive endurance may be seen in an increase in preventable errors as you progress through the section.

MCAT EXPERTISE

The constant overstimulation and fragmented attention required by social media can erode your ability to sustain the deep focus needed for complex cognitive tasks. Reducing your usage may help in retraining your brain for the prolonged concentration demanded by activities like completing a CARS section.

→ Action Step

Like the timing drill above, try gradually increasing the number of CARS passages you do in one sitting. Consider how many you're comfortable with and start with that, but increase the number of passages by one at regular intervals (every week, every other practice session, etc.). If you're building your timing and endurance simultaneously, be sure to adjust the time limit you set yourself to account for any extra passages.

After you start attempting four or more passages at a time, you may consider dropping your frequency of CARS practice per week, especially if you're practicing CARS daily. Just like a marathon runner wouldn't run a marathon every day, you don't want to be completing an entire CARS section daily!

7.2 Effective Review of CARS

Many students find reviewing CARS challenging because the errors feel *subjective* and personal, unlike the clear, content-based errors in the science sections. There's no clear formulaic set of steps to follow, and much of CARS relies on your personal interpretation. This ambiguity can make the path to improvement seem vague and frustrating. The reasoning presented for the correct answer can seem like a matter of opinion, making the review process more like an argument with an invisible test maker rather than a logical puzzle to solve. The challenge is learning to see the evidence-based logic that makes one answer choice correct, even when the differences are subtle.

Additionally, there's a real danger in being overly specific when reviewing CARS; you'll never see this specific passage and question again, which often contributes to the feeling that reviewing CARS is a "waste of time." The solution to this is to learn how to generalize the mistakes made by following the guidelines below, thereby creating *objective* metrics to evaluate your CARS practice.

MCAT EXPERTISE

To get the most out of your review, don't wait too long to review CARS, particularly when reviewing practice tests. Waiting days after completing the practice will not only make you take longer to review since you'll need to reacquaint yourself with the passage and question, you're also less likely to remember your thought processes for each question. Understanding the steps you're taking to answer the questions is the point of practicing CARS!

Why I Missed It (WIMI)

To effectively analyze patterns in your performance, we recommend tracking each question you review in a **Why I Missed It (WIMI)** spreadsheet. Think of this log as a "patient chart" for your CARS skills. Below are some common metrics to include as you begin diagnosing your practice. While this is not an exhaustive list, and you're welcome to include additional metrics, we would recommend avoiding overly specific details about individual passages and questions in WIMI.

Q #	Passage #	Time (s)	Passage Type	Question Type	Question Skill	Passage Evaluation	Q/A Evaluation	Wrong Answer Pathology	Strategy Evaluation
4	1	75	SS	FOC	Paraphrase Detail	-	50/50	FUD	Pacing issue
13	3	55	Hum	RBT	S/W Argument	Mistaken ID	-	DIST	Outline

Table 7.1 Example Why I Missed It (WIMI) Log

Question Details

The first thing you should include in your WIMI are the concrete details about the individual questions that you missed or had to guess on. These details include:

- Question number
- The associated passage number
- The general passage topic (humanities vs. social sciences and their subtopics)
- The AAMC question type and the question skill
- How much time you spent on the question

Passage Evaluation

When it's time to reflect on your performance during your practice, start with how you read and distilled the passage. Now that you've seen all of the questions and their explanations, make note of anything you might have missed while reanalyzing the passage that would have helped you on the questions, then think about the strategies that would have helped you notice those details. Some common errors include:

- **Mistaken Identity**: This is common when there are multiple viewpoints in the passage, and you mistakenly attributed one viewpoint to another's perspective.
- **Misinterpreting Tone**: You didn't identify the author's underlying attitude—such as critical, supportive, or ambiguous—which caused you to misinterpret the purpose or meaning of their statement.
- **Overlooked Keywords**: You missed identifying critical keywords that the author uses to show how various claims are related in the passage.
- **Trees Over Forest**: You got bogged down in the specific details, examples, or complex phrasing within a passage (the "trees") at the expense of understanding the author's main argument and purpose (the "forest").

MCAT EXPERTISE

Because they're structured as tables, spreadsheet tools can be very helpful for analyzing CARS. Consider using a spreadsheet-creating program so you can add to them from multiple devices, sort them by different columns to more easily see trends, and organize them in different ways that best suit your current needs.

Question/Answer Evaluation

After evaluating your read of the passage, the next step is to analyze how you interacted with the questions and the answer choices themselves. Reflect on your thought process for the questions you missed, considering why a specific answer seemed persuasive and why the correct answer was dismissed. This will help you identify flaws in your reasoning. Some common errors in this stage include:

- **Wrong Answer Pathology** of the Answer Chosen: This is described in more detail in Chapter 6, but below is a brief summary of each of the four.
  - **Distortion**: The answer has definitive language when the author's claims were more nuanced; the statement twists or changes the meaning of a claim from the passage.
  - **Faulty Use of Detail**: The answer contains words/phrases taken directly from the passage but doesn't match what the question is asking.
  - **Out of Scope**: The answer choice is a reasonable statement that could be true in the real world but isn't supported by the information in the passage.
  - **Opposite**: The answer contains a few words or even just a modifier that makes the statement contradictory to what the passage supports.
- **Misunderstood Question Stem**: You had difficulty understanding what the question was asking for or misinterpreted the task of the question.
- **Misunderstood Answer Choice**: You focused on some parts of the answer while excluding others or misunderstood the meaning of a word or phrase.
- **Answer Swap/Debate**: You initially selected the correct answer, then second-guessed yourself and changed it to an incorrect one, leading to wasted time.
- **50/50**: You were able to quickly eliminate two incorrect answer choices but found yourself choosing the remaining incorrect answer more often than not.

Strategy Evaluation

Finally, zoom out from individual passages and questions to reflect on your high-level strategy across the entire section. Consider your overall time management, your energy levels from start to finish, and how effectively you used your test-day tools. Pinpointing flaws in the overarching process is essential for making significant gains. Some common strategic errors include:

- **Pacing Issues**: You spent too much time on earlier passages/questions, forcing you to rush or guess on later ones, or (less commonly) nervousness led you to rush through one or more early passage sets, increasing the frequency of avoidable mistakes.
- **Stamina/Focus Fade**: Mental fatigue played a bigger role in the latter half of the section, causing preventable errors. Evidence of this is if you find that the question is straightforward to answer in review.
- **Tool Usage – Outline**: Notes with either too much detail (wasting time and obscuring author intentions) or too little (making it harder to locate specific information in the passage) would be included. Either way, your outline wasn't all that useful when attacking the questions.
- **Tool Usage – Highlight**: Excessive, insufficient, or misplaced highlights fail to clarify the structure of the passage. Regardless of the specifics, the highlights are more distracting than helpful.

How I'll Fix It (HIFI)

When practice and review are complete, the next step is to create a **How I'll Fix It (HIFI)** list, which serves as an action plan for how to correct the errors you're making. While it's possible to do this for each incorrect question you have, use the patterns you've generated in the review to help prioritize which corrections to work on first. Select your 3–5 most common misses from your review sheet and examine the table that follows for some action steps to implement in your next CARS practice set.

WIMI Pattern	HIFI
Passage Topic	• Apply interrogation principles from Chapter 4 to new passages • Alternate between highlighting and outlining to determine which tool is more efficient for you • Read articles on unfamiliar topics for 15 minutes daily to build comfort with diverse topics
Specific Question Type/Skill	• Revisit the corresponding skill chapter(s) to review strategy • Complete Skillbuilder exercises for the specific question skill
Mistaken Identity	• Use an outline to explicitly track multiple perspectives and label the author's own voice • Actively hunt for answer choices that intentionally confuse the author's viewpoint with another mentioned in the text
Misinterpret Tone	• Review the different types of Author keywords found in Chapter 3.3, and consider what each reveals about tone • After each paragraph, ask, "what does the author think about this?" • After reading, write down one word that describes the author's overall attitude about the passage's subject (e.g. critical, supportive, neutral)
Overlooked Keywords	• Review Connection keywords in Chapter 3.1 and Logic keywords in 3.2, and practice connecting parts of the passage by identifying those keywords

WIMI Pattern	HIFI
Trees Over Forest	• Review Chunking and passage architecture principles in Chapter 4.2 to map the primary function of each paragraph, not just its content • While reading, consistently ask, "Why did the author include this?" instead of "What does this say?" • Before starting the questions, write a one-sentence goal statement summarizing the passage's main point
Wrong Answer Pathology - Faulty Use of Detail	• Reread the question *with* the answer choice selected and examine for mismatch
Wrong Answer Pathology - Out of Scope	• Ensure that the selected answer choice is supported by the author/passage, rather than your own common sense or reasoning
Wrong Answer Pathology – Opposite	• Highlight negative or relationship-flipping modifiers in the answer choices (e.g., *un-, except, not, less*)
Wrong Answer Pathology – Distortion	• Watch for modifying language that changes the meaning of text; strong language *can* be a signal that the answer is not supported by the passage
Misunderstood Question	• Slow down and/or double check your rephrase • Consider common rephrases of question skills (like "why" for Describe Purpose)
Misunderstood Answer	• Practice identifying subject and verb, then analyze the words that modify or qualify the claim • Compare strength of the claim in the answer to the passage argument
Answer Swap/Debate	• Stick with your first answer unless you have concrete proof that you misunderstood the question/answer or missed the relevant passage support • Enforce a strict 90-second triage rule: if a question is taking longer, guess strategically and move on
50/50	• When stuck between two choices, identify their primary point of disagreement, then hunt for evidence in the passage that disproves one of them
Pacing Issues	• Log the features of any passage and question set that takes over 10 minutes and triage similar passages to the end during practice • Focus less on the "what" of the passage details, and work on chunking for the "why"; revisit the strategies for interrogation in Chapter 4
Stamina/Focus Fade	• Implement the drill suggestion in Phase 3 of structuring CARS prep in Chapter 7.1
Tool Usage – Outline	• Review Outlining in Chapter 5.1 • Use shorthand and write only the paragraph's function, not its detailed content
Tool Usage – Highlight	• Review Highlighting in Chapter 5.2 • Reduce the number of highlights to essentials to avoid distractions • Choose different points of focus for highlights (architecture, content, perspective) and evaluate whether it's helpful for the questions

Table 7.2 Sample List of How I'll Fix It (HIFI)

The above list presents potential patterns and corresponding action steps for improvement but is not comprehensive. Feel free to utilize them directly, but also consider them as inspiration for generating your own patterns and corrections!

It is important to acknowledge that, particularly early on in your studies, you might identify numerous corrections that could be made. Attempting to implement them all simultaneously could be too great a cognitive load and diminish the effectiveness of your efforts. Instead, a more strategic approach involves selecting one or two key areas for improvement to integrate into your practice. The focus should be on making tangible behavioral adjustments rather than immediate score improvements. By concentrating on small, manageable changes, you can build momentum and achieve more sustainable progress over time.

Thinking Like the Test Maker: Post-Phrasing

Does this scenario sound familiar? You skim through the explanation for a question that you missed, shrug, and think, "I guess I get it." When you miss a practice question, you've actually made two mistakes. Not only were you tempted by a trap answer, but also you looked right at the correct answer and thought, "Nah! Not that one!" To turn today's wrong answers into tomorrow's right answers, you need a proactive technique for reviewing questions. Post-phrasing is that technique.

MCAT EXPERTISE

Make your action steps visible! Write out a short description of 1–2 action steps on a sticky note and put it on your screen to remind yourself of your goals. Once you've mastered them, replace it with a new one!

With **post-phrasing**, you go over both why incorrect answers are wrong and why correct answers are right. This is a different approach from the WIMI and HIFI above in that it's much more in-depth. Post-phrasing is a more elaborate technique of review, with the goal of proactively reviewing questions by dissecting them step-by-step. As such, it's not sustainable to post-phrase every question. Instead, pick out a completed passage and question set that you found particularly challenging.

To post-phrase, open a question you answered incorrectly and make a note of the correct answer. Take the following steps to carefully dissect the question:

1. Reread the passage if necessary.
2. For each question, identify both the question type (Foundations of Comprehension, Reasoning Within the Text, Reasoning Beyond the Text) and skill and write them down. Recall that Kaplan's TRIM method can be optimized to fit each skill; if necessary, briefly review strategy guidelines for the question's skill using the appropriate chapter.
3. Paraphrase the question stem, writing it down. By doing this, you are essentially practicing a formal version of the Rephrase step from TRIM. Your focus here should be to carefully decode what the question stem is asking you to do.
4. Investigate the solution, finishing when you can write out your prediction for the correct response. While you wouldn't write down a prediction on Test Day, the post-phrasing exercise is designed to ensure you are making concrete predictions as part of your Investigation. It's essential to take the time to write your prediction down: many students find that a poorly focused prediction keeps them from finding a match on MCAT questions. The more you practice writing out your predictions during the post-phrasing process, the more routine making predictions will become.
5. Justify why *each* incorrect answer is unsuitable, again by writing it out. Does it fail to match your prediction? Does it have a common wrong answer pathology? Are there other subtle flaws in logic or reasoning that misrepresent the author's arguments? Pay special attention to the wrong answer you actually chose.

Why was this answer tempting? Why is it ultimately wrong? By taking the time to write or type out an explanation of the flaw for each incorrect answer, you'll become better at identifying flaws in future wrong answers.

6. Examine Kaplan's explanation and check how well your reasoning matches up.

You may notice that the description of post-phrasing, thus far, basically describes a regimented and very deliberate use of the Kaplan Method for CARS Questions (TRIM). This is deliberate because, with CARS, you must remember: *Practice alone doesn't make perfect. Perfect practice makes perfect.* Post-phrasing is that perfect practice. You are taking a question that you did not answer correctly, and you are modeling the steps, actions, and strategies that you should have used to get that question right, which reinforces those behaviors for next time.

Lastly, after such a thorough review of a question, what's the best next step? Summarize the results of this detailed, post-phrasing investigation in your spreadsheet! You don't have to post-phrase every question you missed on every practice exam. Instead, save post-phrasing for the questions that really deserve a thorough examination: the ones where you were stumped, where you were stuck between two answers, and the ones where you made a silly mistake that you want to avoid in the future.

Alternatively, a variant of post-phrasing can be used as an exercise to proactively identify wrong answer pathologies in passages you haven't seen yet. Consider practicing with a few passages following the steps below:

1. Find a fresh CARS passage from your Kaplan resources.
2. If you're using an online passage, click through quickly and submit the quiz so the correct answers will be marked for you. If you're working on paper, mark the correct answers by hand. Don't read the explanations; just record the correct answers and set them aside for now.
3. Read and Distill the passage as you normally would.
4. When you work on the questions, do so in a fundamentally different way: as above, the goal here is not to find the right answers (as they are already identified), but to reason why each incorrect answer is wrong. Read the right answer to be sure you understand it, but spend more time identifying the types of wrong answers presented by the other choices.
5. Look at the explanations for each incorrect answer choice and compare them with your notes. If there are any major omissions or other discrepancies in your explanations, be sure to note them prominently. The more you practice, the closer you should find the correspondence between your post-phrasing notes and Kaplan's explanations.

Remember, on the MCAT the right answer is not just the "most correct" answer. Each question has one right answer and three answers with objective flaws, meaning that the right answer is objectively correct because it is the only answer without flaws. Through regular post-phrasing practice, you will begin to see the patterns emerge. What seem now like very subtle flaws will soon start to seem very pronounced. As a result, you will find yourself recognizing the correct answer, the one that doesn't suffer from any flaws, and thinking this one just feels right. Furthermore, taking the time to post-phrase will expand your awareness of how the test is written and what the expectations are for CARS questions. Through post-phrasing practice, you will refine your thought process and your approach to passages and questions, making you better prepared for Test Day.

Conclusion

The path to CARS mastery is a deliberate and iterative process, moving beyond mere practice to encompass skillbuilding, self-diagnosis, and strategic refinement. Just as a surgeon meticulously develops their craft, success in CARS is not an innate talent but a cultivated ability, demanding a growth mindset and the systematic analysis of mistakes. By actively diagnosing thought patterns through techniques like WIMI/HIFI and engaging in the in-depth review of post-phrasing, you can transform errors into invaluable data for improvement.

The remaining chapters of this book focus on specific CARS skills and include some initial practice (both Skillbuilder drills and test-like passage sets) to help kickstart your CARS practice journey. As discussed above, the skill chapters (8–11, 13–15, and 17–20) are recommended for students beginning in Phase 1 but can also be used selectively by students in Phase 2 looking to improve weak skills. The practice chapters are recommended for all students in Phase 2: Chapters 12, 16, and 21 provide targeted practice on the AAMC question types (FOC, RWT, and RBT), while Chapter 22 provides general test-like practice. For additional practice, see your online resources.

Skill and Strategy Summary

Structuring your CARS Prep

- **Phase 1: Skillbuilding** helps you develop your CARS skills through reading skill chapters and completing Skillbuilder exercises.
- **Phase 2: Diagnosis and Troubleshooting** focuses on identifying and correcting patterns of error.
- **Phase 3: Timing and Endurance** addresses pacing and the ability to maintain focus.

Effective Review of CARS

- **Why I Missed It (WIMI)** is a technique used to analyze patterns by tracking the following question and passage metrics:
  - **Question Details:** Basic question data, including passage and question number, passage topic and subtopic, question type and skill, and time spent
  - **Passage Evaluation:** Issues with reading and distilling the passage, including Mistaken Identity, Misinterpreting Tone, Overlooked Keywords, and Trees over Forest
  - **Question/Answer Evaluation:** Issues with questions and answers, including the four wrong answer pathologies, Misunderstood Question Stem, Misunderstood Answer Choice, Answer Swap/Debate, and 50/50
  - **Strategy Evaluation:** Holistic problems, including Pacing Issues, Stamina/Focus Fade, and Tool Usage concerns specific to highlighting or outlining
- **How I'll Fix It (HIFI)** works on creating specific action plans based on the identified patterns.
- **Post-Phrasing** is a more in-depth review technique for understanding features of correct and incorrect answers, allowing more insights into how the test maker designs CARS questions.

UNIT 2

FOUNDATIONS OF COMPREHENSION SKILLS

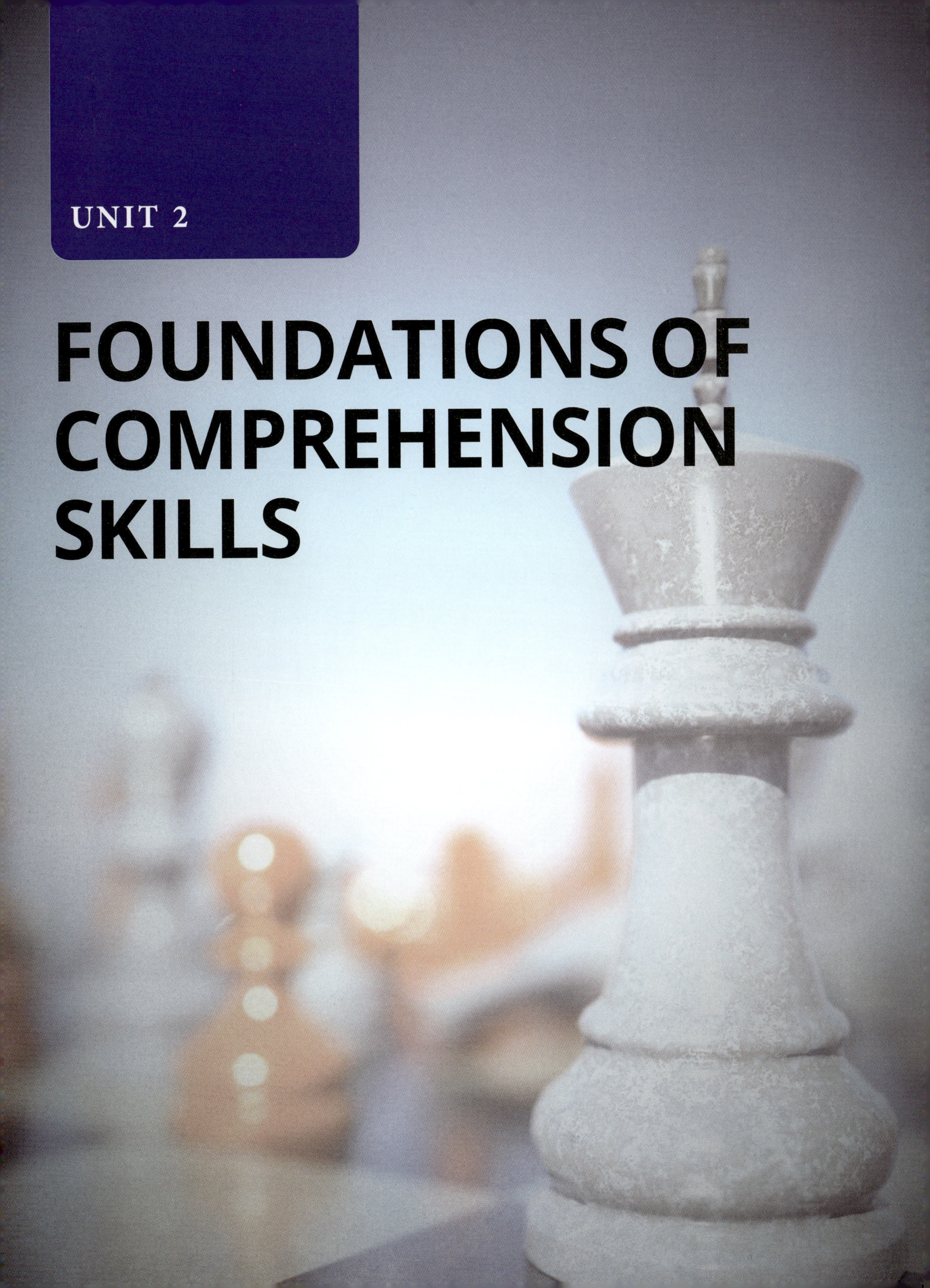

CHAPTER 8

INTERPRET MEANING

In This Chapter

8.1 Skill Description 108

The Immediate Context: Clues Within the Sentence 109

The Broader Context: Clues from the Paragraph and Beyond 110

8.2 Question Variations and Examples. . . . 111

Quote Length.......................... 111

Location Clues......................... 111

Definition Clues........................ 112

Answer Choice Length.................. 113

8.3 Applying the Kaplan Method. 113

Step 1: Type the Question................ 113

Step 2: Rephrase the Stem 114

Step 3: Investigate Potential Solutions 115

Step 4: Match Your Prediction to an Answer Choice............................. 115

8.4 Skillbuilder 115

Skill and Strategy Summary 123

LEARNING OBJECTIVES

After Chapter 8, you will be able to:

- Define the Interpret Meaning skill
- Infer the intent of passage quotations by starting with immediate context and broadening as needed
- Recognize common wordings for questions that test Interpret Meaning
- Apply the Kaplan Method for CARS Questions to Interpret Meaning questions
- Evaluate your current proficiency with the Interpret Meaning skill

FOUNDATIONS OF COMPREHENSION SKILL

Interpret Meaning: Use context to determine what a word/phrase from the passage is intended to communicate.

Approximate frequency: 20% of Foundations of Comprehension questions

Theories of social mobility often focus on individual merit and the acquisition of formal credentials. However, this overlooks the powerful role of communal context in shaping life chances. Some communities are characterized by dense, close-knit social networks where obligations are strong and personal histories are deeply shared. This environment provides a powerful form of social insurance, as individuals can rely on neighbors and kin for mutual aid in times of crisis. It also fosters a profound sense of belonging and solidarity that is essential to human well-being.

Yet this same environment can also be socially viscous. The very density of the local ties that provides security can also inhibit movement. Information about opportunities outside the immediate area may penetrate the community slowly, if at all. An individual who seeks to pursue a different path—whether through higher education or migration—may be perceived as abandoning their obligations, facing subtle pressure to remain. The cohesive social world that offers comfort and support can simultaneously act as a brake on individual ambition that deviates from the communal norm.

In describing a social environment as "viscous," the author intends to suggest one in which:

A. social interactions are frequently hostile and untrustworthy.
B. close community bonds restrain individual advancement.
C. transportation is inhibited by slow-moving traffic circulation.
D. outsiders are unwelcome and universities are underfunded.

8.1 Skill Description

Applying the **Interpret Meaning** skill is like performing a differential diagnosis on a word or phrase. When a physician evaluates a patient, a single symptom like a cough can point to dozens of possible conditions. To arrive at the correct diagnosis, the physician uses context—the patient's history, lab results, and other clinical signs—to rule out possibilities until only the most plausible answer remains.

Words in CARS passages work the same way. A single word can have many potential meanings. Your job is to use the context provided by the author as your diagnostic tool, eliminating the meanings that don't fit and confirming the one the author intends.

Authors in academic fields, from archaeology to architecture, often use words in very specific ways that can differ from their everyday definitions. They do this not to be confusing, but to be precise, to load terms with specific, nuanced meanings that are perfectly suited to their argument. Really, it's not so different from the way that healthcare professionals use clinical terminology to achieve extra precision.

We can see this unique use of language in the sample question at the beginning of the chapter. The word "viscous" in physics refers to a fluid's resistance to flow. In everyday usage, you might think of fluids like honey and molasses, which are thick, sticky, and pour slowly. However, if you stuck to this definition, you'd probably fall for trap answer **(C)**, "transportation is inhibited by slow-moving traffic circulation." But the passage never even brings up the topic of traffic.

MCAT EXPERTISE

When a question asks for the meaning of a particular word as used in the passage, it isn't expecting you to know every dictionary definition of that word, so that you can choose the correct interpretation from among them. In fact, the correct answer may be a definition that doesn't appear in the dictionary at all.

Instead, there will always be clues somewhere in the passage that provide solid evidence of what the author intended. Find those clues and you'll find the right answer.

If you look at the actual context of the paragraph, the author's intention will emerge. The sentence immediately after "viscous" explains: "The very density of the local ties that provides security can also inhibit movement." In other words, the close community bonds that were discussed in P1 also have a downside: they "inhibit movement." Before you think, "hey, isn't that more or less what **(C)** was saying?" consider the further context of the paragraph.

What kind of "movement" are we talking about here? Well, the rest of the paragraph clarifies that it's not literal motion, but more like social mobility, the ability to get ahead in life. The last sentence states pretty directly what the author means by viscous: "The cohesive social world that offers comfort and support can simultaneously act as a brake on individual ambition that deviates from the communal norm." Or, as correct answer **(B)** puts the same idea, "close community bonds restrain individual advancement."

When you Interpret Meaning, your task is to use context to uncover the author's specific meaning. As we saw with the sample question, this sometimes involves looking for clues in several places. But when approaching these questions systematically, you should always start with the sentence where the quoted part of the passage appears.

The Immediate Context: Clues Within the Sentence

The single best place to find clues is the sentence that houses the quoted word or phrase. Sometimes, authors will provide a direct definition right in the flow of their writing, using punctuation as a signpost for the reader.

Imagine a sentence from a passage on linguistics:

> Many languages contain what can be called "linguistic fossils"—vestiges of older grammatical forms that persist in modern speech long after their original logic has faded.

If a CARS question asks what the author means by "linguistic fossils," the sentence itself provides the answer. The author uses a dash to provide an immediate definition: they are "vestiges of older grammatical forms."

Phrases like *in other words, that is,* or other Continuity keywords (see Chapter 3) can also serve as clues. Consider the following example that might feature in a political science passage:

> Jackson argued that the new legislation, despite its seemingly benevolent goals, was ultimately designed to expand the legibility of the populace, that is, to make ordinary citizens' lives more easily monitored, quantified, and controlled by the state.

Suppose a question asked you to interpret the meaning of "legibility of the populace." What does the author want to communicate with this expression? "Legibility" usually just means "readability" but, setting aside people who have tattoos with words, you cannot literally read a person. So this CARS author must be employing a more metaphorical sense of the word when applying it to "the populace."

The author's exact intention is clarified after the Continuity keyword "that is." Increasing the legibility of people would mean they are "more easily monitored,

MCAT EXPERTISE

When you see a question that quotes a specific word or phrase and asks what it means, scan the sentence it's in for these key punctuation marks:

- Dashes [—]
- Parentheses [( )]
- Colons [:]
- Semicolons [;]

These various marks (all of which function like Continuity keywords, as discussed in Chapter 3) are often used to set off direct definitions, restatements, examples, or explanations, which can serve as excellent predictions for the intended meaning of the quoted part of the passage. Commas [,] are another potential clue for Interpret Meaning questions, but they are more common than these other marks and used for many other purposes, making them a less reliable guide.

quantified, and controlled by the state." So "legibility of the populace" in this context means something more like "surveillability," or the capacity of the government to surveil people.

This interpretation also helps to explain why the author contrasts expanding legibility with "seemingly benevolent goals" by using the Contrast keyword "despite" (see Chapter 3) earlier in the sentence. Notwithstanding the common stereotype about doctors' handwriting, legibility is usually considered to be a good thing. However, the author makes it clear with this contrast that "legibility of the populace" is bad.

Even without clear punctuation or keyword clues, the sentence's own descriptive language can redefine a term. Consider this example from a passage on art history:

> The artist's later work was characterized by a startling violence, his canvases attacked with energetic, almost frantic, brushstrokes and a clashing color palette that seemed to shatter the placid conventions of the era.

To interpret the word "violence" here, you must ignore the common definition of physical harm. The sentence itself provides the necessary context immediately after the comma. The descriptive phrases about "energetic, almost frantic, brushstrokes" and a "clashing color palette" function as a direct explanation of what the author means by "violence" in this artistic context. The clues redefine the term as an aggressive, intense, and convention-breaking style.

MCAT EXPERTISE

With more challenging Interpret Meaning questions, the only relevant clue from the passage might be a description of what the definition is *not*, revealed by a Contrast keyword. When a contrast is your only clue, just take the opposite as your prediction for the term's definition.

The Broader Context: Clues from the Paragraph and Beyond

Sometimes, a single sentence isn't enough. The author might build a definition over the course of an entire paragraph. In these cases, you must connect ideas from multiple sentences to construct the full meaning.

For example, a passage on sociology might state:

> The digital world operates on a unique economy of attention. In this system, influence is not measured in dollars, but in likes and shares. Users "spend" their creative energy to produce compelling content in the hopes of "earning" engagement, which functions as a kind of social currency. Those who accumulate more of this currency are granted a larger platform and a more powerful voice.

To understand the phrase "economy of attention," you need to synthesize all the clues. The author isn't talking about money. The paragraph explains that in this "economy," creative energy is "spent," engagement is "earned," and likes function as "currency." By putting these pieces together, you can correctly infer that an "economy of attention" is a system in which social standing is gained by competing for the limited resource of audience engagement.

Sometimes you may need to expand beyond the paragraph that contains the quote to the surrounding ones, particularly if the quote appears early or late in the paragraph. For example, if the quote appears in the last sentence of the paragraph, and then the next paragraph contains a Continuity keyword, especially one at the very beginning of its first sentence, then the important clues will probably be in that subsequent paragraph.

There are some cases in which you may need to draw on multiple paragraphs, perhaps even ones that are far apart. This typically only occurs when a term gets used repeatedly throughout the passage. If you discover that you're dealing with a question that requires this kind of more extensive research, it's okay to put a pause on that question and come back after answering the other questions in the set, or even to make an educated guess based on any partial clues you may have uncovered and move on.

8.2 Question Variations and Examples

While the core skill of Interpret Meaning remains the same, these questions can vary in four significant ways: the length of the text taken from the passage, the location clues provided, how much of the definition is provided, and the length of the answer choices. In addition to these variations, be aware that the use of quotation marks is the default, which is why we refer to the text from the passage as the "quoted text," but sometimes the passage text will appear without quotes.

Quote Length

The length of the quoted text in an Interpret Meaning question varies along a spectrum. At the short end are questions that zoom in on a single term, consisting of one or a few words.

EXAMPLE QUESTION STEMS

As used in the passage, the word "artifact" (paragraph 4) most nearly means:

In the context of paragraph 2, the term "heavy" refers to:

What does the author intend to suggest by using the term epistemic humility?

At the other end of the spectrum, a question might ask you to interpret the meaning of a longer quotation from the passage, consisting of a phrase or even an entire sentence.

EXAMPLE QUESTION STEMS

The author uses the phrase "the long shadow of the frontier" (paragraph 1) to indicate:

What does the author mean by the statement, "A city's downtown is less a place on a map and more a conversation between generations" (paragraph 4)?

These questions might quote more text, but they aren't necessarily more difficult. Just use the same approach with them, looking for clues from the immediate sentence outwards.

Location Clues

Another common variation concerns the presence or absence of paragraph references, which will impact how easy it is to find the quoted text in the passage.

Paragraph Reference

Most Interpret Meaning questions will give you a specific paragraph number, which allows you to narrow your search. In rare cases, a question may cite multiple paragraphs.

EXAMPLE QUESTION STEMS

In the context of the final paragraph, the word "legibility" is intended to signify:

The passage author's claim that "the hermeneutics of suspicion undermines the possibility of class solidarity" (paragraph 2) suggests the belief that:

As used in paragraphs 3 and 4, what does the term aestheticism mean?

Passage-Wide Reference

Occasionally, a question might ask how a term is used in the passage as a whole, which may require you to consider multiple instances of the word in different paragraphs.

EXAMPLE QUESTION STEMS

Throughout the passage, the author uses the term "power" to refer to:

The frequent mention of "guardrails" in the passage implies that the author believes:

No Location Clue

Sometimes the question may not tell you where to find the word. This requires you to scan the passage to locate the term yourself.

EXAMPLE QUESTION STEMS

As used in the passage, what does the author mean by the term "utilitarianism"?

The passage implies that investiture is:

Definition Clues

Another noteworthy variation is how much of the definition you have to supply. Sometimes you'll need to provide the whole thing, while other questions will give you some clues about where to start, asking you to fill in the remainder.

Supply the Full Definition

This is the most common format. The question asks what the quoted text means, and the answer choices are complete definitions.

EXAMPLE QUESTION STEMS

"Biopolitics" (paragraph 6) most nearly means:

The phrase "a dissonant harmony" (paragraph 2) is best interpreted as meaning:

Complete a Partial Definition

Less frequently, the question stem will include a clue by providing part of the definition and asking you to complete the thought. The answer choices will be words or short phrases that logically finish the sentence presented in the stem.

EXAMPLE QUESTION STEMS

The author's use of "narrative" (paragraph 1) suggests that a person's self-concept is essentially:

The "old guard" (paragraph 3) describes a group of politically influential people who:

Answer Choice Length

Finally, keep in mind that the answer choices can also vary in length, which may affect the difficulty of the question. In some questions, each answer choice might only be a single word, with the correct answer being the closest synonym of how the author uses the term. In other, more challenging questions, you may have four complete sentences as answer options, each a complex statement in its own right.

As a general rule, questions with shorter answer choices are more straightforward. Longer answer choices require you to carefully unpack up to four distinct definitions, adding another layer of analysis to your task.

8.3 Applying the Kaplan Method

Let's take a look at how to apply the Kaplan Method for CARS Questions (Type-Rephrase-Investigate-Match) to the skill of Interpret Meaning. For basics on the TRIM method, return to Chapter 6.

Step 1: Type the Question

Your first step is to read the question stem thoroughly and glance at the answer choices to try to assess the question type and difficulty and make a triaging decision. Always try to identify at least the broad skill category: Foundations of Comprehension (surface questions), Reasoning Within the Text (deep questions), or Reasoning Beyond the Text (new info questions). Remember that even when the question stem does not indicate the specific skill being tested with 100% certainty, this step will still help to focus your approach to the subsequent steps, letting you identify the correct answer choice more quickly.

Identifying the Skill

You can usually type a question as testing the Interpret Meaning skill by looking for a reference to actual words from the passage, often in quotation marks, accompanied by meaning-related phrasing: "mean" and "meaning" are the most frequent, though another common pattern is use of the verb "to be" ("is," "are," etc.). There is frequently, but not always, a reference to a specific paragraph as well. Return to Section 8.2 above for variations on typical wordings.

Deciding When to Attack

Interpret Meaning is a Foundations of Comprehension skill. This means it is a surface-level skill that relies only on your understanding of what the text explicitly says. As such, your strategy should almost always be to attack them *now*.

The only times you may wish to save them for *later* in the question set is if the quoted part of the text is particularly long, or similarly if the answer choices are too long. One other case when you should triage these questions for later is if there are no location clues and you don't know where to start looking. Working on other questions in the meantime will give you additional opportunities to find that quoted text while earning points.

Interpret Meaning questions are often quick points you can confidently secure before moving on. They may even shore up your understanding of the author's argument by clarifying key terms, empowering you to tackle future questions with a stronger grasp of the passage.

BRIDGE

Questions that ask what the author means by a particular quotation almost always test the Interpret Meaning skill. However, questions that ask about what the author implies or suggests about a particular phrase or concept, without quoting from the passage directly, might test the Interpret Meaning skill but could also test the Paraphrase Detail skill (if the meaning of the phrase or concept is stated directly in the passage) or the Make Deduction skill (if more complex reasoning is required to deduce what the author is implying). See Chapter 10 for more on Paraphrase Detail and Chapter 15 for Make Deduction.

Step 2: Rephrase the Stem

After you know you're being tested on the Interpret Meaning skill, you need to translate the question into a concrete task or set of tasks. This means shaping the test maker's language into a simple mission for yourself. With Interpret Meaning questions, you primarily need to identify two things: what and where the quoted text is.

When the question actually uses quotation marks, the "what" is easy: it is inside the quotes. If quotation marks are missing, look for a technical or abstract term, which may even be preceded in the question by "the term" or "the word."

Once you know what you're looking to define, next you'll need to figure out where to look. These questions often identify specific paragraphs for you, which can help to narrow down your search, but you will ultimately want to find the specific sentence that contains the quoted text. So your task can be restated as something like: "Go to the part of the passage that contains this term and reread that sentence and any surrounding sentences until I can define it in the way the author uses it."

For example, if the question stem is:

> What does the author mean by the statement, "A city's downtown is less a place on a map and more a conversation between generations" (paragraph 4)?

Your rephrased task becomes:

- Go to paragraph 4 and find that specific quote about a city's downtown, then reread that sentence and the ones around it to figure out exactly what the author means by calling downtown a "conversation between generations."

This step turns you from a passive reader into an active searcher with a clear goal.

Step 3: Investigate Potential Solutions

With your mission clear, you can now turn to the passage to find the answer. For this skill, your investigation will be highly targeted: you want to find the quoted term or phrase, starting with the sentence that contains it and expanding outwards to sentences that come before and/or after as needed. Paragraph references will narrow down this search if provided, but otherwise you may need to rely on your choice of tool, outlining or highlighting, to locate the source of the quote.

Remember that you are looking for clues about what the quoted text means, so watch out for Continuity keywords, punctuation marks like dashes and colons, or nearby descriptive language. You may find that the author simply restates the idea in simpler language in the same sentence or an adjacent one. Even if you don't find a synonym, at minimum you should find some ideas related to the author's intended meaning that can point you in the right direction.

Your ultimate goal is to predict the text's meaning. If the quoted text is a single term, define it in your own words. If it's a phrase or sentence, come up with your own paraphrase of what the author is trying to say. You can use those clues from the surrounding context as a starting point for your prediction, but keep in mind that answer choices often use language that is only similar (but not identical) to the passage's.

Step 4: Match Your Prediction to an Answer Choice

Questions that test the Interpret Meaning skill almost always allow you to make a prediction, so try not to end your Investigation until you have a clear one in mind. Once you have that, it's just a matter of finding the equivalent idea in the answer choices.

One way to test that you have found the match to your prediction is to replace the quoted text from the passage with the wording from the answer choice and see if it makes sense in context. This technique is most likely to work when dealing with shorter answer choices, so it's not one you can always use.

If you cannot find a match, you will need to use the process of elimination. But watch out for the **dictionary definition trap**, a wrong answer pathology that is unique to Interpret Meaning. If the answer choice simply reproduces the most common definition of the quoted text, the first one you would see when you checked the dictionary, it's probably wrong, especially when dealing with words that have widely-known, common meanings.

Interpret Meaning questions are not intended to test your vocabulary or how well you can memorize the dictionary. They are intended to test if you can decipher meaning through context, so a common definition will ensnare test takers who haven't adequately practiced this skill.

8.4 Skillbuilder

Use the following shortened passage to practice the Interpret Meaning skill. The reading is scaffolded to reinforce good active reading habits and to let you devote more of your attention to practicing your critical thinking skills. It includes Active Reading Checks with each paragraph to evaluate how well you're uncovering important passage information at every level. Answer both the Active Reading Check and the CARS question that accompanies each paragraph before continuing. You can check your answers on the next page before you move on to paragraph 2, and the same for paragraph 3.

This page is intentionally blank. Chapter continues on the next page. ▶ ▶ ▶

Paragraph 1

The distinction between democracy and oligarchy is best understood not as a sharp line but as a blurred one. Indeed, most modern, developed "democracies" exhibit many characteristics of so-called civil oligarchy, where the formal institutions of republican rule coexist with powerful elite networks that exert disproportionate influence. In this blended state, democratic processes and institutions continue, but are consistently steered by economic elites to protect their own interests. Civil oligarchies are mediated through established legal frameworks. They limit arbitrary authority, but also restrict dissent and competition to formally sanctioned channels—at once perpetuating class inequalities and permitting gradual social change.

Active Reading Check for Paragraph 1

By putting "democracies" in quotation marks, what is the author likely suggesting?

A. That the word's usage is questionable
B. That the word is being defined
C. That the author is quoting someone else

1. Based on the first paragraph, the author uses the term "civil oligarchy" to refer to a society in which:

A. rules about civility restrict dissent and competition.
B. elites are composed of civilians rather than military leaders.
C. democracy is mediated through republican institutions.
D. the wealthy dominate through a system of laws.

Active Reading Check for Paragraph 1: (A)

(A) The author notes that these "modern, developed 'democracies' exhibit many characteristics of so-called civil oligarchy" where elites "exhibit disproportionate influence" and "protect their own influence." This reference to oligarchy, a different political system, suggests that the author questions whether these governments are true democracies and indicates that the quotation markers are used to signal skepticism (a technique known as "scare quotes").

(B) While quotation marks can be used to set off a term for definition, the author's skeptical tone here indicates this is not a definition but a critique. Moreover, there is nothing in the text immediately before or after the word "democracies" that could be interpreted as a definition.

(C) There is no specific external source mentioned in the passage, nor is there any indication that the author is quoting such a source. Therefore, these quotation marks must be used for a purpose other than quoting another person.

Question 1: (D)

Answer Choice Explanations for Question 1

(A) The passage defines the "civil" nature of the oligarchy as being "mediated through established legal frameworks," not as being related to polite behavior or "civility." Indeed, there is no discussion of civility anywhere in the passage.

(B) While the elites in such a system may be civilians, the passage never makes this claim, or even mentions the distinction between the military and civilians.

(C) The author states that "developed 'democracies' exhibit many characteristics of so-called civil oligarchy, where the formal institutions of republican rule coexist with powerful elite networks." This sentence structure suggests that "republican rule" is a characteristic of democracies, while "civil oligarchy" shifts at least some influence to "elite networks." This choice fails to make any connection to that elite element.

(D) This choice accurately summarizes the author's description. The passage states that the system is "mediated through established legal frameworks" (a system of laws) and that it is "consistently steered by economic elites" to perpetuate "class inequalities" (the wealthy dominate).

Detailed Explanation for Question 1

Skill: Because it requires you to combine various descriptive details provided throughout the first paragraph and come up with a valid definition of a key term as it is used by the author, this question tests the Interpret Meaning skill.

Question: You are being asked to identify the best characterization of "civil oligarchy" as it's presented in the passage. Review the author's description first, then match it to the answer choice that best captures its essential features.

Passage: The author cites several key characteristics of a "civil oligarchy" in paragraph 1. First, it involves "powerful elite networks that exert disproportionate influence," who are later specified as "economic" elites. Second, this influence is not random but structured, "mediated through established legal frameworks." Thus, elites protect their interests and perpetuate "class inequalities." Summarizing this in the form of a prediction, the correct choice should talk about a system in which the rich use the legal system to maintain their power. Look proactively for a paraphrase of this idea among the available options.

Answer: The prediction emanating from the passage is closely paraphrased in **(D)**, "the wealthy dominate through a system of laws." **(A)** and **(B)** both misinterpret the word "civil" by applying meanings that are not supported by the context. **(C)** describes a republic but misses the central oligarchic element of control by a wealthy elite.

Paragraph 2

Civil oligarchy, however, can easily devolve into what has been termed "sultanistic oligarchy." Ironically, this is often driven by grassroots sentiment, cleverly exploited by a populist demagogue. The resultant autocracy is typically defined by the near-total fusion of the head of state's personal interests with the functions of government. Formal institutions become hollow shells as the leader treats state resources as personal property and bypasses laws, courts, and other institutions with arbitrary decrees or "executive orders." Power is no longer a shared project of the wealthy but an intensely personal one, where officials are appointed and promoted based on sycophancy and fealty. Individual rights are routinely violated and public discourse is both suppressed and contaminated by propaganda and outright prevarication.

Active Reading Check for Paragraph 2

According to the author, how can a civil oligarchy turn into a sultanistic one?

A. An elite group decides to transfer power to a single, charismatic person.

B. A popular movement overthrows the existing hierarchy and restores democracy.

C. An opportunist manipulates the public to seize personal control.

2. The author uses the expression "hollow shells" (paragraph 2) to describe:

A. structures that are delicate and easily broken.

B. things that exist in name but lack substance.

C. resources whose value has been depleted.

D. barriers intended to protect those inside.

Active Reading Check for Paragraph 2: (C)

(A) The passage describes the devolution into sultanistic oligarchy as a consequence of a *breakdown* of the "shared project of the wealthy," rather than a *planned* transfer of power by them.

(B) Although the passage says that the rise of a sultanistic oligarchy is often "driven by grassroots sentiment," it also states that the result is an "autocracy," not a "restore[d] democracy."

(C) This accurately reflects the passage's claim that the change is typically "driven by grassroots sentiment, cleverly exploited by a populist demagogue." Definitionally, a populist demagogue is someone who opportunistically manipulates public sentiment to gain power.

Question 2: (B)

Answer Choice Explanations for Question 2

(A) The words "hollow shell" in the passage refer to the "formal institutions" of government. The subject of how delicate such institutions are is not dealt with in paragraph 2. Instead, the author talks about how, in a sultanistic oligarchy, their functions are usurped by the leader.

(B) The author states that "Formal institutions become hollow shells as the leader treats state resources as personal property and bypasses laws, courts, and other institutions," suggesting that a "hollow shell" has been robbed of something essential or important—in this case, important institutional controls that the leader ignores.

(C) The metaphor applies to "formal institutions," not to physical or economic resources. Moreover, it describes a loss of ostensible function, not a loss of value.

(D) While one meaning of "shell" is a protective barrier, the author states that institutions become "hollow shells" as part of the problematic and "arbitrary" behavior of a government where "individual rights are routinely violated." The idea that these "hollow shells" are "intended to protect" is too positive of an interpretation to match the passage.

Detailed Explanation for Question 2

Skill: This question tests the Interpret Meaning skill because it asks you to determine the meaning of a common metaphor within the particular context of the passage.

Question: The question asks what a particular expression signifies in context. Go back to the passage and decipher what exactly the words "hollow shells" are meant to refer to, and why that description is appropriate. Then, look for the answer choice that matches.

Passage: According to paragraph 2, "*Formal institutions* become *hollow shells* as the leader treats state resources as personal property and bypasses laws, courts, and other institutions with arbitrary decrees." The phrase in question, therefore, refers specifically to formal institutions such as courts, which are "bypass[ed]" in favor of the leader's "arbitrary decrees." In other words, these institutions retain their outward appearance (a shell), but are emptied of their actual authority and substance (hollowed out). Look for something like this among the answer choices.

Answer: **(B)** is a direct paraphrase of the prediction. Although **(A)** is a potential *consequence* of being "hollow," it isn't the fact of hollowness itself. Moreover, there is no discussion of fragility, one way or the other, in this paragraph. **(C)** misidentifies what is being described (institutions, not resources) and what has been lost (power or function, not value). **(D)** suggests a protective purpose, which is directly contradicted by the passage's description of a repressive regime.

Paragraph 3

A society's position along this spectrum carries profound implications. A drift towards greater civil oligarchy erodes democratic legitimacy but, due to the oligarchs' shared interest in systemic continuity, it typically maintains a degree of stability and responsiveness to the public interest. However, such a drift also makes the rise of sultanistic oligarchy more likely, and this further shift marks a critical degradation, replacing even the corrupted infrastructure of elite norms with radical uncertainty and institutional brittleness. Though both may wear a democratic mask, a civil oligarchy, with its manipulated structural coherence, offers a relatively durable environment where interests are negotiated and change is mediated through recalibrations among elites. A sultanistic oligarchy, on the other hand, with power concentrated and capriciously exercised behind a more transparent facade, fosters extreme institutional fragility. It's less about managing an inequitable system than perpetuating personal dominance, and inevitably leads to overt repression. Remaining democratic forms become increasingly farcical, and the society grows more and more vulnerable to the whims of its leader, often culminating in state failure or violent upheaval.

Active Reading Check for Paragraph 3

According to the author, what is one important difference between civil oligarchy and sultanistic oligarchy?

A. A sultanistic oligarchy is more unstable.
B. A sultanistic oligarchy is more common.
C. A sultanistic oligarchy is less corrupt.

3. What does the author most likely mean by calling sultanistic oligarchy "more transparent" than civil oligarchy?

A. The true nature of the government is less effectively concealed.
B. Institutions have been reformed to allow for greater oversight.
C. Societal structures are flimsier and more subject to public pressure.
D. The ruling system is less complex and easier to understand.

Active Reading Check for Paragraph 3: (A)

(A) The paragraph repeatedly contrasts the "degree of stability" and "durable environment" of a civil oligarchy with the "radical uncertainty," "institutional brittleness," and "extreme institutional fragility" of a sultanistic oligarchy.

(B) Although the passage describes the potential progression from civil to sultanistic oligarchy, it provides no information about which system is more common.

(C) The passage describes sultanistic oligarchy as a "critical degradation" from the "corrupted infrastructure" of a civil oligarchy, implying it is more, not less, corrupt.

Question 3: (A)

Answer Choice Explanations for Question 3

(A) (The passage says both oligarchic systems "wear a democratic mask," but sultanistic oligarchy has a "more transparent facade"—a facade that is easier to see through. In other words, a sultanistic oligarchy's authoritarian nature is not hidden as effectively as a civil oligarchy's.

(B) This represents a drastically different sense of "transparency" (related to open government and accountability) than that intended by the author. The passage describes sultanistic oligarchy as less—not more—accountable than civil oligarchy.

(C) Paragraph 3 suggests that sultanistic oligarchies are more likely to be overthrown by "violent upheaval" than civil oligarchies are, which could be a sign that sultanistic oligarchies are "flimsier and more subject to public pressure." However, this idea is not relevant to the phrase "transparent facade," which refers to the surface or appearance of the sultanistic oligarchies rather than the instability that results from them.

(D) The passage does not suggest that rule by a single individual is less complicated than dominance by an entire social class. Also, this idea refers to the nature of the "ruling system," while "transparent facade" refers to the "democratic mask" that *hides* the repressive reality of this system.

Detailed Explanation for Question 3

Skill: Because it requires you to figure out precisely what "facade" the author is referring to, and what is meant by saying that this facade is "more transparent" in a sultanistic oligarchy, this question tests the Interpret Meaning skill.

Question: This question asks you to explain what the author means by saying that a sultanistic oligarchy is "more transparent." First, you need to identify which aspect of oligarchy is being discussed, and then decide which sense of the word "transparent" is intended.

Passage: In particular, the author says it is the sultanistic oligarchy's "facade" that is "more transparent." The word *facade* is defined as a deceptive outward appearance. This perfectly fits the author's claim, earlier in paragraph 3, that both types of oligarchy hide behind a "democratic mask." Furthermore, the actions of a sultanistic leader—bypassing laws, ruling by decree, overt repression (paragraph 2)—all involve the "degradation" of these "democratic forms" (paragraph 3). This is much harder to disguise than the subtle, procedural manipulation of a civil oligarchy. Therefore, the "mask" worn by the sultanistic ruler is easier to see through, or "more transparent," and the autocratic reality behind the mask is more visible.

Answer: The prediction that the true, undemocratic nature of the government is more obvious in a sultanistic oligarchy is an excellent match for **(A)**: "The true nature of the government is less effectively concealed." This is almost surely the correct choice, but you can quickly check the other options to make sure you're not missing anything. **(B)** confuses the meaning of "transparent" in this case, and is contradicted by the passage. **(C)** correctly identifies fragility but misattributes the cause to public pressure rather than the leader's whims; it also doesn't really employ any plausible metaphorical sense of the word "transparent." **(D)** also misses the point; the "facade" is not the governmental system itself, but the "democratic mask" that it wears. **(A)** is definitely the right answer.

Skill and Strategy Summary

Skill Description

- The **Interpret Meaning** skill is your ability to understand what words mean within the context in which they're used.
    - Interpret Meaning accounts for about 20% of Foundations of Comprehension questions.
- When using this skill, you start with the immediate context of the sentence that contains the quotation, gradually broadening to adjacent sentences, the rest of the paragraph, and beyond, as needed.
    - Continuity keywords, including punctuation marks like dashes and colons that function the same way, point to passage clues about the intended meaning.

Question Variations and Examples

- Interpret Meaning questions can vary in the following ways:
    - Quote Length: The text from the passage is usually in quotes (but not always) and can range from one word to an entire sentence.
    - Location Clues: Typically one paragraph is cited, but sometimes none or multiple.
    - Definition Clues: Questions occasionally include part of the definition in the stem.
    - Answer Choice Length: Choices vary like quotations do, from single words to whole sentences.

Applying the Kaplan Method

- Step 1: Type the Question
    - Recognize Interpret Meaning by inclusion of quotations and meaning-related language.
    - As surface questions (Foundations of Comprehension), answer them *now*, most of the time.
    - Save for *later* if the quotation in the question is long or the answer choices are long, or if you have no idea where to find the quotation in the passage.
- Step 2: Rephrase the Stem
    - Include *what* you need to interpret (the quotation) and *where* you can find it (the paragraph) in your rephrase.
- Step 3: Investigate Potential Solutions
    - Start with the sentence that contains the quotation featured in the question and expand outwards as needed.
    - End this step with a prediction in your own words of the quotation's intended meaning.
- Step 4: Match Your Prediction to an Answer Choice
    - Substitute your suspected match into the original context to see if it has the intended meaning, if possible.
    - Beware the **dictionary definition trap**: the correct answer is usually not the most common definition.

CHAPTER 9

RECOGNIZE OPINION

In This Chapter

9.1 Skill Description 126
Distinguishing Opinions from Facts....... 127
Identifying Indirect Opinions 128
9.2 Question Variations and Examples.... 129
Scope of Subject........................ 129
Source of Opinion...................... 130
Location Clues......................... 131
Directness of Answer Choices........... 131
9.3 Applying the Kaplan Method........ 132
Step 1: Type the Question............... 132
Step 2: Rephrase the Stem 133
Step 3: Investigate Potential Solutions 134
Step 4: Match Your Prediction to an Answer Choice............................. 134
9.4 Skillbuilder 135
Skill and Strategy Summary 141

LEARNING OBJECTIVES

After Chapter 9, you will be able to:

- Define the Recognize Opinion skill
- Distinguish opinions from facts
- Grasp opinions that are expressed indirectly
- Identify common wordings for questions that test Recognize Opinion
- Apply the Kaplan Method for CARS Questions to Recognize Opinion questions
- Evaluate your current proficiency with the Recognize Opinion skill

FOUNDATIONS OF COMPREHENSION SKILL

Recognize Opinion: Identify what the author or someone else feels about a passage idea based on word choice or other context clues.

Approximate Frequency: 20% of Foundations of Comprehension questions

The debate over urban historical preservation often pits the desire for continuity against the pressures of development. The preservationist impulse stems from the desire to safeguard a city's architectural heritage and maintain a healthy connection to its past. This has led to the codification of historic districts, governed by commissions that enforce strict adherence to prescribed aesthetic standards. From the composition of mortar in brickwork to the permissible color palettes for facades, these regulations are designed to halt the visual signature of time, preserving a neighborhood as a specific, idealized version of itself. The goal is to create a consistent and historically legible landscape, shielding cities from the perceived chaos of contemporary construction.

Yet a city is not a static artifact to be kept under glass; it is a dynamic, living organism, a constantly evolving tapestry. When preservation efforts focus too rigidly on maintaining a particular historical state, they create a facsimile of a neighborhood rather than a living one. The subtle, organic changes that mark a community's genuine evolution—its adaptations and accretions, the messy and unpredictable layers of history—are replaced by a curated veneer of historical authenticity. This approach can inadvertently sanitize the very character it seeks to protect by favoring a clean, museum-like consistency over the more complex, and perhaps more truthful, narrative of a place that is still being written.

The author's characterization of historical preservation efforts suggests they believe that these actions are:

A. an effective method for documenting past architectural styles.
B. partially justified as a way to limit current urban development.
C. primarily motivated by political ideology.
D. well-intentioned but deeply artificial.

9.1 Skill Description

Using the **Recognize Opinion** skill is like assessing a patient's tone of voice and body language as you interview them. These behaviors signal their attitude towards the symptoms and events they describe, revealing additional information they might not even be aware of. Brief and tired-sounding responses from a typically energetic patient might be an important clue to their condition, even if they never bring up tiredness as an issue. Similarly, changes in posture might indicate an orthopedic problem that only a physician would recognize. Clues like these help to paint a more complete picture of a patient's situation than you would be able to get from reading a transcript of their comments.

The authors of CARS passages won't narrate the text for you, but they do the next best thing, indirectly telling you how they feel through precisely chosen language that reveals attitudes without stating them outright. Some words indicate positive or negative opinions, while others specify whether the author feels strongly about their beliefs or is not fully committed to them. With practice, you can use these clues to construct a mental portrait of the author and imagine the tone of their voice and the expression on their face as they discuss different details.

MCAT passages are full of information, but CARS questions are much more likely to focus on the author's opinions (their personal and subjective beliefs) than on other details. That means the Recognize Opinion skill is a crucial guide to information that CARS questions are highly likely to ask about. Reading for opinions also makes it easier to understand the passage as a whole. It doesn't matter if a passage expresses many opinions or few, or whether those opinions are indirect or overtly stated: when they do appear, you should pay attention to opinions in a CARS passage.

The sample question at the beginning of this chapter shows us why. It asks for the author's opinion about historical preservation. The first paragraph of the passage mentions that people want to "safeguard a city's architectural heritage," which sounds a bit like **(A)**. Or you might notice that the end of paragraph 1 discusses the idea of "shielding cities from the perceived chaos of contemporary construction," which resonates with **(B)**. But do either of these really reflect how the author feels?

The goal of saving "architectural heritage" is described as the source of the "preservationist impulse," so we know that people in favor of historical preservation would probably agree that **(A)** is true, that preservation efforts do a good job of documenting architecture. But there's nothing in the passage that indicates the author agrees. Similarly, the passage states that protecting cities from overactive urban development is "the goal" of people who favor historical preservation, meaning that the author doesn't necessarily agree with **(B)**.

Instead of relying on paragraph 1 and its description of the pro-preservation viewpoint, search for the opinion clues in the second paragraph. In paragraph 2, the author writes that preservation can "focus too rigidly" on capturing a specific point in history, leading to a "facsimile of a neighborhood" and a "curated veneer of historical authenticity."

This language (particularly "too rigidly," "facsimile," and "veneer") suggests that the author doesn't approve of historical preservation because it can lead to a superficial representation of the past, one that isn't true to the evolution of urban spaces. This matches the correct answer **(D)**, which calls historical preservation "deeply artificial," despite being "well-intentioned," as it is indeed described in paragraph 1.

As we can see with this example, the author is the "main character" of any CARS passage, and so their personal beliefs are almost always the most important opinions in the text. The opinions of other people in the passage are also significant: as soon as you understand that the author begins the passage by speaking in the voice of the "preservationist impulse," you realize that you shouldn't use any of the information there to answer questions about how the author themself feels.

On top of that, you might occasionally see a question about what these other viewpoints think. Even when you don't see questions about other viewpoints, though, tracking which paragraphs represent which perspectives will enhance your understanding of the passage as a whole. And a sound holistic understanding of the passage reduces the likelihood that you fall into wrong answer traps on many questions.

This chapter will teach you the clues and techniques necessary to notice when someone in a passage expresses an opinion. This will simultaneously enhance your understanding of the passage and your preparation for Recognize Opinion questions, as well as other questions that involve elements of opinion. There are two main aspects of the Recognize Opinion skill: determining which details are opinions and locating opinions that the author expresses indirectly.

Distinguishing Opinions from Facts

While opinions appear regularly in many CARS passages, they're typically outweighed by factual information. Distinguishing between facts and opinions is a key aspect of the Recognize Opinion skill, because opinions are always more likely to be the topic of test questions. The fundamental difference is that factual claims are objective and that opinions are subjective. Consider the following statement:

> The population of China is greater than the population of Scotland.

This is a **factual claim**, because it is either objectively true or false (true, in this case). The same with this next statement:

> Darius the Great of the Achaemenid Empire died in 486 BCE.

This is also a factual claim, even if you are not familiar enough with ancient history to recognize whether it's true. The year that any particular person passed away is an objective fact. Now consider a very different kind of statement:

> Soft cheeses such as Camembert are more delicious than hard cheeses such as Pecorino Romano.

This claim is purely subjective: it depends on your personal taste and which flavors and textures you prefer in your cheese. If you are lactose intolerant, you may not have an opinion at all. This subjective nature is what makes a statement an **opinion**. Opinions can cover many topics beyond personal preferences, however:

> Britain should not have invaded the United States in 1812.

Warfare between nations is a much more serious matter than a person's favorite foods, but serious issues don't necessarily have an objective resolution. Unpack the statement above and consider why someone might have made this claim. Perhaps they believe that Britain did not have a proper legal or moral basis for invading another country. Perhaps they thought that the practical outcome of the invasion would be negative for Britain, the United States, or both. All these judgments are fundamentally subjective, because they depend on things that can never be "fact-checked": personal values or preferences. For this reason, statements about what "should" be done are almost always opinions.

Identifying Indirect Opinions

When a physician diagnoses a patient, some signs are associated with obvious symptoms that point to a specific condition. Other indicators are beneath the surface, may not involve any visible symptoms, and are only noticeable to a practiced eye. Opinions in CARS passages are similar: they can be expressed directly or only hinted at. While certain kinds of statements always convey an opinion, as described above, most opinions in CARS passages are communicated in a more subtle way. When you can consistently identify these subtle opinions, you will be a true master of the Recognize Opinion skill.

These indirect opinions are typically expressed through Author keywords, which are discussed in Chapter 3. These keywords can indicate the opinions of any person discussed in the passage, not just the author. Positive keywords and Negative keywords indicate whether someone approves or disapproves of what they are discussing. Amplifying keywords suggest a stronger or more extreme opinion, while Limiting keywords indicate a weaker or more qualified opinion. Consider a sentence that could appear in a CARS passage.

> Ngo's latest novel, with its unflinching depiction of family dynamics, represents an absolute victory over the critics who questioned her capacity for more grounded narratives.

KEY CONCEPT

In everyday conversation, it is common to refer to statements as "facts" if you believe they are true, and to deny that a statement is a "fact" if you believe it is false. However, for the purposes of the MCAT, factual claims can be either true or false: they are factual because they deal with objective reality.

Similarly, you may personally agree with some opinions expressed in CARS passages and disagree with others. Whether a statement is true or false does not determine whether it addresses facts or opinions. And in CARS passages, you should generally treat author claims as if they are true for the purpose of answering questions, because the author is the ultimate authority.

MCAT EXPERTISE

Because the passage is written in the author's voice, all statements (both facts and opinions) reflect what the author believes, unless the statement is specifically described as coming from someone else.

The Amplifying keyword "absolute" indicates that the author feels very strongly about their positive evaluation of Ngo's novel as a "victory." Contrast this with the following example:

> The XBS group's findings, while only somewhat beneficial, did offer a new perspective on the recent grain shortage.

Although the Positive keyword "beneficial" shows that the author has a positive attitude toward the group's findings, the Limiting keyword "somewhat" shows that they do not feel very strongly about it.

While these previous examples involve Positive or Negative keywords that are separate from the Amplifying or Limiting keywords that modify them, sometimes a single keyword can capture both effects:

> The scientific community regarded the Stein research team's experimental design as a competent approach to the problem.

The term "competent" serves the function of both a Positive keyword and a Limiting keyword, indicating that the scientific community has a mildly favorable view of the experimental design. So in combination—or in some cases, alone—these different types of keywords can show how much the author or another figure approves or disapproves of specific passage concepts.

9.2 Question Variations and Examples

On the MCAT, questions that test the Recognize Opinion skill will ask about different kinds of opinions and frame the issue in different ways. They typically vary along the following dimensions: the scope of the opinion's subject, the source of the opinion, the presence or absence of location clues, and the directness of the answer choices.

Scope of Subject

The most significant variation hinges on how specific of a subject the question is asking about.

Specific Concept

The most common type of questions testing the Recognize Opinion skill ask about a specific concept mentioned in the passage.

EXAMPLE QUESTION STEMS

Based on paragraph 3, what would most accurately describe the author's attitude toward Frank Gehry's designs?

The author apparently believes that the historical practice of alchemy was:

The specific concept inquired about may be a minor detail mentioned at only one point in the passage, or it may be discussed throughout the passage and connected to the main

KEY CONCEPT

Opinions commonly involve claims about:

- personal preferences
- value judgments
- recommendations or suggestions
- issues that are too complicated to be evaluated objectively

Facts commonly involve claims about:

- specific events
- trends and relationships that can be tested scientifically

MCAT EXPERTISE

Amplifying keywords can indicate that a statement:

- is certain or universal (*must, all, always, invariably, inevitably*)
- deserves emphasis (*indeed, above all, particularly, especially*)

Limiting keywords can:

- put limits on time or place (*currently, at times, in some cases, in this instance*)
- indicate that a statement is partially true (*to some extent, in a manner of speaking, in some sense*)
- indicate doubt about whether a statement is true (*potentially, possibly, could, might, may*)

theme. It requires familiarity with the passage to distinguish between these two situations, as they have almost indistinguishable question stems.

Passage-Wide Idea

Sometimes, the question asks about broader subject matter that involves the entire passage. Topics include the author's (or another figure's) opinion about the overall subject matter, the author's expectations about the reader, or the overall tone of the passage.

EXAMPLE QUESTION STEMS

Based on the passage, the author feels that her readers are largely:

The passage is most likely to have been written for:

Which of the following characterizations of the passage and its author are the most accurate?

Source of Opinion

The individual or group whose opinion the question asks for also varies.

Author Opinion

The overwhelming majority of Recognize Opinion questions ask about the author's beliefs, emphasizing that the author is the most significant viewpoint in any CARS passage. Questions testing other skills reflect this importance as well.

EXAMPLE QUESTION STEMS

The author would probably agree with the claim that the "reader-response" school of literary criticism is:

The author's attitude toward the subject of the passage would best be described as:

Non-Author Opinion

Occasionally, questions will instead ask for the opinion of another individual, group, or organization mentioned in the passage, making it essential to track the origin of each belief.

EXAMPLE QUESTION STEMS

Based on the first paragraph, which of the following statements best reflects the attitude of A. J. P. Taylor toward the diplomatic efforts of the late 1930s?

Simone de Beauvoir's critique of Sartre's concept of radical freedom is portrayed as being rooted in a sense of:

Questions that ask for opinions other than the author's typically focus on a specific concept from the passage, rather than the passage as a whole.

Location Clues

Recognize Opinion questions that ask about specific concepts from the passage can also be categorized based on whether they indicate where the concept is discussed.

No Paragraph Reference

In this most common format, the question stem does not indicate where the concept is discussed, requiring that you skim the passage and locate it yourself.

EXAMPLE QUESTION STEMS

Which of the following best describes the author's attitude toward the early, chaotic paintings of the Abstract Expressionists?

The author implies that Roosevelt's private correspondences about the New Deal expressed her:

Paragraph Reference

For these variants, the question stem directly states the paragraph that mentions the concept in question.

EXAMPLE QUESTION STEMS

Based on paragraph 2, what language would most accurately describe the author's perspective on Chicago's new zoning ordinances?

The language used in the first paragraph to describe the reintroduction of wolves to Yellowstone National Park indicates that the author regards the project as:

A direct paragraph reference in the question stem typically indicates the first place that the author mentions the concept in question. However, the concept may be mentioned in subsequent paragraphs as well, so take this into account when formulating a prediction for this variant.

Directness of Answer Choices

The answer choices for Recognize Opinion questions fall into two broad categories based on how direct the opinions are. For any single question, all of the answer choices will usually fall into the same category.

Indirect Opinions

Questions with these answer choices are much more common. They rely heavily on the Author keywords described earlier in this chapter to convey an opinion about the subject of the question through tone. These choices tend to be three or fewer words in length, but are sometimes longer.

EXAMPLE QUESTION

The author's treatment of the Futurist movement's core principles can best be described as one of:

A. unreserved praise.

B. detached curiosity.

C. profound disapproval.

D. mild confusion.

Direct Opinions

Questions with these answer choices are much less common. These choices involve the kinds of statements that logically must be opinions, as described earlier in this chapter: value judgments, personal preferences, recommendations, and so on. These answer choices often lack clear Author keywords and tend to be longer than those that express indirect opinions.

EXAMPLE QUESTION

Based on paragraph 1, with which of the following statements about "gamification" would the author be most likely to agree?

A. Schools should focus on substantive learning goals over superficial rewards.

B. All school districts should adopt these gamified platforms to boost student engagement.

C. Educators must reject digital tools and return to purely traditional teaching methods.

D. Further implementation should be paused until studies on its efficacy are conducted.

The question stem is not a reliable indicator of which kind of answer choices are associated with a Recognize Opinion question, but glancing at the choices themselves can reveal this information and potentially inform your prediction.

9.3 Applying the Kaplan Method

Step 1: Type the Question

As described in Chapter 6, the first step of answering any CARS question is to read the question stem, determine the type and difficulty, and decide whether the question is worth attempting right away. Always at least try to assign the question to one of the three broad skill categories: Foundations of Comprehension (surface questions), Reasoning Within the Text (deep questions), or Reasoning Beyond the Text (new info questions). As discussed earlier, this step will orient you strategically even when the question stem does not indicate the skill being tested with complete certainty.

Identifying the Skill

Questions that ask for the author's or another figure's subjective beliefs about concepts discussed in the passage usually test the Recognize Opinion skill. Such question stems often reveal their subjective nature by referring to a "perspective," "view," "attitude," or "reaction." Question stems that ask for a general description of the author, the tone of the passage as a whole, or a figure's attitudes toward the subject matter or the audience also typically indicate a Recognize Opinion question.

Deciding When to Attack

Because Recognize Opinion is a Foundations of Comprehension skill, questions that test it rely on the direct interpretation of information stated in the passage. So you should almost always attack them *now*.

However, you might wish to save a Recognize Opinion question until *later* in the question set if it asks about an idea or figure that you do not recall from your reading and that you are unable to quickly locate in the passage, which will typically occur when the question stem addresses a very minor detail without a paragraph reference. In the process of answering other questions, you may encounter the part of the text that such a question refers to and therefore be in a better position to answer it later.

Many of the other skills tested in CARS questions are connected to the opinions expressed in the passage. Clarifying these opinions while answering a Recognize Opinion question can help to prepare you for these other questions, providing another reason to attack Recognize Opinion questions as soon as you encounter them.

MCAT EXPERTISE

Questions that ask what the passage implies about someone's beliefs may test the Recognize Opinion skill, but could instead test the Paraphrase Detail skill (if these beliefs are directly stated in the passage) or the Make Deduction skill (if deducing the opinion requires more complex reasoning rather than following direct cues like Author keywords). The Paraphrase Detail skill is discussed in Chapter 10 and the Make Deduction skill is discussed in Chapter 15.

Step 2: Rephrase the Stem

After determining that a question is testing the Recognize Opinion skill, you must translate it into a specific task. For this skill, that involves two pieces of information: the topic of the opinion and the source of the opinion.

The topic is what the question is asking for an opinion about. As discussed earlier in this chapter, it can be a specific concept from the passage or something as broad as the passage's overall tone or the author's implied attitude toward the reader.

The source is the individual or group who is providing the opinion. When the source is not directly named in the question stem, it is almost always the author, as with question stems that read "The passage was most likely written for:" or "Which of the following best captures the overall tone of the passage?"

Once both of these elements are identified, the final phrasing of the task depends on the specificity of the topic. If the question asks for an opinion about the passage as a whole, phrase the task as "Use your distillation of the passage to identify what the source believes about the topic." If the topic is a specific detail and the question stem does not mention which paragraph it is discussed in, phrase the task as "Locate where the topic is discussed, and read the surrounding text for direct opinions and Author keywords to identify what the source believes about the topic." For example, if the question stem is:

> Based on the passage, what is the author's attitude toward the prescriptivist grammarians' arguments?

Then your rephrased task is:

- Scan the passage and locate where "prescriptivist grammarians" are discussed, then read around and determine the essence of their argument, looking for any direct opinions from the author or Author keywords that reveal their perspective on the topic.

It can feel challenging to get a hold of opinions because we've seen that they are often expressed through hints and subtle choice of words, rather than direct statements. But a plan focused on the specific clues that reveal these attitudes will locate them efficiently.

Step 3: Investigate Potential Solutions

Next, follow the instructions in your rephrased task. For the Recognize Opinion skill, the scope of text that you need to investigate can vary widely. For questions that ask about the entire passage, such as the overall tone or the author's opinion toward a concept that is discussed throughout the text, the best source for an accurate prediction is your outline or highlighting from the Distill step of Kaplan's PCRD method, as discussed in Chapter 5. Your distillation has a good chance of containing broad opinions that address the passage as a whole and can be analyzed much more quickly than the passage itself.

If the Distill step did not reveal the opinions you need to answer the question, then scan the passage for Author keywords connected to the topic and source that the question is asking about. You often won't have to scan through the whole passage to find the desired opinion.

For questions that ask about a specific topic, either go directly to the paragraph indicated in the question stem, or (if there is no paragraph reference in the stem) use your memories from the Read step and your work from the Distill step to locate the part of the passage that discusses the topic. For topics that are details within the passage, the direct opinions or Author keywords that indicate the opinion are usually located in a narrow part of the passage: either the same sentence as the topic reference, or the sentence immediately before or after.

Regardless of whether the topic is specific or passage-wide, your final goal is to make a prediction of the opinion that the source (the author or other figure in the passage) would have about this topic. Summarize this opinion with a simple phrasing that reflects a direct opinion such as a value judgment or recommendation, using simple Author keywords.

Because it is almost always possible to make a useful prediction for Recognize Opinion questions, try to have one phrased in your mind before moving on to the answer choices.

Step 4: Match Your Prediction to an Answer Choice

The last step is to find an opinion in the answer choices that matches your prediction. The choices for Recognize Opinion questions, particularly short ones, often include the same kinds of Author keywords that regularly appear in

BRIDGE

When using the rephrased task to investigate the passage, it's most helpful to look for the "rarest" idea mentioned in the task; that is, the idea that seems like it was mentioned the least frequently in the text. This increases your chances of quickly locating the precise part of the passage that will help you to answer the question. This technique is discussed at greater length in Chapter 10, where it is a major part of applying the Paraphrase Detail skill.

MCAT EXPERTISE

You should usually avoid reading the answer choices in detail before making a prediction because it distracts from the analysis needed to answer CARS questions accurately. However, glancing at the length of the answer choices can help you to make more accurate predictions for Recognize Opinion questions.

Short answer choices usually reflect indirect opinions and suggest that you should phrase a brief prediction based on 1–2 Author keywords that capture the opinion you located in the passage. Answer choices longer than a few words are more likely to reflect direct opinions; if they are framed as recommendations or suggestions, phrase your prediction the same way.

CARS passages. Keywords do not capture all the nuances of opinion conveyed in CARS passages, but comparing the Author keywords that the passage uses to the Author keywords used in the answer choices is a valuable technique to quickly focus on plausible options. Give serious consideration to an answer choice that uses keywords matching the value (positive or negative) and intensity (strong or weak) of your prediction.

In contrast, trap answer choices will often match either the value or intensity of the correct opinion, but not both. The most common pattern is the **Distortion** answer trap, especially when the passage expresses a weak opinion (often through the use of Limiting keywords) and an incorrect answer choice takes the form of a similar opinion that is too extreme. Be suspicious of answer choices that exaggerate opinions in this way. Incorrect answer choices may also use convoluted language, such as double negatives, to obscure the opinion that they are communicating.

If you cannot find a match for your prediction, eliminate any of the answer choices that directly contradict opinions you recall from the passage. Then look for Author keywords or direct opinions in the passage to support the remaining choices, until you find validation for one of them.

9.4 Skillbuilder

Use the following shortened passage to practice the Recognize Opinion skill. The reading is scaffolded to reinforce good active reading habits and to let you devote more of your attention to practicing your critical thinking skills. It includes Active Reading Checks with each paragraph to evaluate how well you're uncovering important passage information at every level. Answer both the Active Reading Check and the CARS question that accompanies each paragraph before continuing. You can check your answers on the next page before you move on to paragraph 2, and the same for paragraph 3.

Paragraph 1

The Library of Alexandria was more than a vast repository of scrolls; it was arguably the preeminent center of intellectual life in the ancient world. The Library was established in the 3rd century BCE under the Ptolemaic dynasty as the pursuit of a remarkable scholarly ambition: to collect a comprehensive record of human knowledge at the time. This institution functioned not only as a collection of texts, but also as a research center with lecture halls, meeting rooms, laboratories, and observatories. The scale of this Hellenistic endeavor suggests a profound commitment to inquiry. Its legacy persists in the Western intellectual tradition as a benchmark for a particularly fertile period of scholarship.

Active Reading Check for Paragraph 1

Why does the author begin by stating the Library was "more than a vast repository of scrolls"?

A. To suggest that the number of scrolls the Library contained is often underestimated

B. To emphasize that the Library did more than store information and was a center of research

C. To introduce the idea that the main inter-esting feature of the Library was its size

1. The author's attitude toward the Library of Alexandria can best be described as one of:

A. deep admiration.

B. conditional appreciation.

C. scholarly neutrality.

D. cautious skepticism.

Active Reading Check for Paragraph 1: (B)

(A) The words "more than" indicate that this phrase is meant to emphasize that the Library was important for more reasons than just the number of scrolls that it contained, rather than correcting a misconception about the quantity of scrolls it contained.

(B) After stating that the Library was "more than a vast repository of scrolls," the author describes it as "arguably the preeminent center of intellectual life in the ancient world." The paragraph lists more details later, including the Library's role as a "research center." So this opening emphasizes that the Library's true significance came from its role as a place of active scholarship.

(C) The author explicitly states that the Library was "more than a vast repository," signaling that its size or capacity for storage was *not* its defining feature.

Question 1: (A)

Answer Choice Explanations for Question 1

(A) The author uses a series of very positive phrases to describe the Library in paragraph 1, calling it "arguably the preeminent center of intellectual life," its goal a "remarkable scholarly ambition," and its scale a sign of a "profound commitment." So it's clear that the author has a deep sense of respect for the Library.

(B) The author's appreciation in the first paragraph is expressed without any reservations and without the sense that it depends on meeting other conditions, so it cannot be described as "conditional."

(C) A neutral stance would involve objective language. The author's use of terms like "remarkable" and "profound" in paragraph 1 demonstrates a clear positive opinion of the subject, not neutrality.

(D) The author does not express any doubt or skepticism regarding the achievements or significance of the Library in this passage. The tone is consistently positive and respectful.

Detailed Explanation for Question 1

Skill: This question requires you to provide a general description of the author's personal attitude towards something discussed in the passage, so it tests the Recognize Opinion skill.

Question: The question asks you to describe the author's attitude towards the Library of Alexandria. Review the first paragraph and analyze the author's word choice and tone as they describe the Library, condensing what you find into a concise characterization of their viewpoint.

Passage: The first sentence describes the Library as "arguably the preeminent center of intellectual life," and throughout the first paragraph, the author consistently uses language that indicates a very high opinion of it. The author refers to the Library's "remarkable scholarly ambition" and "profound commitment to inquiry." Finally, the author claims that its legacy serves as a "benchmark for a particularly fertile period of scholarship." Words like "preeminent," "remarkable," and "profound" all convey appreciation of the Library, so you should predict that the correct answer will reflect a very positive attitude.

Answer: The prediction that the author holds the Library in high regard means their attitude is best summarized as "deep admiration," as stated in **(A)**.

Paragraph 2

The narrative of the Library's end is often distilled into a theatrical account of its destruction in a single fire, frequently associated with Julius Caesar's campaign in 48 BCE. While historical sources suggest that Caesar's actions did cause a fire that destroyed scrolls in a portside warehouse, many scholars now question whether this event was responsible for the ruination of the entire Library. One noteworthy piece of evidence is that the geographer Strabo, who wrote several decades after the fire, mentioned visiting the Mouseion—the larger research institution to which the Library was attached—implying its continued operation. The persistence of the story of the fire in popular imagination tends to obscure the reality of the Library's mysterious fate.

Active Reading Check for Paragraph 2

What is the main purpose of mentioning the geographer Strabo?

A. To provide evidence that the Library complex was still in use after Caesar's fire

B. To suggest that the fire started in the Mouseion, not the portside warehouse

C. To demonstrate that an important scholar studied at the Library

2. The author apparently views the theory that a fire destroyed the Library as:

A. a complete fabrication about Julius Caesar that lacks any factual basis.

B. a dramatic story about the establishment of the Ptolemaic dynasty.

C. a well-documented historical fact that has been misinterpreted by the public.

D. an ultimately misleading portrayal of historical events.

Active Reading Check for Paragraph 2: (A)

(A) The passage states that Strabo visited the Mouseion, which was part of the Library's research institution, "several decades after the fire." The author uses this piece of information to indicate that the Library had "continued operation" and cast doubt on the theory that the fire destroyed the Library.

(B) The author does not suggest that the fire began in the Mouseion, and they do not question the story that the fire "destroyed scrolls in a portside warehouse."

(C) While it is possible that Strabo was an important scholar, the author doesn't suggest this directly. And providing a general example of the Library's visitors does not seem to serve the author's larger purpose in paragraph 2; instead, they use Strabo to make a point about the Library's continued existence after the fire.

Question 2: (D)

Answer Choice Explanations for Question 2

(A) The author states in paragraph 2 that "Caesar's actions did cause a fire that destroyed scrolls in a portside warehouse," demonstrating that this theory does have at least some basis in fact.

(B) Paragraph 1 mentions the founding of the Library under the Ptolemaic dynasty in the 3rd century BCE, so that dynasty was established a long time before the fire attributed to Julius Caesar's campaign, which was in 48 BCE according to paragraph 2.

(C) Paragraph 2 states that "many scholars now question" the theory that a fire destroyed the Library, and the author mentions Strabo as evidence that supports these doubts. So the author frames it as a questionable story, not a well-documented fact.

(D) The author calls the fire theory a "theatrical account" and states that its persistence "tends to obscure the reality of the Library's mysterious fate," indicating that the author believes it gives a false impression of the Library's disappearance.

Detailed Explanation for Question 2

Skill: This question asks you to determine the author's personal viewpoint on one of the theories from the passage, so it tests the Recognize Opinion skill.

Question: The question asks how the author views the theory that a single fire destroyed the Library. Your task is to analyze the language the author uses to describe this theory in paragraph 2, looking for keywords that reveal their opinion.

Passage: The author introduces the theory of the fire as a "theatrical account," a phrase that suggests it is more dramatic than factual. After acknowledging that there was a fire during Julius Caesar's campaign, the author casts doubt on the theory that the fire destroyed the Library by stating that "many scholars now question" it, and by presenting Strabo's visit to the Mouseion several decades later as a "noteworthy" piece of conflicting evidence. The paragraph's concluding sentence delivers the author's main judgment: the "persistence of the story . . . tends to obscure the reality of the Library's mysterious fate." This indicates that the author believes the story is an obstacle to understanding what really happened to the Library. So the correct answer will describe the theory as an inaccurate portrayal of the Library's destruction.

Answer: The author's argument that the fire story is a "theatrical account" that "tends to obscure the reality" points directly to the conclusion that it is a distorted version of history. The author's main issue with the narrative is not that it is entirely baseless, but that it is a simplification that gets in the way of a more complex truth. Based on this, **(D)** is the choice that best captures the author's specific opinion.

Paragraph 3

The more probable, if less sensational, explanation is that the Library experienced a protracted decline. Its vitality appears to have diminished over several centuries, stemming from a confluence of factors including inconsistent royal patronage and prolonged political instability. These factors coincided with shifting cultural priorities that were at times hostile to open scholarly inquiry. It was therefore not a sudden inferno that extinguished the intellectual fire of Alexandria, but a slow erosion of the civic and financial support that had sustained it. The fading of the Library represents an incalculable loss, a cautionary tale not of a singular destructive act, but of a civilization slowly turning its back on the very principles that made it great.

Active Reading Check for Paragraph 3

According to the passage, what is the author's view regarding the ultimate cause of the Library's fading?

A. The cause was likely a single, catastrophic event.
B. The cause was likely a gradual loss of societal support.
C. The cause is a mystery with no likely explanation.

3. The author's overall treatment of the Library of Alexandria's fate can best be characterized as:

A. ambiguous.
B. enthusiastic.
C. regretful.
D. dispassionate.

Active Reading Check for Paragraph 3: (B)

(A) The author explicitly argues against this idea in the third paragraph, stating that it was "not a sudden inferno" that destroyed the Library.

(B) The author begins paragraph 3 by identifying the "more probable" cause as a "protracted decline" resulting from a "slow erosion of the civic and financial support that had sustained it." This matches the idea of a gradual loss of societal support.

(C) Although paragraph 2 mentions "the Library's mysterious fate," the author dedicates the paragraph to presenting what the author believes is the "more probable ... explanation." Therefore, the author would not claim that the cause is a mystery.

Question 3: (C)

Answer Choice Explanations for Question 3

(A) An ambiguous treatment would be open to multiple different interpretations. This does not fit with the author's definite point of view. The author clearly expresses the "more probable" cause of the Library's decline and how they feel about these events.

(B) This choice mischaracterizes the author's tone regarding the Library's end. While the author is enthusiastic about the Library's importance in history, the tone that the author uses to describe its fate is somber, not excited.

(C) The author uses phrases like "incalculable loss" and "cautionary tale" when describing the Library's end to communicate a strong sense of sadness for what was lost.

(D) The word dispassionate means "without passion or feeling." This word is contradicted by the author's use of opinionated language throughout the passage, which demonstrates a passionate treatment of the topic rather than objective detachment.

Detailed Explanation for Question 3

Skill: Because the task is to identify an adjective that best describes the author's tone when discussing a concept from the passage, it tests the Recognize Opinion skill.

Question: The question asks for the word that best describes the author's attitude toward the "fate" of the Library. This requires you to assess the emotional tone of paragraphs 2 and 3 as the author discusses theories about the Library's disappearance.

Passage: In paragraph 2, the author introduces the common view that the Library was destroyed in a single fire. The author describes this theory as "a theatrical account," presents evidence against it, and concludes that the theory regarding the fire "tends to obscure the reality of the Library's mysterious fate."

Paragraph 3 opens with the claim that a drawn-out decline is the "more probable" explanation, indicating that the passage is shifting to a discussion of the author's beliefs about the Library's fate. They use strongly opinionated language in the last sentence of paragraph 3, describing the Library's end as an "incalculable loss, a cautionary tale ... of a civilization slowly turning its back on the very principles that made it great." The correct answer will match this deep sense of sadness over the Library's decline.

Answer: **(C)** most accurately matches the author's sorrow over the demise of the Library of Alexandria.

Skill and Strategy Summary

Skill Description

- The **Recognize Opinion** skill is the ability to identify the subjective beliefs of the author or other figures mentioned in a passage.
  - Recognize Opinion accounts for about 20% of Foundations of Comprehension questions.
- This skill involves distinguishing opinions, like value judgments and recommendations, from objective facts.
- Many opinions are expressed indirectly through Author keywords that indicate a speaker's positive and negative attitudes, as well as how strong those feelings are.

Question Variations and Examples

- Recognize Opinion questions can vary in the following ways:
  - Scope of Subject: The opinion is usually about some specific topic but can also concern something general like the intended audience or overall passage tone.
  - Source of Opinion: The author's opinions are most tested, but occasionally those of other viewpoints discussed in the passage.
  - Location Clues: Specific paragraph references are rare with this skill.
  - Directness of Answer Choices: Indirect opinions reflecting author word choice are much more common in answer choices than statements of direct opinion.

Applying the Kaplan Method

- Step 1: Type the Question
  - Identify Recognize Opinion questions through subjective language such as "perspective," "view," or "attitude."
  - As surface questions (Foundations of Comprehension), answer them *now*, most of the time.
  - Save them for *later* if they ask for an opinion about topics you don't know how to locate in the passage.
- Step 2: Rephrase the Stem
  - Include *what* the opinion is about (the topic) and *who* holds that opinion (the source) in the rephrase.
- Step 3: Investigate Potential Solutions
  - For passage-wide opinions, use your distillation (outline or highlights) to form a prediction.
  - For opinions on specific topics, locate the relevant section of the passage and check the surrounding text for direct opinions or Author Keywords to use in forming a prediction.
- Step 4: Match Your Prediction to an Answer Choice
  - Compare the charge (positive/negative) and intensity (strong/weak) of the keywords in your prediction to those in the answer choices.
  - Avoid the **Distortion** answer trap, where an incorrect answer choice exaggerates a mild opinion expressed in the passage.

CHAPTER 10

PARAPHRASE DETAIL

In This Chapter

10.1 Skill Description 144
Search for the Rarest Concept 145
Isolate the Relevant Information 146
Paraphrase Effectively 147
10.2 Question Variations and Examples . . . 148
Description of the Detail 148
Location Clues 149
Number of Details Requested 150
Present or Absent Details 151
Stated or Implied Information 152
10.3 Applying the Kaplan Method 152
Step 1: Type the Question 152
Step 2: Rephrase the Stem 153
Step 3: Investigate Potential Solutions 154
Step 4: Match Your Prediction to an Answer Choice 154
10.4 Skillbuilder 155
Skill and Strategy Summary 161

LEARNING OBJECTIVES

After Chapter 10, you will be able to:

- Define the Paraphrase Detail skill
- Locate information in passages that is relevant to questions
- Restate passage information in simpler language
- Recognize common wordings for questions that test Paraphrase Detail
- Apply the Kaplan Method for CARS Questions to Paraphrase Detail questions
- Evaluate your current proficiency with the Paraphrase Detail skill

FOUNDATIONS OF COMPREHENSION SKILL

Paraphrase Detail: Recognize a specific piece of information that is stated or strongly implied at one location in the passage.

Approximate Frequency: 40% of Foundations of Comprehension questions

The jurisprudential debate concerning constitutional interpretation is largely dominated by two opposing hermeneutic approaches. One approach, the doctrine of the "Living Constitution," advocates for a dynamic and flexible interpretive method. Its supporters contend that constitutional principles cannot be perpetually tethered to the historical context in which they were written; rather, they must be adapted in light of evolving societal mores, technological advancements, and unforeseen modern challenges. Accordingly, the Constitution's language should be read as a set of broad principles whose application must be informed by present-day values to remain relevant and just. Critics, however, contend that such jurisprudential flexibility risks eroding the distinction between interpretation and legislation, effectively empowering judges to engage in policymaking untethered from the foundational text they are sworn to uphold.

In contrast, the philosophy of originalism posits that the semantic content of the constitutional text is fixed at the time of its enactment. In public discourse, originalism is often framed as a focus on discovering the subjective and often private "original intent" of the drafters, a variant that is related but distinct from its core meaning. Properly speaking, this view argues that any legitimate interpretation must be constrained by the text's original public meaning—that is, the meaning that a reasonable, informed citizen would have understood the words to convey at the time of ratification. Adherents believe that this interpretive discipline is necessary to prevent judicial rulings based on contemporary political preferences, thereby preserving a stable and predictable rule of law that is independent of the judiciary's own normative considerations.

The passage suggests that originalism is characterized by interpretations of the Constitution that:

A. shift in response to changing societal values.
B. preserve its meaning as generally understood at the time of its creation.
C. reflect the personal motivations and beliefs of its authors.
D. adhere strictly to the dictionary definition of the terms it uses.

10.1 Skill Description

Employing the **Paraphrase Detail** skill is like searching through a patient history to find a specific test result necessary to diagnose their condition. Based on some prior experience with this patient and an understanding of how patient histories are typically organized, you can often quickly locate the information you need. Since physicians are regularly obliged to locate individual details in a larger set of data, it's no coincidence that the MCAT tests you on this skill as well.

Sometimes, a piece of information that turns out to be essential for diagnosing a complex medical condition seems unimportant before new symptoms or additional test results reveal its true significance. Similarly, a number of CARS questions ask about details that initially appear minor: the ones that don't have any such clues pointing to them. Even if you do an excellent job reading and distilling the passage, as described in Chapters 2–5, you'll regularly encounter questions about information that is unlikely to be included in your outline notes or highlighting. This is where Paraphrase Detail comes in: it is the skill of locating what the author suggests about specific topics and expressing those claims in simple language.

The sample question at the beginning of this chapter, which asks about the principles that characterize "the judicial philosophy of originalism," illustrates how to accomplish this dual task. In the first paragraph of the passage, there is a statement that "the Constitution's language should be read as a set of broad principles whose application must be informed by present-day values," which is very similar to **(A)**. However, paragraph 1 is devoted to discussing the "Living Constitution" doctrine, not the philosophy of "originalism" that the question asks about.

Originalism is the focus of paragraph 2 instead. Reviewing that part of the passage, your attention might be drawn to the statement that "originalism is often framed as a focus on discovering the subjective and often private 'original intent' of the drafters," which looks like it matches **(C)**. However, does this way of describing originalism reflect the reality of the situation, as the author sees it? The phrasing of "often framed as" is noncommittal, and it's essential to make sure that you have enough context to be sure that you've captured the desired detail.

Reading further in paragraph 2, the passage clarifies that the interpretation that points to **(C)** is "distinct from its [orginalism's] core meaning," confirming that this isn't the appropriate description. The passage finally states that "properly speaking," originalism "argues that any legitimate interpretation must be constrained by the text's original public meaning," which closely matches the idea expressed by **(B)** and confirms that this choice is correct. As this sample illustrates, applying the Paraphrase Detail skill requires that you focus on the exact idea that the question asks for, locate where it is discussed in the passage, and recognize the answer choice that expresses this detail.

Reading and writing are acts of communication, and another person will never use precisely the same language as you to describe a particular idea or situation, even if you are both effective communicators and have similar backgrounds. As both a medical student and later a physician, you will constantly need to absorb ideas expressed by other medical professionals and communicate them in your own words.

This task is equally important on the MCAT. The ability to express complex passage claims in simple terms is the best measure of whether you understand those claims well enough to answer questions about them. It protects you from misunderstandings that could lead you to select incorrect answer choices.

Since the Paraphrase Detail skill involves identifying information that is directly stated or implied, the logic involved may seem straightforward compared to most other types of CARS questions. However, in order to locate and paraphrase information quickly and accurately, you must perform a few specific tasks.

Search for the Rarest Concept

Almost every question that tests the Paraphrase Detail skill mentions one or more passage concepts and then asks you what the author claims about a particular topic. If you can determine which part of the question stem is the best clue, then locating the information that Paraphrase Detail questions are asking for will be a lot easier. This is particularly important when the stem involves multiple concepts that could potentially serve as clues.

The correct answers to these questions are always drawn from one location in the passage, and concepts in the question stem that are rarely mentioned in the passage are much more likely to point to this exact part of the text. On the other hand, tracking concepts from the question stem that are discussed throughout the passage would force you to look in a variety of locations, and most of these locations would not contain any helpful information. So use your work from the Read and Distill steps to identify the "rarest" concept in the stem, then base your passage search on it.

BRIDGE

Searching for the rarest concept is also a useful approach for questions that test other skills. Whenever the question stem refers to ideas from the passage, this approach will increase your chances of quickly locating the part of the text that is most relevant to the question.

Imagine that the question stem is:

> Based on the passage, which of the following did Ira Gitler consider an essential component of the bebop style of jazz?

There are two specific concepts mentioned: Ira Gitler and bebop jazz. Depending on the passage context, either of them could be the rare concept that we're looking for. If the passage focuses on the jazz critic Ira Gitler and his opinions on various different forms of jazz, then bebop is the rare concept. Searching for that word will probably direct you to a specific paragraph, bypassing other paragraphs that discuss other forms of jazz.

In contrast, suppose that bebop is the topic of the entire passage. Then Gitler is the rare concept, and scanning the passage for his name will likely take you to the necessary location to make a strong prediction. The same principles apply if the question stem includes a specific paragraph reference; this extra piece of information simply narrows the search, letting you look for the rare concept in one part of the passage.

Isolate the Relevant Information

After you find where the passage mentions the concept you're searching for, you must identify the text that addresses the specific detail the question is asking about, separating it from the surrounding text. Sometimes, the detail you need is located in the same sentence as the concept you searched for, but not always.

The rare concept clue is a signpost, not the destination. It efficiently guides you to the correct location in the passage, but the sentence containing the clue may not contain the answer itself. Often, the answer is located in the sentence immediately before or after the one that mentions the rare concept.

Suppose that this question stem is associated with a passage that discusses multiple 19th-century art movements:

> According to the passage, the central feature of the Hudson River School's artistic philosophy was:

MCAT EXPERTISE

Searching for a common concept rather than a rare one may eventually lead to the correct passage claim, but the rare concept approach will always be faster. The Kaplan strategies for applying each CARS skill are designed to optimize accuracy and speed simultaneously to maximize your score.

The rare concept in the passage is the specific name "Hudson River School," and so this is the most efficient term to search for. Suppose that you scan the passage for that phrase and find that it only appears in the following sentence:

> The most prominent American art movement of the mid-19th century was the Hudson River School, a group of painters based in New York.

This sentence provides some information about the Hudson River School but does not suggest anything about their artistic philosophy, so it is missing the information you need to answer the question. Because this sentence appears to introduce the School, it's extremely unlikely that there is any useful information earlier in the passage, so look at the next sentence instead. Suppose that reads:

> The most prominent American art movement of the mid-19th century was the Hudson River School, a group of painters based in New York. Their work was defined by a belief that the American landscape was a divine creation, and they sought to depict the natural world with a kind of reverent, detailed grandeur that emphasized its sublime and untamed qualities.

This sentence does not use the phrase "artistic philosophy" or refer to its "central feature," as the question stem does, but it describes what their work "was defined by," which is a close match for what the question is requesting. So now you've isolated the information you need to make a prediction, and the rare concept clue pointed the way.

The important detail can also appear before the sentence containing the rare concept from the question stem. Consider a stem that reads:

> The author states that the primary purpose of the potlatch ceremony was to:

In this example, the potlatch ceremony is the only specific concept mentioned in the question stem and so it must be the rarest concept as well. Suppose that the only appearance of this term is in the following sentence from the passage:

> This complex ceremonial practice is known as a potlatch.

This sentence also lacks the information the question is asking for, but the Continuity keyword "this" implies that the potlatch was discussed in more detail earlier, so look at the previous sentence:

> Among certain Indigenous societies of the Pacific Northwest, a leader's social rank required constant public validation through elaborate festivals involving the redistribution or even destruction of vast amounts of personal wealth. This complex ceremonial practice is known as a potlatch.

This sentence describes a leader who conducts "elaborate festivals," so this must be the "ceremonial practice" that the following sentence refers to. In addition to testing your ability to locate information that is directly stated in the passage, Paraphrase Detail questions also ask you to make straightforward deductions like this. Since this sentence also describes the purpose of these festivals (validation of the leader's social rank), you have isolated the information that the question is asking for.

MCAT EXPERTISE

When CARS question stems refer to passage concepts without directly quoting the text, these concepts are often phrased differently than they appear in the passage. Don't overemphasize minor differences in word choice: if the ideas in the question stem and passage are similar, ask yourself whether the change in phrasing indicates a clear difference in meaning that reflects the way the author uses language in the passage. If not, then the distinction probably doesn't matter.

Sometimes, even the rarest concept in the question stem will be mentioned in multiple parts of the passage, potentially far apart from one another. In these cases, treat each reference to that concept as a separate part of the text to be investigated. Look for the detail the question asks for in the sentences surrounding the reference to the concept clue. If the target detail is not stated or directly implied in that part of the passage, move on to the next place that the concept clue is mentioned and repeat the process until you locate the information you need.

Paraphrase Effectively

Once you locate the detail that the question is asking about, it is also important to rephrase it in simple language. Information in CARS passages is often expressed in an academic writing style that employs long, complex sentences and uncommon vocabulary.

Your role at this point is like that of a skilled translator. A translator doesn't just swap words one-for-one; they understand the core meaning of a phrase in one language and then express that same meaning clearly and naturally in the new language. You must do the same with academic CARS writing and translate it into simpler and more direct terms.

The following questions can be useful to simplify the information you've isolated:

- Who is performing an action, and what are they doing?
- What is the main quality being described?
- What is the primary cause and effect?

The answers to these questions provide a simpler picture of what the isolated information is describing, which can help you to break down long multi-part sentences into one or two core ideas. If the isolated information includes technical terms or jargon that are defined in the passage, use the passage context to replace those terms with their simple meaning. Also, replace any unusual words with equivalent language that you would use in everyday writing and conversation. The result should be a short phrase or sentence that sounds like it could have come from an email you wrote to a friend or colleague.

Consider one of the question stems discussed earlier in this chapter, which asked for "the central feature of the Hudson River School's artistic philosophy." We isolated the relevant information from the passage:

> [The Hudson River School's] work was defined by a belief that the American landscape was a divine creation, and they sought to depict the natural world with a kind of reverent, detailed grandeur that emphasized its sublime and untamed qualities.

Now, let's translate this academic language into simpler terms, piece by piece. These artists' "work was defined by" their "belief that the American landscape was a divine creation," so they saw nature as sacred. The phrase "reverent, detailed grandeur" suggests that these artists painted with great respect and detail. The "sublime and untamed qualities" of nature that they emphasized could be expressed more simply as "wild" or "awe-inspiring."

MCAT EXPERTISE

The author is the ultimate source of the passage information that is addressed in Paraphrase Detail questions, but these details may involve statements by other people, groups, or organizations as well.

By combining these simplified pieces, you can formulate a clear and effective paraphrase:

> *The Hudson River School painters thought nature was sacred, wild, and worthy of being captured in detail.*

You will become more comfortable and effective applying the Paraphrase Detail skill as you repeatedly practice the steps of isolating and rephrasing the requested information.

10.2 Question Variations and Examples

There are several ways that Paraphrase Detail questions vary: the description of the requested detail, the clues about the location of that detail, the number of details that are requested, whether the question requests present or absent information, and whether the detail is stated or implied.

Description of the Detail

The most significant variation is the amount of information that you are given about the detail in question. Sometimes the question stem will partially phrase the detail and ask you to complete the statement, while other Paraphrase Detail questions will ask for the entire detail.

Complete a Partial Detail

Many question stems will include part of the requested detail, with the answer choices completing the statement.

Roman Numerals

Occasionally, questions present three statements labeled with Roman numerals, and the answer choices are different combinations of one or more of these statements. The correct answer choice includes all of the Roman numeral statements that answer the question accurately and no statements that are incorrect.

EXAMPLE QUESTION

The passage suggests that the theory of Keynesian economics (paragraph 3) proposes managing aggregate demand with:

I. government spending.

II. taxation rates.

III. production quotas.

A. I only

B. II only

C. I and II

D. II and III

These variations reward an approach that focuses on evaluating the accuracy of each Roman numeral statement. By discarding answer choices that do not include accurate statements (or include inaccurate ones), you will reach the correct answer by the process of elimination.

Present or Absent Details

While most Paraphrase Detail questions ask for claims that appear in the passage, some ask for a claim that does not appear.

Details Included in Passage

This is the most common variation. These questions ask for what the passage or author states or implies.

EXAMPLE QUESTION STEMS

The passage suggests that the main distinction between social norms and laws is that laws are:

According to the passage, the primary purpose of the peer review process in academic publishing is to:

Details Not Included in Passage

In this rare variation, questions ask for information that is not present in the passage.

EXAMPLE QUESTION STEMS

Which of the following is NOT in accord with the information presented in the passage?

Which of the following is neither stated nor implied by the author?

Variations that ask for information absent from the passage are typically also
the Open-Ended Detail variation, so they will not include any description suggesting the topic of the correct or incorrect answer choices.

Stated or Implied Information

The last common variation of Paraphrase Detail questions depends on the logic needed to decide what is true according to the passage. While many questions testing this skill simply require you to locate information that is stated explicitly in the passage, it may also be necessary to determine what the author believes even when they do not state it directly. An idea that the author indirectly implies is called an **inference**. In Paraphrase Detail questions, however, the logic necessary to determine what the author believes will be straightforward and based on a specific part of the passage.

Stated Details

This variation asks about details directly included in the passage. The answer choices will still paraphrase that information, expressing it in different words, but they will reflect an idea plainly stated in the text.

Simple Inferences

This variation asks for an idea that is not expressed directly in the passage, regardless of wording. Instead, there is a specific statement in the passage that clearly implies that this claim is true, without directly stating it.

The question stem and the answer choices do not reliably indicate whether the question is testing stated examples or direct inferences. For example, questions that include the language "according to the passage" in the stem typically have a correct answer that is directly stated, but sometimes the correct answer will be implied instead. Similarly, questions that use phrases like "the author implies" may involve stated details as well as direct inferences. So the simplest and best strategy is to approach these Paraphrase Details questions with the expectation that the correct answer may be directly stated or implied, and that you will know which after you isolate the necessary information.

MCAT EXPERTISE

Questions that ask for statements that are absent from or inconsistent with the passage in some way can test a variety of CARS skills, but they have some characteristics in common. The process of elimination is more likely to be the best strategy for these variations, since it is often challenging to predict the claim made by the correct answer choice. However, predictions can still be useful in these questions, since any statement that contradicts the central ideas of the passage is likely to be correct.

BRIDGE

Inferences are discussed in greater detail in Chapter 15 on the Make Deduction skill. Keep in mind, however, that the discussion there also includes more complex inferences than those tested in Paraphrase Detail questions.

10.3 Applying the Kaplan Method

Step 1: Type the Question

Your first move when tackling any CARS question is to read the question stem to assess what skill it tests and decide if you should answer it immediately. You should always attempt to classify the question into one of three general categories: Foundations of Comprehension (surface questions), Reasoning Within the Text (deep questions), or Reasoning Beyond the Text (new info questions). As noted previously, this initial step makes it easier to find the correct answer, even when you are not certain which specific skill is being evaluated.

Identifying the Skill

Questions that ask for information that is true "according to the author" usually test the Paraphrase Detail skill. Question stems that ask for what is or is not stated in the passage, or consistent with the passage, almost always test this skill as well.

Deciding When to Attack

Paraphrase Detail addresses the Foundations of Comprehension and so it's a surface skill. These questions depend entirely on your understanding of what the passage states directly. So for most variations of questions that test this skill, you should attack them *now*. However, there are some variations that you may wish to save for *later*:

- **Open-Ended Detail**: These questions provide no information about the detail you're looking for, often requiring you to scan more of the passage and use the process of elimination. Such tactics are effective but can be more time-consuming, potentially justifying saving these questions for the end of the set.
- **Details Not Included in Passage**: These questions ask for information that the author does not state in the passage, so the more time-consuming process of elimination is typically the best way to approach them.
- **Roman Numerals**: Questions that involve Roman Numeral statements require you to evaluate the accuracy of multiple claims, so they are usually more time-consuming.

BRIDGE

Questions that ask what the author implies or suggests may test the Paraphrase Detail skill, but may also test the Recognize Opinion skill (if the implied idea is a subjective belief) or the Make Deduction skill (if determining the implied claim requires more complex reasoning than a direct inference). The Recognize Opinion skill is discussed in Chapter 9, and the Make Deduction skill is discussed in Chapter 15.

Step 2: Rephrase the Stem

After determining that a question tests the Paraphrase Detail skill, you must rephrase the task in simpler language. For this skill, the key element of the question stem is a description of the information that is being requested. As discussed above, most Paraphrase Detail questions include such information, and it is common for the question stem to begin the statement that the correct answer choice will complete.

If the topic is a specific detail and the question stem does not mention which paragraph it is discussed in, then begin by identifying the rarest concept mentioned in the stem, as discussed in Section 10.1. You will use this concept as the focus of your search. Consider this question stem:

> According to the author, what initial technological development was most responsible for the Industrial Revolution?

Let's imagine that your reading and distillation showed that the whole passage is devoted to the Industrial Revolution. In that case, the rarest concept mentioned in the question stem is this "initial technological development." Your task is then to follow that clue, identify the requested information, and paraphrase it. So your rephrase could read as follows:

- Scan the passage for any mention of early technology, then read around that sentence and potentially the ones immediately before and after to capture the complete passage idea. Then paraphrase it in your own simple words.

If the question stem provides a paragraph reference, incorporate it into the beginning of your rephrase with language like "Scan paragraph 2 for …" If the question is an open-ended variation that doesn't describe the relevant information at all, an appropriate rephrase might be:

- Evaluate each answer choice in order, scanning the passage for information that confirms or disproves that choice.

Step 3: Investigate Potential Solutions

Continue the process of answering the question by beginning your rephrased task. For the majority of Paraphrase Detail questions, which ask for a single detail and describe the information you need to locate, this is a focused task as described in Section 10.1 of this chapter.

Follow any rare concept clues and scan either the whole passage or a particular paragraph, depending on the references in the question stem. Once you isolate the relevant information, paraphrase it in simpler language to form your prediction, and move on to the answer choices. For this skill, it typically will not be helpful to glance at the answer choices before making a prediction.

For questions that do not request a single idea from the passage, such as ones that are open-ended, involve Roman numeral statements, or ask for information that is not stated, you can conduct a similar process. The clues about what to look for are provided in the answer choices instead.

Just like a question stem, the answer choices can include rare concepts that are probably discussed in only a few parts of the passage. Instead of predicting what the correct answer will likely say, you can use the same strategies of locating, isolating, and paraphrasing information to determine whether the passage validates each answer choice.

For example, suppose that an answer choice reads "diplomatic exchanges trailed off prior to the Opium Wars" in a passage that only mentions those wars in one part of the text. This is a clue to go directly to that part and determine whether the passage confirms that this choice is true.

MCAT EXPERTISE

Answer choices that put ideas from the passage in incorrect contexts are common in questions that test many different CARS skills. The best vaccine against these choices is to avoid relying on single words or concepts as indicators that an answer choice is correct. Consider the entire choice as a whole, rather than focusing on specific words. A word or phrase that you expect to see in the correct answer never proves that an answer choice is correct.

Step 4: Match Your Prediction to an Answer Choice

If the question stem led to a specific prediction, the last step of Kaplan's TRIM method is to match that prediction to an answer choice. This task employs a different aspect of your ability to paraphrase: rather than generating one yourself, you must now identify the answer choice that accurately paraphrases the prediction.

Incorrect answer choices in Paraphrase Detail questions will regularly mention people, places, and ideas discussed in the passage, but in a statement that does not match what the passage states about these concepts. Another common trap is an "extreme" answer, a kind of **Distortion** wrong answer pathology discussed in Chapter 6. These choices exaggerate a stated detail in some way or contain a claim that can't be definitively inferred from the text, even if they seem plausible in real-life terms.

If you cannot find a match for your prediction, eliminate any of the answer choices that directly contradict details you remember appearing in the passage. Then consider each of the remaining answer choices in turn and use the same locate and paraphrase strategy to seek information in the passage that validates that particular choice. Continue this process until you find clear support for one of them.

Paraphrase Detail questions that ask for information that is not included or implied by the passage are a trap in themselves. Compared to more common questions testing this skill, they reverse which choices are correct and incorrect. So when you notice this, highlight the word indicating that you're dealing with this variation (typically "not" or "least") to remind yourself of exactly what the question is requesting. That way, you'll avoid selecting a choice that follows the **Opposite** wrong answer pathology discussed in Chapter 6.

10.4 Skillbuilder

Use the following shortened passage to practice the Paraphrase Detail skill. The reading is scaffolded to reinforce good active reading habits and to let you devote more of your attention to practicing your critical thinking skills. It includes Active Reading Checks with each paragraph to evaluate how well you're uncovering important passage information at every level. Answer both the Active Reading Check and the CARS question that accompanies each paragraph before continuing. You can check your answers on the next page before you move on to paragraph 2, and the same for paragraph 3.

Paragraph 1

Many high schools offer advanced math classes, such as honors or Advanced Placement course options. The benefits to students who take such classes are numerous, enabling those with either a preference for the subject or a desire to challenge themselves to engage with rigorous material and potentially earn college credit while still in high school. Math classes at many middle schools are available with honors options as well. In fact, the benefits of offering advanced math education to students can begin as early as the middle grades of elementary school.

Active Reading Check for Paragraph 1

What is the author's primary goal in paragraph 1?

- **A.** To describe which high school math courses are available to students
- **B.** To introduce benefits of advanced education in math at different age levels
- **C.** To contrast honors and Advanced Placement courses

1. Which of the following claims about students aligns most closely with the author's ideas?
   - **A.** Students who are indifferent toward math may still choose to take an advanced math class for the challenge.
   - **B.** Students will avoid advanced math classes unless they have a strong preference for the subject.
   - **C.** Students are more inclined to take advanced math classes in high school than they are in middle school.
   - **D.** Students will only choose to take an advanced math class if they can earn college credit for it.

Active Reading Check for Paragraph 1: (B)

(A) The author mentions two broad types of advanced math classes, honors and Advanced Placement, but does not describe the specific courses available.

(B) The author first introduces advanced math education at high schools and then mentions middle and elementary schools, so their focus in paragraph 1 is on advanced math education at multiple grade levels.

(C) While both of these types of courses are mentioned as examples of advanced math classes, the author never "contrasts" them by showing how they are different.

Question 1: (A)

Answer Choice Explanations for Question 1

(A) The author describes students who take advanced math classes as having "either a preference for the subject or a desire to challenge themselves." Therefore, it can be inferred that desire for challenge alone may be enough for a student to take an advanced math class.

(B) The author never discusses why students might avoid advanced math classes. Instead, the author provides reasons why students might choose to take advanced math classes, and preference is only one of the possible reasons given.

(C) The passage does not suggest that these two age groups have a different level of interest in advanced math classes.

(D) The author mentions college credit as a possible benefit, but never suggests that it is the only reason students choose to take advanced math. Paragraph 1 mentions other possible motivations as well.

Detailed Explanation for Question 1

Skill: This question tests the Paraphrase Detail skill because it requires determining what is stated in the passage or directly implied.

Question: The question stem focuses specifically on claims about students. Search the passage for any such claims so that you'll be prepared to recognize the correct answer.

Passage: The first thing that the author states about students is that those who take advanced math classes receive numerous benefits. One of the benefits is that students who either have a preference for math or just want to challenge themselves can engage with rigorous material. Another benefit is that these students may be able to earn college credit while still in high school. Lastly, the author mentions that the benefits can start as early as elementary school. The correct answer will likely be connected to one of these points about the benefits that students receive from studying advanced math.

Answer: Students' choices or preferences show up repeatedly in the answer choices. **(A)** claims that students who do not prefer math may still choose an advanced math class for a challenge. The passage describes students who take advanced math as having "either" a preference "or" a desire for challenge, which indicates that a student may choose an advanced math class even if only one of the stated reasons applies. Therefore, **(A)** matches the author's idea that a student may choose to take advanced math for the challenge alone.

Paragraph 2

For students in third and fourth grade, the ability to move at a more rapid pace while learning mathematics, when appropriate for a given student, can help alleviate boredom in the classroom. Once a student has mastered the multiplication tables, for example, permitting them to advance to new topics right away can excite interest and prompt students to envision themselves as successful in future studies involving math. With a wide variety of career options in STEM—science, technology, engineering, and mathematics—fields, there are numerous possibilities open to students once their interest is piqued. Given the potential payoff later in life, effort must be made to encourage all students to engage with increasingly challenging topics in mathematics.

Active Reading Check for Paragraph 2

In paragraph 2, the author focuses on the benefits of:

A. taking advanced math at specific grade levels.
B. advancing in math compared to other subjects.
C. their own career path.

2. According to the passage, the main reason to encourage students of all ages to take on difficult math is:

A. the assurance of future academic success in mathematics.
B. the immediate need to alleviate student boredom in the classroom.
C. the long-term career opportunities available in certain fields.
D. the inherent intellectual value of engaging with difficult subjects.

Active Reading Check for Paragraph 2: (A)

(A) While high school, middle school, and elementary school are all mentioned in the first paragraph, paragraph 2 focuses on the advantages of offering advanced math to third and fourth grade students specifically.

(B) The author never mentions areas of study other than math or compares the benefits of advancing in different subjects.

(C) The author never states their own career path, so they do not promote its benefits.

Question 2: (C)

Answer Choice Explanations for Question 2

(A) The second paragraph states that advancing to new topics *can* "prompt students to envision themselves as successful in future studies involving math," but the passage never claims that this success is guaranteed.

(B) The second paragraph mentions that accelerated learning can "help alleviate boredom," but only "when appropriate for a given student," not necessarily as the primary benefit for students of all ages.

(C) The last sentence of paragraph 2 directly mentions a "potential payoff" as the reason "to encourage all students to engage with increasingly challenging topics in mathematics." The sentence immediately before clarifies that this payoff is the "wide variety of career options in STEM … fields."

(D) The passage does not address the inherent intellectual value of challenging oneself with difficult material; it addresses specific and tangible future benefits instead.

Detailed Explanation for Question 2

Skill: By asking for a piece of information directly stated in the passage, this question tests the Paraphrase Detail skill.

Question: The question stem asks about the reason behind a particular author recommendation, encouraging all students to take on difficult math courses. Locate where this idea appears in the passage and identify the justification presented for it.

Passage: The importance of encouraging students to take on these courses is mentioned in the last sentence of paragraph 2: "Given the potential payoff later in life, effort must be made to encourage students of all demographics to engage with increasingly challenging topics in mathematics." The "potential payoff" mentioned in this sentence is probably the reason for this engagement that the question is asking for. The nature of this "payoff" is clarified in the previous sentence, where the "wide variety of career options in STEM" means that "there are numerous possibilities open to students once their interest is piqued." So the correct answer choice will likely refer to the career possibilities made available through this pursuit of math.

Answer: **(C)** is a close match for this idea, while all the other choices refer to concepts that are either unrelated to the value of pursuing difficult math or not addressed in the passage at all.

Paragraph 3

So how else can we facilitate interest in mathematics among younger students? First, all students must be given the message that everyone can learn these skills and improve with practice. The mindset of learning through effort is empowering and effective. Second, activities that introduce an element of fun should be incorporated into the classroom. For example, students can apply math topics by creating a game, designing a poster, or drawing a comic in which characters use what the students have recently learned. When such projects are completed as a group, students also have the opportunity to explain what they have learned to their peers, solidifying understanding and assisting one another so that learning is enhanced.

Active Reading Check for Paragraph 3

How does the author answer the question at the beginning of the paragraph?

A. With advice on student mindset and classroom activities
B. By suggesting a focus on art instead of math
C. By advising teachers to start with easy questions

3. The passage suggests that young students who believe that everyone is able to learn math skills will be:

A. more likely to develop an interest in mathematics.
B. less likely to pursue a career in a STEM field.
C. more likely to enjoy working on projects in groups.
D. less likely to fall asleep in class.

Active Reading Check for Paragraph 3: (A)

(A) The author first states that all students must be given a message related to mindset and, second, recommends fun activities for the classroom.

(B) While the author does recommend some art-related activities as a way to introduce fun into the classroom, they are described as a way to apply math rather than to replace it. The author answers the question with both fun activities and a recommended message for students.

(C) While paragraph 3 advises teachers to find various ways to make learning math feel more achievable to students, starting with questions that are inherently easy is not one of them.

Question 3: (A)

Answer Choice Explanations for Question 3

(A) In paragraph 3, the author first asks how to facilitate interest in math among younger students and then answers that question by claiming that students must first be told that everyone can learn these skills. So if students believe this claim, they are more likely to develop an interest in math.

(B) According to paragraph 2, the STEM career options are open to students once their interest in math is stimulated. If a student then believes that it is possible for everyone to learn math skills, they would probably be *more* likely to pursue a STEM career rather than less likely to do so.

(C) The paragraph states that working on projects in groups gives students an opportunity to explain what they have learned and boost understanding. However, the author does not make any claims about what will make students more likely to *enjoy* the group work.

(D) The passage claims that moving at a more rapid pace in learning mathematics can alleviate boredom. While that might help students avoid falling asleep, it is not mentioned by the author in the context of believing that everyone can learn math skills.

Detailed Explanation for Question 3

Skill: This question tests the Paraphrase Detail skill because it requires recognizing something unstated but directly implied by the passage. In this case, the unstated idea is that the message about everyone being able to improve in math is an essential part of facilitating interest in math.

Question: The question asks about a specific group of young students: those who believe that everyone is able to learn math skills. Your task is to determine what can be expected of those students based on the passage.

Passage: The author claims in paragraph 3 that students "must be given the message that everyone can learn" math skills. This claim is a response to the author's question in the previous sentence about how to facilitate or promote interest in math among young students. The use of the words "First" and "must" indicates that the author thinks sharing this belief with the students is a necessary step in encouraging this interest.

Answer: Based on the connection the author makes between sharing this belief with students and facilitating their interest in math, students who adopt this belief must be more likely to respond to efforts directed at developing an interest in math, matching choice **(A)**.

Skill and Strategy Summary

Skill Description

- The **Paraphrase Detail** skill is the ability to locate information that is specifically stated or directly implied in the passage.
  - Paraphrase Detail questions account for about 40% of Foundations of Comprehension questions.
- This skill involves searching for a specific detail, often by looking for the "rarest concept" from the question stem as a clue.
- Once the relevant text is located, the skill requires you to restate that information in simpler language to form a prediction.

Question Variations and Examples

- Paraphrase Detail questions can vary in the following ways:
  - Description of the Detail: Questions may ask you to complete a partial detail, provide a guided description of the detail, or (rarely) be open-ended with no description.
  - Location Clues: Stems may provide a paragraph reference or no reference at all; no reference is more common.
  - Number of Details: Questions usually ask for a single detail but can involve multiple details, potentially in a Roman numeral format.
  - Present or Absent Details: Most questions ask for information included in the passage, but some ask for information that is not present.
  - Stated or Implied Information: The correct answer may be explicitly stated in the passage or be a straightforward inference from the text.

Applying the Kaplan Method

- Step 1: Type the Question
  - Identify Paraphrase Detail questions with phrases like "according to the author," "the passage states," or "consistent with the passage."
  - As surface (Foundations of Comprehension) questions, they should generally be answered *now*.
  - Save them for *later* if they are open-ended, ask for information not in the passage, or use Roman numerals, as these variations can be more time-consuming.
- Step 2: Rephrase the Stem
  - Your rephrase should focus on the description of the requested information.
  - Identify the rarest concept mentioned in the stem to use as the focus of your search in the passage.
- Step 3: Investigate Potential Solutions
  - For most questions, scan the passage for the rare concept clue, isolate the relevant sentence(s), and paraphrase the information to make a prediction.
  - For open-ended or Roman numeral questions, use the answer choices themselves to provide the clues for what to look for in the passage.

- Step 4: Match Your Prediction to an Answer Choice
  - Compare your prediction to the answer choices to find the one that is an accurate paraphrase.
  - Avoid common traps like answer choices that use concepts from the passage in an incorrect context **(Faulty Use of Detail)** or choices that use extreme language to exaggerate a claim from the passage **(Distortion)**.

CHAPTER 11

SUMMARIZE TEXT

In This Chapter

11.1 Skill Description 164

Convert Your Passage Distillation to a Main Idea 165

11.2 Question Variations and Examples. . . 167

Scope of Summary. 167

Information in the Stem 168

11.3 Applying the Kaplan Method. 169

Step 1: Type the Question. 169

Step 2: Rephrase the Stem 169

Step 3: Investigate Potential Solutions 170

Step 4: Match Your Prediction to an Answer Choice. 171

11.4 Skillbuilder. 171

Skill and Strategy Summary 178

LEARNING OBJECTIVES

After Chapter 11, you will be able to:

- Define the Summarize Text skill
- Convert passage distillations to the main idea of paragraphs or entire passages
- Recognize common wordings for questions that test Summarize Text
- Apply the Kaplan Method for CARS Questions to Summarize Text questions
- Evaluate your current proficiency with the Summarize Text skill

FOUNDATIONS OF COMPREHENSION SKILL

Summarize Text: Articulate the main idea of the passage or of a part of it.

Approximate Frequency: 20% of Foundations of Comprehension questions

The value of semantic indeterminacy in aesthetic objects is often misunderstood, seen as a failure of communicative intent rather than a deliberate strategy. The impulse to distill a singular, definitive meaning from a work of art stems from a desire for cognitive closure, yet this very impulse is what such works seek to subvert. It is not that the artwork fails to signify, but rather that its signification is predicated on a multiplicity of potentials. The work's refusal to resolve into a digestible message is precisely its mechanism of engagement, compelling the observer to inhabit a space of interpretive possibility rather than passively receiving a predetermined concept. This orchestrated ambiguity is thus a functional component, not a deficit.

This dynamic fundamentally recasts the role of the observer from that of a mere recipient to an active co-creator of meaning. The interpretive act becomes less an archeological excavation of the artist's original intent and more a collaborative performance, where the viewer's own perceptual and cultural frameworks are brought into dialogue with the work's structural cues. This process complicates any simple dichotomy between affective response and cognitive appraisal, as the intellectual labor of navigating ambiguity is itself a source of aesthetic experience. Ultimately, while this engagement is deeply personal, it is not purely subjective; the artwork provides the necessary constraints, guiding the interpretive dance without dictating its final form.

The primary argument of the passage is that:

- **A.** the deliberate ambiguity in certain artworks serves to actively involve the viewer in the co-creation of meaning.
- **B.** the emotional response to a work of art is more significant than its cognitive appraisal.
- **C.** truly great art is defined by its resistance to any form of clear interpretation.
- **D.** the refusal of certain artworks to provide a clear message is a deliberate technique for engaging the viewer.

11.1 Skill Description

Applying the **Summarize Text** skill is like diagnosing a complex, mysterious illness. As a physician, you could face a mountain of data associated with such a patient: a detailed chart and years of lab results, as well as various symptoms and other self-reported anecdotes. While some of this information contains direct clues, other parts may prove to be only loosely connected or entirely unrelated to their illness.

Rather than memorizing all of this information, you must filter through it to identify the pieces that collectively point to the underlying cause of the patient's condition. The ability to distill a complex case down to its essential issue is the bedrock of effective diagnosis, allowing you to see the big picture without getting lost in the details.

Similarly, capturing the essence of a CARS passage (or part of one) involves identifying the most important information by distinguishing between major and minor ideas. Each passage or paragraph has a central message that may be broken down into pieces and distributed throughout a text full of facts, opinions, examples, and digressions. In order to understand a passage more clearly, you must piece together these scattered elements and uncover the core takeaway.

The sample passage from the beginning of the chapter can illustrate this process. If you read only part of the passage before considering the answer choices, **(D)** is very tempting. It serves as an excellent summary of the first paragraph, which introduces the idea that semantic indeterminacy is a "deliberate strategy." However, this choice fails to include the consequence of that strategy, the transformation of the viewer into a "co-creator of meaning," which is the central topic of the second paragraph. A main idea must encompass the entire argument.

(B) is a classic trap that preys on the repetition of ideas from the passage. A reader might notice words like "affective response" and "aesthetic experience" and jump to the conclusion that the author is prioritizing emotion over logic. This fails to grasp the author's actual point, which is that the two are intertwined and cannot be separated into a simple hierarchy.

The incorrect answer choices for this question highlight common summarization pitfalls, each representing a plausible but ultimately incomplete or distorted reading of the author's main point. To arrive at the correct answer, you must apply the Summarize Text skill by synthesizing the key information in both paragraphs. The first paragraph establishes that ambiguity is a deliberate, functional strategy for engagement. The second paragraph explains that this strategy's function is to make the viewer an "active co-creator of meaning." **(A)** is the only option that accurately links this cause (deliberate ambiguity) with its effect (involving the viewer in co-creation), thereby capturing the central argument of the entire passage.

The Summarize Text skill is directly tested by questions that ask for the main idea or central theme of the passage or a single paragraph, but it also provides the context you'll need to answer nearly every other type of question. Summarizing helps you to understand the logical structure of the author's arguments, why they used a specific tone or example, and many other aspects of the passage. For this reason, it is one of the most important CARS skills. This chapter will provide you with a systematic approach to consistently identify the main point of any CARS passage.

Convert Your Passage Distillation to a Main Idea

The Summarize Text skill is the ability to identify the main idea or central theme of the passage as a whole, or sometimes of one part of it. Just as a diagnosis isn't simply a list of a patient's symptoms, a passage's main idea isn't just a list of the topics it covers. Instead, the main idea is the central argument or message that connects all those topics and details into a coherent whole.

Determining that central point is closely connected to the Distill step of Kaplan's PCRD method, which involves locating the most important information in a passage. Chapter 5 introduced two main approaches to distilling passages: outlining, where you produce a short written note for each paragraph, and highlighting, where you directly mark a few words/phrases in each paragraph. Either of these techniques is a very effective foundation for summarizing the whole passage or one paragraph, but we will use outlining as an example here.

Chapter 3 discusses several types of keywords that are particularly useful for identifying the most important information in a passage, including Logic keywords that point to conclusions or counterarguments and Author keywords (especially Amplifying keywords) that indicate strong opinions. These are powerful clues that an idea or claim is significant and therefore probably connected to the main idea. Names or ideas that are mentioned repeatedly throughout the passage are also likely to be part of the main idea.

Main ideas can be nuanced and subtle, with two passages that come from the same field of study having very different themes or theses. To illustrate this, and to give you an opportunity to use the Summarize Text skill yourself, consider a different passage on the arts. Distill this new passage using the approach to outlining discussed in Chapter 5 and try to articulate the passage's main idea, then compare your results to the following analysis:

Art Deco sculpture is often interpreted by formalist critics as a celebration of the machine age and modernity. Proponents of this view point to the style's characteristic use of sleek, industrial materials like chrome and steel, as well as its streamlined, geometric forms. Sculptures from this period frequently depict figures embodying speed, technological prowess, and an optimistic vision of a future defined by human achievement. This interpretation frames Art Deco not merely as an aesthetic choice, but as a confident ideological statement about progress and the power of industry to reshape the world in a heroic image.

Many cultural historians prefer to argue that Art Deco represents a fundamentally conservative and even anxious retreat into classicism. This perspective emphasizes the style's deep neoclassical roots, noting that its idealized, monumental figures are direct descendants of Greek and Roman statuary. The modern materials are merely a superficial costume for an ancient impulse: to impose a sense of order, permanence, and timeless value onto a rapidly changing and uncertain world. The sleek surfaces, therefore, are seen as an attempt to contain the chaos of modernity within a rigid, traditional form.

Chapter 5 describes two versions of outlining: the first is passive, focusing almost exclusively on content. The second is functional, digging deeper into the role or purpose of the key details that would be included in a content outline. Functional outlining is superior preparation for most types of questions, including those testing the Summarize Text skill.

A passive reading of the passage above might produce a content outline that captures the topic of each paragraph but misses the story of the text:

P1. Art Deco and modernity

P2. Art Deco and classicism

An active reader, on the other hand, interrogates the text to uncover the author's purpose for including each paragraph. In the passage above, the architecture of the passage hinges on how the paragraphs related to one another, and the beginning of each paragraph serves as a crucial clue to this relationship:

Art Deco sculpture is often interpreted by formalist critics as . . .

Many cultural historians prefer to argue that Art Deco represents . . .

These phrases suggest that each paragraph represents the view of a different group of experts, the "formalists critics" in paragraph 1 and the "cultural historians" in paragraph 2. Further exploration of the passage reveals the nature of these perspectives.

Positive Author keywords in paragraph 1, such as "celebration," "prowess," "optimistic," "confident," and "heroic," indicate that formalist critics view Art Deco sculpture as a dramatically hopeful vision of modern times and the future. The language in paragraph 2 is more mixed: "anxious," "uncertain," and "chaos" are not emphatically Negative keywords, but they indicate a sense of instability that cultural historians believe Art Deco will "attempt to contain" through a "retreat into classicism." This deeper analysis shows how fundamentally different the two paragraphs' perspectives are.

KEY CONCEPT

A passage's topic is not the same as its main idea. The **topic** is what the passage is about: its subject matter. Topics are typically only a few words at most and address the ideas discussed in a paragraph or passage, such as "social networking."

The **main idea** is the specific, central claim that the author makes about the topic: for example, "dense social networks can both help and hinder people."

This analysis shows that the author introduces a common interpretation of Art Deco sculpture in the first paragraph only to challenge it with a competing theory in the second. The overall goal is not just to describe two theories, but to reveal a central tension among those who study the Art Deco movement. So a functional outline might look like:

P1. formalists: Art Deco sculpture celebrates modernity

P2. cultural historians: roots in retreat to classicism

Goal: contrasts two competing views of Art Deco sculpture

This deeper understanding of the passage's structure prepares you to determine the main point of either paragraph or the passage as a whole. The outline note for each paragraph already conveys the main idea of that paragraph in shorthand, so they can be slightly expanded into a concise description:

Main idea of P1: Formalist critics think Art Deco sculpture has a hopeful message about progress and the future.

Main idea of P2: Cultural historians believe Art Deco sculpture strives for classical style due to the disorder of the modern world.

The overall passage goal can be directly restated as the main idea of the whole passage, by shifting from *why* the author wrote the passage to *what* the takeaway message is:

Main idea of passage: Formalist critics and cultural historians have very different interpretations of what the style of Art Deco sculpture signifies.

In this way, the Distill step of Kaplan's PCRD Method is a direct pipeline to identifying the central thesis of any CARS paragraph or passage. If you distilled the passage through highlighting rather than outlining, you can use a very similar approach. But instead of deriving the main idea from outline notes, you'll get it by assembling the picture formed by the words and phrases you highlighted.

11.2 Question Variations and Examples

As one of the most straightforward skills, Summarize Text does not have many variations, but there are a few significant ones.

Scope of Summary

Questions vary based on how much of the passage they ask you to summarize. Some address the passage as a whole, while others focus on a smaller part of the text.

Entire Passage

The majority of Summarize Text questions ask about the main point of the entire passage, requiring you to synthesize information from each paragraph and identify the author's overarching argument or theme.

EXAMPLE QUESTION STEMS

The main topic of the passage is:

The main idea of the passage is that the decline of the Mayan Classic Period was:

Which of the following statements best conveys the main point of the passage?

What is the central thesis of the passage?

Single Paragraph

This rare variant narrows the focus to a single paragraph, but the task is the same: you still need to distinguish the main point from supporting details.

EXAMPLE QUESTION STEMS

What is the main point of the second paragraph?

Which of the following statements best summarizes the third paragraph?

Questions that ask for a summary of a single paragraph are typically phrased as full sentences, so the answer choices are complete sentences also. They also typically provide no clues about the main idea that they ask you to identify.

Information in the Stem

Summarize Text questions can also differ in how much information they provide in the stem itself. Some give you a significant head start by beginning to state the main idea.

Stem is Open-Ended

These variants ask you to identify the main idea or central theme without providing any information about its nature.

EXAMPLE QUESTION STEMS

What is the main idea of the passage?

Which of the following statements most accurately expresses the central thesis of the passage?

Which of the following best describes the main point of the final paragraph?

Stem Begins the Summary

These questions present part of the main idea in the stem, while the answer choices complete that claim in various ways.

EXAMPLE QUESTION STEMS

The central thesis of the passage is that baroque and classical music:

The main point of the passage is that the field of bioethics:

This variation is unlikely to include questions that ask about a single paragraph, typically asking about the entire passage instead.

11.3 Applying the Kaplan Method

Step 1: Type the Question

Your first task for any CARS question is to analyze the question stem. This allows you to assess the skill being tested and decide whether to answer the question *now* or save it for *later*. Always try to classify the question into one of three broad categories: Foundations of Comprehension (surface questions), Reasoning Within the Text (deep questions), or Reasoning Beyond the Text (new info questions). As mentioned before, this quick classification helps guide you toward the correct answer, even when the specific skill involved isn't immediately obvious.

Identifying the Skill

You can identify Summarize Text questions by looking for stems that ask for the major takeaway of the passage or a paragraph. Key phrases to look for include "main idea," "main point," "central thesis," and "best summarizes." Questions that use this language are very likely to test the Summarize Text skill.

Deciding When to Attack

As Summarize Text questions fall under Foundations of Comprehension, they test your direct understanding of the information explicitly stated in the passage, and so you should generally attack them *now*. As mentioned earlier in this chapter, effective passage distillation is very helpful in answering these questions. Consequently, it's particularly sensible to tackle them right away if you feel that you have a strong understanding of the passage from the Read and Distill steps of the PCRD method. These steps are discussed in detail in Chapters 4 and 5. The variations of Summarize Text questions that ask about a particular paragraph are often even more straightforward, as they let you limit your analysis to a smaller part of the text.

Answering a Summarize Text question right away and confirming your understanding of the main idea early can help to answer other questions more confidently. However, if you found yourself particularly confused or unsure about the overall point of the passage, it is reasonable to consider saving a Summarize Text question for *later*. Answering a few questions focused on specific details can help you piece together the author's argument and make a question about the main idea easier to answer.

BRIDGE

Some questions that ask about the entire passage test a different skill than Summarize Text:

- Questions that ask for the author's general attitude toward the audience or the passage topic, or that ask who the passage was written for, test the Recognize Opinion skill (discussed in Chapter 9). Unlike Summarize Text questions, these focus on the author's unstated views *about* the passage rather than breaking down the message of the passage itself.
- Questions that ask about the overall "purpose" of the passage test the Describe Purpose skill (discussed in Chapter 13). Unlike Summarize Text questions, which ask *what* main point the author is trying to make, Describe Purpose questions ask *why* the passage was written. The purpose is the author's goal: to explain, to criticize, to advocate, to compare, etc.

Step 2: Rephrase the Stem

Once you know that you're being tested on the Summarize Text skill, you must reword the question stem in a way that helps you focus on the task. While the stems for this skill are generally straightforward, the Rephrase step can still help to express the specific ways that you determine the main point or theme of a passage, as discussed in Section 11.1.

For example, when a question stem says something like:

> What is the main point of the passage?

It can be rephrased as:

- Review the most important information from your outline or highlighting of the passage, then combine it into a single short sentence that captures the author's main message.

This rephrase would work for many Summarize Text questions, not just the original example. However, if you struggled to create a good distillation of the passage, you might rephrase these questions a little differently:

- Use Author and Logic keywords as well as repeated concepts to identify the most important information from each paragraph of the passage, then connect these in a single statement.

Summarize Text questions that ask about a single paragraph can be rephrased very similarly, but with language directing you to search for clues only in that particular paragraph. As with questions that ask about the whole passage, you should adjust your rephrase depending on how well your distillation went for that particular paragraph.

MCAT EXPERTISE

A useful rephrase will often be longer than the original question stem, particularly when the stem is quite short. This lets the rephrase clearly communicate how to accomplish the task that the question is directing you to complete.

If question stems provide some information about the main idea they're asking for, this should be directly incorporated into the rephrase. For example, for the question stem:

> The central thesis of the passage is that the Mayan Classic Period was:

It could be rephrased as:

- Revisit your distillation of the passage and use your outline or highlights to identify the author's main message about the Mayan Classic Period.

Step 3: Investigate Potential Solutions

With a clear mission from your rephrased stem, you can now return to the passage to formulate a prediction. For Summarize Text questions that ask about the whole passage, your primary tool is your distillation, either an outline or highlights. If you identified an overall goal for the passage, you can translate this purpose about *why* the passage was written into a main idea of *what* the author communicated, as discussed in Section 11.1. This main idea is your prediction.

If the passage goal is not part of your distillation, address your highlights or outline notes for each paragraph, and attempt to synthesize these smaller ideas. Ask yourself "What is the common thread that connects all of these paragraph summaries? What is the one idea that they all build up to or support?" The answer to that question is the main idea of the passage and also serves as your prediction. Act like a journalist writing a headline for an article: be concise yet comprehensive.

For questions asking you to summarize a single paragraph, rely on your distillation in a more focused way. Either use the outline note as the direct source for a prediction, or navigate directly to the paragraph cited in the stem and assemble your highlights into a summary. If your distillation isn't helpful, scan the paragraph again. Pay close attention to the opening sentence and the concluding sentence, as these often contain the main point. Identify the paragraph's primary function: Does it introduce a problem? Provide a key piece of evidence? Refute a counterargument? Once you've identified its role, state its core message in your own words. That statement is your prediction.

Step 4: Match Your Prediction to an Answer Choice

As you review each answer choice, compare it to your predicted summary of the passage or paragraph. Any answer choice that includes similar concepts is worth considering more closely, but these simple similarities do not necessarily indicate that a choice is correct.

The most common traps for Summarize Text questions fall under the **Faulty Use of Detail** wrong answer pathology. Since the main point is the *most* important claim made by the text, there are many other statements, even important ones, that do not qualify as the passage's central idea. These choices can be tempting because they accurately reflect something that the author said, and may even be a significant part of the passage, but are *too narrow* to summarize the text as the question asked. Ultimately, these answers are details masquerading as a main idea. Even questions that ask about a single paragraph can still include wrong answer choices that focus too narrowly on a minor detail from that paragraph.

When a Summarize Text question requests the main point of the whole passage, avoid narrow answer choices by asking, "Is this choice connected to what's going on in almost every paragraph?" Answer choices are typically too short to directly include concepts from each paragraph, but the main idea of a passage will relate to almost every part.

A less common trap that also falls under Faulty Use of Detail is when an answer choice is *too broad* to match the passage. Even in questions that ask about the whole passage, a wrong answer choice could make a sweeping generalization that goes beyond the specific topic of the passage. It might be a plausible statement about the general topic ("art interpretation is subjective"), but it isn't the specific, nuanced point the author is making.

Questions that ask for a summary of a particular paragraph offer even more opportunities for answer choices that are too broad, so evaluate the choices based only on the information within the specified paragraph. Incorrect answers will often involve significant ideas from other parts of the passage.

MCAT EXPERTISE

It is almost never advantageous to look at the answer choices for Summarize Text questions before putting a prediction for the main idea into words. The choices to questions that test this skill are typically structured the same, so there is rarely information to be gained by reviewing them. It's more helpful to generate your own summary of the passage or paragraph without being influenced by the language of the choices.

11.4 Skillbuilder

Use the following shortened passage to practice the Summarize Text skill. The reading is scaffolded to reinforce good active reading habits and to let you devote more of your attention to practicing your critical thinking skills. It includes Active Reading Checks with each paragraph to evaluate how well you're uncovering important passage information at every level. Answer both the Active Reading Check and the CARS question that accompanies each paragraph before continuing. You can check your answers on the next page before you move on to paragraph 2, and the same for paragraph 3.

Paragraph 1

On the eleventh hour of the eleventh day of the eleventh month in 1918, an armistice sought to end the "war to end all wars," but ultimately failed to establish peace in German society. The trauma of industrial warfare persisted in the insidious horror of the "Spanish Flu" as the germs of resentment, economic instability, and extremism spread. Influenza's invisible transmission and the utter failure of medicine to contain its devastation created widespread, visceral anxiety. It reinforced the post-war sense that the world was governed not by reason, but by malevolent chaos. Where the war had shattered the myth of the rational nation-state, the pandemic attacked the integrity of the individual body itself, transforming it into a site of unpredictable fever, decay, and collapse. The diseased populace of a defeated nation was predisposed to an art movement reflecting the world's absurdity.

Active Reading Check for Paragraph 1

The first paragraph most seamlessly sets up a second paragraph about:

A. the economic and political instability that allowed for the rise of the Nazi party in post-war Germany.

B. the specific characteristics of an art movement that channeled the widespread sense of absurdity.

C. the public health and medical innovations that arose in response to the pandemic's devastation.

1. Which of the following statements best expresses the main idea of the first paragraph?

A. The senseless trauma of the flu pandemic and sociopolitical turmoil after World War I left Germany receptive to art of the absurd.

B. Medicine's failure to contain the "Spanish Flu" after World War I reinforced the perception in German society that the world was governed by chaos.

C. The trauma of modern warfare inevitably spreads resentment and extremism in defeated nations.

D. Germany's post-war art movement was a political protest against the state's failure to manage the pandemic and economic instability.

Active Reading Check for Paragraph 1: (B)

(A) Paragraph 1 mentions that "resentment, economic instability, and extremism" spread after the war, but presents these as contributions to the atmosphere of irrationality rather than the focus. Attention turns decisively toward a cultural response in the final sentence, making it unlikely that the passage will backtrack to detail political history.

(B) After providing the historical context, paragraph 1 concludes that the German populace was "predisposed to an art movement reflecting the world's absurdity." This establishes the expectation that the passage will continue by elaborating on the characteristics of this art movement.

(C) The "utter failure of medicine to contain" the flu is presented in paragraph 1 as a factor in the overall breakdown of order. Since the argument's trajectory points toward a cultural response to this chaos, a pivot to public health interventions would be an unexpected departure.

Question 1: (A)

Answer Choice Explanations for Question 1

(A) This statement correctly links all of the key components of the paragraph's argument: the "trauma of industrial warfare [that] persisted in the insidious horror of the 'Spanish Flu,'" and the resulting chaotic environment that predisposed people to "an art movement reflecting the world's absurdity."

(B) While the paragraph does state that the "utter failure of medicine" reinforced a sense that the world was governed by "malevolent chaos," this is only a supporting detail. This choice omits the "trauma of industrial warfare," its political ramifications, and the paragraph's main conclusion about an "art movement."

(C) The paragraph mentions that "the germs of resentment… and extremism spread," but this is presented as part of the post-war context, not the paragraph's main argument. This choice makes a broad generalization that goes beyond the text and misses the central points about the pandemic and the resulting artistic response.

(D) This statement distorts the relationship between details in the passage to present the "art movement" as a direct "protest" against specific government failures rather than simply "reflecting the world's absurdity," as the passage indicates.

Detailed Explanation for Question 1

Skill: The Summarize Text skill is tested in this question by asking for the main idea of an entire paragraph.

Question: The question asks you to find a statement that reflects the overarching message of the first paragraph as a whole while avoiding those that misrepresent the argument's connections or scope.

Passage: Paragraph 1 begins by establishing the dual societal traumas of "industrial warfare" and pandemic disease and connects these events to a resulting sense that the world was governed by "malevolent chaos." This leads to the conclusion that the post-war German populace was "predisposed to an art movement reflecting the world's absurdity." Look for an answer choice that correctly represents all of the key links in the paragraph's chain of causality.

Answer: Only **(A)** encapsulates the cause-and-effect relationship with the phrase "senseless trauma" to efficiently describe both the state of public senselessness and its triggers (war and pandemic) as bringing about receptivity to "art of the absurd."

Paragraph 2

Dadaism spread like a "virgin microbe," according to Tristan Tzara, at a conference in the city of Weimar where the new German constitution was drafted. Dada artists in Berlin developed a potent aesthetic of "dysfunctional physiology." George Grosz and Otto Dix drew caricatures of war-mutilated veterans and corrupt officials, their bodies propped up by crude prosthetics or visibly rotting from within. Grosz described his painting *The Funeral* as "an infernal procession of dehumanized figures, their faces reflecting alcohol, syphilis, the plague . . ." The photomontages of Hannah Höch went a step further, literally dissecting images of public figures and reassembling them into scrambled, unsettling anatomies with mechanical parts. Their art rejected any notion of classical beauty or idealized humanity to render the human form as a grotesque hybrid of broken flesh and faulty machinery.

Active Reading Check for Paragraph 2

The Dadaists' depiction of the human form suggests they viewed people primarily as:

A. a new kind of being, evolving beyond biological limits through technology.

B. vessels of resilient beauty amid the ravages of the modern world.

C. merely another broken component in a chaotic and malfunctioning society.

2. The second paragraph is best summarized by which of the following statements?

A. The Dada movement in post-war Germany rejected classic figures to portray the human body as a deformed mechanism.

B. The work of Berlin Dada artists like George Grosz and Otto Dix exaggerated the decay of sick and wounded bodies.

C. Dadaism was transmitted from its Weimar conference to become the most prevalent artistic style across Germany.

D. The goal of Berlin Dada artists was to realistically depict the effects of illness and war injuries on the human body.

Active Reading Check for Paragraph 2: (C)

(A) Although paragraph 2 mentions "mechanical parts" and "prosthetics," it describes them as components of "unsettling anatomies" and "faulty machinery." This suggests dysfunction and decay, not a positive evolution beyond biological limits.

(B) Paragraph 2 says Dadaists "rejected any notion of classical beauty" to depict grotesque dysfunction and decay, the very opposite of beautiful resilience.

(C) Dadaism's "dysfunctional physiology" aesthetic is described in paragraph 2 as portraying human figures as a "grotesque hybrid of broken flesh and faulty machinery," supporting the view of people as deteriorating parts of a defective social machine.

Question 2: (A)

Answer Choice Explanations for Question 2

(A) This statement brings together the paragraph's key ideas: the Dadaists' rejection of "classical beauty" for an aesthetic that rendered the human form as a "grotesque hybrid of broken flesh and faulty machinery."

(B) This is a supporting detail, not the main idea. It focuses only on the work of Grosz and Dix while omitting Höch, the mechanical motif, and the rejection of classical beauty.

(C) Paragraph 2 starts by mentioning the viral-like spread of Dadaism, but the author doesn't focus on quantifying its popularity, instead going on to describe its "potent aesthetic of 'dysfunctional physiology.'"

(D) While paragraph 2 says Dadaist depictions of the human form were not "idealized," they also were not "realistic" as reflected in descriptions like "caricatures," "scrambled," and "grotesque hybrid," indicating an exaggerated and symbolic approach.

Detailed Explanation for Question 2

Skill: This question assesses the Summarize Text skill by asking which statement reduces down a whole paragraph into its essential message.

Question: To recognize the best summary of the second paragraph, reflect on the author's goal for including that part of the passage.

Passage: The second paragraph describes a set of artistic choices that define the Berlin Dada movement's "dysfunctional physiology" style. Examples by Grosz, Dix, and Höch support the conclusion in the final sentence that they generally favored disturbing representations of the human body as failing mechanisms instead of traditional depictions of beauty. A good summary should encapsulate this takeaway.

Answer: **(A)** paraphrases the concluding sentence that sums up paragraph 2 by capturing both the Dadaist rejection of "classic figures" and their choice to "portray the human body as a deformed mechanism."

Paragraph 3

Ironically, the Dadaist embrace of absurdity and rejection of logic was actually a reasoned diagnosis of social pathology. The broken bodies they depicted were the demonstrable result of a civilization that had irrationally resorted to industrial slaughter and bureaucratic dehumanization. Challenging the concept of art itself by compiling disparate images and repurposed materials allowed a radically different expression of reality than previous art forms. The supposedly rational society that built industrial cities and armies had, in the Dadaist view, produced only sick, fragmented citizens. Wounded bodies disturbed the facade of peace, and sick bodies disturbed the facade of modern medicine. Art of the grotesque was therefore not merely an attempt to shock; it displayed specimens of the twin plagues of physical disease and sociopolitical decay festering beneath the promise of progress.

Active Reading Check for Paragraph 3

According to the third paragraph, the Dadaists' "rejection of logic" could paradoxically be considered a "reasoned diagnosis" because their art:

- **A.** focused on expressing and appealing to emotion rather than reasoning.
- **B.** deliberately reflected absurdity in response to the perceived senselessness of war and disease.
- **C.** proposed a new system of logical and moral principles to replace those that had failed society.

3. The passage author's overall thesis is that the German Dadaism movement:

- **A.** rejected classical ideals of beauty by creating shocking caricatures of mutilated and festering figures.
- **B.** embraced chaos and irrationality primarily as a means of escaping the horrors of modern life.
- **C.** challenged traditional notions of art and artistry to provoke and disrupt rather than create aesthetically pleasing objects.
- **D.** depicted dysfunctional bodies as a critique of post-war society afflicted by disease and sociopolitical corruption.

Active Reading Check for Paragraph 3: (B)

(A) Paragraph 3 says Dadaism was "not merely an attempt to shock" but rather a "reasoned diagnosis" that "displayed specimens." Such analytical methods contradict the idea that the artists intended for an emotional rather than rational response.

(B) The absurdity of Dadaist art is "ironically ... a reasoned diagnosis of social pathology," according to paragraph 3, because it logically mirrors the irrationality of the "twin plagues of physical disease and sociopolitical decay."

(C) While paragraph 3 states that Dadaism challenged old concepts, it presents the movement as a "diagnosis of social pathology," not a cure or a proposal for a new system.

Question 3: (D)

Answer Choice Explanations for Question 3

(A) This choice accurately describes the Dadaist aesthetic detailed in paragraph 2. However, it is an incomplete summary of the overall thesis because it omits the author's main argument from paragraph 3 that this art functioned as a "reasoned diagnosis" of society.

(B) Paragraph 3 states that Dadaism was a "reasoned diagnosis" meant to "display" societal plagues, which is a form of confrontation, not escapism.

(C) While the passage supports that Dadaism provocatively challenged artistic norms by rejecting "classical beauty" and "challenging the concept of art itself," the author's central point is that they did this as a "diagnosis of social pathology."

(D) This statement correctly links the Dadaist method ("depicted dysfunctional bodies") to the analytical purpose ("a critique of post-war society") that is developed across all three paragraphs.

Detailed Explanation for Question 3

Skill: This question assesses the Summarize Text skill by asking for the overall thesis, or main idea, of the entire passage.

Question: This question asks for the "overall thesis" of the passage as a whole, which requires identifying a statement that synthesizes the essence of the author's argument across all three paragraphs.

Passage: Paragraph 1 establishes the societal trauma from war and disease. Paragraph 2 describes the Dadaist aesthetic of depicting "dysfunctional" and "grotesque" bodies. The crucial link comes in paragraph 3, which argues this aesthetic was not just absurd but a "reasoned diagnosis" of the "twin plagues of physical disease and sociopolitical decay." A statement of the author's thesis must therefore connect the Dadaist art style to its function as an examination of societal sickness.

Answer: **(D)** connects the artistic style described in paragraph 2 ("depicted dysfunctional bodies") with the purpose explained in paragraph 3 ("a critique of post-war society") to examine the historical context set up in paragraph 1 ("disease and sociopolitical corruption"). **(A)** and **(C)** capture only a limited part of the author's argument while **(B)** misrepresents their conclusion.

Skill and Strategy Summary

Skill Description

- The **Summarize Text** skill is the ability to identify the main idea or central theme of a passage or a single paragraph.
  - Summarize Text questions account for about 20% of Foundations of Comprehension.
- Creating an effective summary requires you to distinguish the author's central message from minor details.
- Your passage distillation, whether an outline or highlights, serves as the foundation for this task.
  - To find the main idea of a single paragraph, you can expand on your outline note or highlights for that paragraph.
  - To find the main idea of an entire passage, you must synthesize the main ideas of all the paragraphs or rephrase the passage's overall goal.

Question Variations and Examples

- Summarize Text questions vary in the following ways:
  - Scope of Summary: Questions usually ask about the entire passage but sometimes target a single paragraph.
  - Information in the Stem: Some questions are open-ended, while others begin the summary in the stem and require you to complete the thought.

Applying the Kaplan Method

- Step 1: Type the Question
  - Identify Summarize Text questions through keywords like "main idea," "central thesis," or "best summarizes."
  - As surface questions, you should generally answer them *now*.
- Step 2: Rephrase the Stem
  - Your rephrase should incorporate the specific scope (passage or paragraph) and any information already provided in the stem.
- Step 3: Investigate Potential Solutions
  - For passage-wide summaries, synthesize your outline notes or highlights.
  - For paragraph-specific summaries, use your outline note or highlights for that paragraph or reread it.
- Step 4: Match Your Prediction to an Answer Choice
  - Compare your prediction to the options to find the best match.
  - Watch out for common traps in which the answer choice is too narrow (often **Faulty Use of Detail**) *or* too broad.

CHAPTER 12

FOUNDATIONS OF COMPREHENSION PRACTICE

How to Use This Chapter

This practice chapter contains two full MCAT passages and question sets, designed to help you practice answering Foundations of Comprehension (FOC) questions using the skills discussed in Chapters 8–11. While FOC questions make up only 30% of the questions you will see on Test Day, the passage sets within this chapter contain *only* FOC questions. Use the strategies discussed in Chapters 1–6 to Read and Distill the passages and answer the associated questions. Then, use the answer explanations at the end of the chapter to review your practice (information on how to review your practice can be found in Chapter 7).

Passage 1 (Questions 1–6)

After World War II, U.S. Director of Policy Planning George F. Kennan's strategy had been to try to bring about changes, over time, in the Soviet concept of international relations: to convince Russian leaders that their interests could be better served by learning to live with a diverse world rather than trying to remake it in their own image. Kennan had rejected both war and appeasement to accomplish this; it could only be done, he thought, through a long-term process of "behavior modification"—responding positively to whatever conciliatory initiatives emanated from the Kremlin, while firmly countering those that were not.

Kennan took the position that it was equally as important to reward the Kremlin for conciliatory gestures as it was to resist aggressive ones. This meant being prepared to engage in such negotiations that would produce mutually acceptable results. The Truman administration conveyed the appearance of being willing to discuss outstanding issues with Moscow, but Kennan believed that several of its major actions between 1948 and 1950—among them the formation of the North Atlantic Treaty Organization (NATO)—would reinforce Soviet feelings of suspicion and insecurity, and hence, would narrow opportunities for negotiations.

The initiatives for the North Atlantic Treaty came from the Western Europeans themselves and reflected the uneasiness they felt over the disparity in military power in Europe. The Russians had thirty divisions in Eastern and Central Europe alone; comparable combined US, British, and French forces came to fewer than ten divisions. Thus, the Western Union countries (Great Britain, France, and Benelux), together with the United States and Canada, agreed on the outlines of a treaty providing that an attack on any one of them would be regarded as an attack upon all.

Kennan had not been involved in the initial discussions, but he expressed his reservations about the course the administration chose to follow. He asserted that the Europeans had mistaken what was essentially a political threat for a military one, and that they consequently risked "a general preoccupation with military affairs, to the detriment of economic recovery." Kennan additionally claimed that outside the immediate North Atlantic, any alliance extended to only some countries would render the rest more vulnerable. Last, Kennan contended that an alliance made up of Western European nations would amount to "a final militarization of the present dividing-line through Europe," and that "no alteration, or obliteration, of that line could take place without having an accentuated military significance." Such a development might be unavoidable, but the policy goal remained "the eventual peaceful withdrawal of both the United States and the U.S.S.R. from the heart of Europe."

These were not isolated concerns. There was worry in Washington that emphasis on rearmament would delay recovery; indeed, one condition attached to the administration's military assistance program for Western Europe was that economic revival would continue to have first priority. The question of how to include some countries without appearing to write off others also caused a great deal of agonizing. In the end, the administration stretched the concept of "North Atlantic" to encompass Italy, but refused to extend it to Greece, Turkey, Iran, or to form a comparable pact with non-communist countries of the Western Pacific. There was less concern about Kennan's third point simply because most observers already regarded division, by mid-1948, as an accomplished fact. Despite its reservations, the administration went on to establish NATO and initiate a program of military assistance to its members. Kennan came to see, regretfully, that because of the military insecurity of Europeans there were few alternatives.

1. The passage implies that Kennan's "behavior modification" approach to changing the Soviet concept of international relations was:
   A. a strategy that would fail if the Kremlin always made conciliatory gestures.
   B. a balanced approach that was unlikely to generate rapid results.
   C. a logical outgrowth of his extensive background in behavioral psychology.
   D. an extension of American strategy during World War II.

2. The passage suggests that the impetus for the formation of NATO was:
   A. the information that a Russian attack on Western Europe was impending.
   B. the understanding that no nation could withstand a Russian attack without assistance.
   C. the desire to aid the Western European economic recovery while providing military support.
   D. the fear that the Soviets would try to capitalize on their military advantage.

3. The central thesis of the passage is that the formation of NATO was:
   A. a military manifestation of Kennan's strategy to reward allies and punish aggressors.
   B. a straightforward and unanimously supported response to Soviet aggression.
   C. a policy decision that was ultimately deemed necessary in response to European security anxieties.
   D. an economic plan designed to prioritize the financial recovery of Western Europe over military rearmament.

4. The passage suggests that the Truman administration was not worried about Kennan's objection that NATO would amount to "a final militarization of the present dividing-line through Europe" because:
   A. they believed that it would be possible to alter the line through negotiations of peaceful withdrawal.
   B. they wanted to maintain a strong American military presence in Europe.
   C. they felt it was too late to prevent the solidification of the dividing line.
   D. neither of Kennan's other two objections to NATO had given them cause for concern.

5. According to the passage, what is the most likely meaning of Kennan's claim that any future change to the dividing line would have "an accentuated military significance" (paragraph 4)?
   A. Changes to the border would be impossible unless they were approved by a consensus of military leaders.
   B. Any diplomatic effort to change the border would be perceived as an act of military strategy.
   C. Any attempt to alter the borders would require a large increase in the size of nations' militaries.
   D. The military power of nations not included in the alliance would become more effective.

6. The passage implies that, with regard to the reservations expressed by Kennan about NATO, the administration was:
   A. often in agreement but ultimately undeterred.
   B. unresponsive to his proposals for improvement.
   C. able to counter each of his criticisms.
   D. forced to carefully reexamine its objectives.

Passage 2 (Questions 7–13)

The United States currently retains less than half of the 215 million acres of wetlands that existed at the time of European settlement. Wetland conversion began upon the arrival of Europeans, who possessed not only their traditional antipathy to wetlands, but also the will and technology to dry them out. Later, in the mid-nineteenth century, the federal government awarded nearly 65 million acres of wetlands to 15 states in a series of Swamp Land Acts. But the most rapid conversion occurred between the mid-1950s and mid-1970s, when an estimated 450,000 acres per year were lost, primarily to agriculture.

This conversion has meant the loss of a wide range of important wetland functions. Wetlands protect surrounding dry land by inhibiting downstream flooding and preventing erosion along coasts and rivers, and they aid the environment as a whole by the removal or assimilation of pollutants. They also support scores of endangered species, including birds, mammals, amphibians, plants, and fishes. The incalculable loss of these ecosystems is paramount, but humans can also mourn the personal loss of aesthetics and pristine natural spaces. These and other public benefits have been sacrificed to agricultural forestry and industrial and residential development enterprises of all kinds, even while most of the conversion goals might have been obtained with far less wetland loss through regional planning, stronger regulation, and greater public understanding of wetland values.

Despite the growing willingness of the government to respond, wetland protection faces significant obstacles. The Emergency Wetlands Resources Act allocates only $40 million per year in federal funds, supplemented by relatively modest state funds, for wetland purchase, so acquisition will always be limited by severe budget constraints. Ultimately, the wetlands that are protected will be a small percentage of the approximately 95 million acres remaining today. Wetland acquisition by private environmental groups and land trusts adds qualitatively important, but quantitatively limited, protection.

A surprising solution to explore may involve the recruitment of the business sector. Some private developers have recognized that their business can protect selected wetlands and still profit. Recreational developments in Florida have benefited from wetland and habitat protection that preserves visual amenities near their facilities or from the promotion of carefully curated tourism. It is doubtful, however, that these businesses' decisions to save wetlands would have occurred without strong government regulation; the marketplace does not generally recognize the public benefits of wetlands.

The currently favored strategy is to protect every wetland in threatened areas with stringent permit guidelines that do not distinguish by wetland types or arbitrary values. This approach may be environmentally desirable, but it has failed to produce meaningful results, and about 300,000 acres of wetlands continue to be lost each year. A more promising strategy is to develop a regional management approach focused on valuable wetlands in selected areas that are under intense pressure. Regional wetland evaluations could more accurately identify critical systems that meet particular local and national needs and prevent abandonment of any wetlands without careful review of the trade-offs. There is no general federal authority to conduct such planning for wetland system protection, but there are several authorities under which a program to anticipate and prevent wetland losses on an area-wide basis has the potential to be developed.

7. In paragraph 1, the author of the passage seems to believe that:
   - A. wetland conservation efforts were initiated through transfer to the states.
   - B. wetland conservation began with the arrival of Europeans to the United States.
   - C. wetlands can be converted to agricultural purposes through currently available means.
   - D. wetlands were better appreciated by the Europeans than they were in the mid-19th century.

8. Which of the following is NOT mentioned in the passage as contributing to the rapid loss of wetlands in the United States?
   - A. Innovations implemented by European settlers
   - B. Increased reclassification to combat climate change
   - C. Developments such as real estate complexes
   - D. Conversion of wetlands for agricultural uses

9. The author uses the word "authority" (paragraph 5) to refer to:
   - A. a person with extensive or specialized knowledge of a subject.
   - B. a person or organization having power to take action.
   - C. the acquisition of information from a reliable source.
   - D. the power to influence others due to one's expertise on a topic.

10. Which of the following best summarizes the fifth paragraph?
    - A. Permitting guidelines must continue to be developed in order to reduce ongoing losses of wetlands.
    - B. The government should abandon protection of less valuable wetlands to focus exclusively on those with the highest ecologic potential.
    - C. The current strategy for wetland protection has failed to stop the annual loss of hundreds of thousands of acres.
    - D. A shift from the current all-encompassing protection strategy to a targeted regional management approach is needed.

11. Which of the following does the author state as beneficial functions of the wetlands?
    - I. Supporting communities of endangered amphibians
    - II. Providing renewable forestry options
    - III. Erosion and flood control
    - A. III only
    - B. I and II only
    - C. I and III only
    - D. I, II, and III

12. The author can best be described as a proponent of:
    - A. developing new strategies and improving current efforts to prevent wetland losses.
    - B. maintaining the current stringent permit guidelines to protect conservation areas.
    - C. promoting development of wetlands for visual amenities and aesthetic benefits.
    - D. current government incentives to induce wetland conservation through private business funding.

13. The author apparently thinks that the effects of wetland loss on humans are:
    - A. more significant than the loss of plant life.
    - B. meaningful in more than just tangible ways.
    - C. deserved results of mismanagement.
    - D. less impactful than many believe.

Answers and Explanations

Passage 1 (Questions 1–6)

Question 1: (B) – Paraphrase Detail

Explanation for Question 1

According to paragraph 1, "behavior modification" was Kennan's advocated method to improve international relations with the Soviets. It relied on "responding positively to whatever conciliatory initiatives emanated from the Kremlin, while firmly countering those that were not," and is described as "a long-term process." This balance between positive and negative responses over time matches closely with **(B)**.

Wrong Answer Explanations

(A) Conciliatory gestures would mean that the Soviets are taking actions that the Western nations approve of, so this would likely indicate that the strategy was succeeding rather than failing.

(C) This choice ascribes an extensive background to Kennan that was never mentioned (or even hinted at) in the passage.

(D) American strategy during World War II was not explicitly described in detail, so it cannot be determined if this could be an extension of that strategy.

Question 2: (D) – Paraphrase Detail

Explanation for Question 2

The formation of NATO is first mentioned in paragraph 3 where the passage states that the "initiatives for the North Atlantic Treaty came from the Western Europeans themselves and reflected the uneasiness they felt over the disparity in military power in Europe." Paragraph 3 also states that Russia had more divisions present in Europe than combined Western forces, which would be a reason for the uneasiness. Therefore, it can be inferred that the Western Europeans requested the North Atlantic Treaty because of their concerns that Russia would act on their greater military numbers, which matches **(D)**.

Wrong Answer Explanations

(A) An attack by Russia was possible, but there was no evidence that information was available that showed the attack was actually about to happen.

(B) Even though certain Western European countries feared an invasion, the idea that no nation could withstand a Russian attack is simply too strong and is never indicated in the passage.

(C) Paragraph 4 states that Kennan was concerned that "general preoccupation with military affairs" would be "to the detriment of economic recovery." Paragraph 5 indicates that the administration was also concerned that "that emphasis on rearmament would delay recovery." Therefore, the formation of NATO happened despite concerns that it would harm economic recovery rather than out of a desire to aid the recovery.

Question 3: (C) – Summarize Text

Explanation for Question 3

Paragraphs 1 and 2 describe Kennan's preferred strategy, which was to influence Russia over time by a process of "behavior modification." However, paragraph 3 describes the Western Europeans' "uneasiness" about the size of the Russian military presence in Europe. Paragraph 4 lists Kennan's "reservations" about the formation of NATO, and paragraph 5 describes the Truman administration's decision to proceed with the formation of NATO in spite of concerns, ending with Kennan's acceptance that "because of the military insecurity of Europeans there were few alternatives." Therefore, the passage's central thesis is that NATO was formed despite concerns because it was believed to be a necessary response to European security worries. **(C)** is correct.

Wrong Answer Explanations

(A) The passage presents Kennan's preferred strategy as "'behavior modification'—responding positively to whatever conciliatory initiatives emanated from the Kremlin, while firmly countering those that were not" (paragraph 1). This strategy involved positive and negative responses to the same entity, Russia, in response to actions, not military action that varied towards allies and aggressors.

(B) The passage's main purpose is to detail the significant internal debate and reservations surrounding NATO's creation, particularly the detailed objections raised by George Kennan. The decision was complex, not straightforward, and support was not unanimous.

(D) NATO is presented as a military alliance that held "that an attack on any one of them would be regarded as an attack upon all" (paragraph 3). Economic recovery was a competing priority that, according to Kennan, was actually threatened by the "general preoccupation with military affairs" that NATO would create (paragraph 4).

Question 4: (C) – Paraphrase Detail

Explanation for Question 4

The author summarizes Kennan's concerns about "a final militarization of the present dividing-line through Europe" as the third reservation discussed in paragraph 4 (after potential harm to economic recovery and leaving countries outside of the alliance more vulnerable). Paragraph 5 states that the administration had "less concern about Kennan's third point simply because most observers already regarded division, by mid-1948, as an accomplished fact." To summarize, they accepted the division of Europe as something that had already happened. **(C)** is correct.

Wrong Answer Explanations

(A) This choice contradicts one of Kennan's opinions from the end of paragraph 4, that "no alteration, or obliteration, of that line could take place without having an accentuated military significance." Paragraph 5 does not indicate that the Truman administration disagreed and thought peaceful withdrawal was possible.

(B) There is no evidence in the passage that the Truman administration desired a strong American military presence in Europe at all.

(D) The administration appeared to agree with Kennan on the first two points because they made their military support conditional on the goal "that economic revival would continue to have first priority" and are described as "agonizing" over which countries to include. Therefore, they were not unconcerned about Kennan's other objections.

Question 5: (B) – Interpret Meaning

Explanation for Question 5

This phrase is found at the end of a sentence in paragraph 4 where the passage summarizes Kennan's final objection to NATO. According to the author, Kennan contended that "the Europeans had mistaken what was essentially a political threat for a military one" and that the alliance would amount to "a final militarization of the present dividing-line through Europe." The phrase "accentuated military significance" is indicated to be a consequence of this "final militarization." Kennan's view is that "no alteration, or obliteration, of that line could take place" without the Soviets interpreting it as a military move because NATO's formation reduces the possibility of resolving tensions with the Soviets through peaceful political means. **(B)** accurately captures this meaning: diplomatic efforts would be reinterpreted as acts of military strategy.

Wrong Answer Explanations

(A) The passage does not describe the creation of a new formal procedure for requiring military leaders to approve border changes. While civilian governments like the United States' Truman administration are discussed in the passage, specific military leaders are not mentioned.

(C) The passage states that Kennan believed that "no alteration, or obliteration, of that line could take place without having an accentuated military significance." However, rather than addressing the requirements or causes of changing the border (perhaps including a larger military), Kennan is discussing the effects or consequences, the way the change would be perceived by those outside NATO. The term "significance" suggests the way that something is interpreted.

(D) Kennan's concern about the vulnerability of non-member countries is a distinct point from his argument about how the dividing line itself would be perceived after NATO's formation. If anything, Kennan was concerned that these countries would be more vulnerable, not more effective militarily.

Question 6: (A) – Recognize Opinion

Explanation for Question 6

Paragraph 5 states that there was "worry in Washington that emphasis on rearmament would delay recovery" and also that the debate over "how to include some countries without appearing to write off others also caused a great deal of agonizing." Paragraph 5 also states that there was "less concern about Kennan's third point." Taken together, these statements indicate that the Truman administration agreed with Kennan on two of his three points, but that it still decided to go ahead with the treaty "despite its reservations." This prediction matches nicely with **(A)**: the administration was often in agreement with Kennan but ultimately undeterred by the reservations that he had.

Wrong Answer Explanations

(B) This choice indicates that Kennan had specific proposals for improvement, but the passage primarily describes his reservations. Kennan had a general strategy in "behavior modification," but no specific proposals are discussed in the passage.

(C) The passage indicates that the administration created a condition that "economic revival would continue to have first priority." This indicates that they agreed with Kennan's first concern and supported it, so they clearly did not counter each criticism.

(D) The passage never discussed a way that the administration reexamined its objectives.

Passage 2 (Questions 7–13)

Question 7: (C) – Recognize Opinion

Explanation for Question 7

In paragraph 1, the author describes the history of wetland conversion. The author first states that conversion "began upon the arrival of Europeans with their traditional antipathy to wetlands and with the will and technology to dry them out." The word "later" implies that the transfer of wetlands to the states continued the process. Finally, the author claims that "the most rapid conversion occurred between the mid-1950s and mid-1970s, when an estimated 450,000 acres per year were lost, primarily to agriculture." Because wetlands were converted to agriculture use in recent history, the author likely believes that the means to do so are still available, as stated in **(C)**. Nothing in the passage suggests that the author believes this capacity was lost.

Wrong Answer Explanations

(A) The transfer of wetlands to the states through the Swamp Land Acts is presented as something that happened "later" in the process of wetland conversion. There is no indication that the author thinks that this transfer was done to conserve wetlands.

(B) According to the author, wetland *conversion* began with the arrival of Europeans, not wetland *conservation*.

(D) The author states that the Europeans had a "traditional antipathy to wetlands" but never describes an attitude in the mid-19th century, when the federal government awarded nearly 65 million acres to states. Therefore, it cannot be determined whether the Europeans appreciated wetlands more, although "antipathy" makes that unlikely.

Question 8: (B) – Paraphrase Detail

Explanation for Question 8

Because the question asks what was NOT mentioned in the passage, it is necessary to find three answer choices that are mentioned in the passage and eliminate them. For **(A)**, the "technology" of European settlers are mentioned in paragraph 1 and can be paraphrased as "innovations." Paragraph 2 mentions "industrial and residential development enterprises of all kinds," which eliminates **(C)**. Finally, conversion of wetlands "primarily to agriculture" is listed at the end of the first paragraph, which eliminates **(D)**. The passage never mentions combatting climate change, so **(B)** is correct.

Wrong Answer Explanations

(A) Paragraph 1 states that wetland conversion "began upon the arrival of Europeans, who possessed ... technology to dry them out."

(C) Paragraph 2 attributes the sacrifice of wetlands to "industrial and residential development enterprises of all kinds," which would include developments such as real estate complexes.

(D) Paragraph 1 mentions the rapid conversion of wetlands between "between the mid-1950s and mid-1970s, when an estimated 450,000 acres per year were lost, primarily to agriculture."

Question 9: (B) – Interpret Meaning

Explanation for Question 9

The word "authority" is used in the following sentence from paragraph 5: "There is no general federal authority to conduct such planning for wetland system protection." The verb "conduct" indicates that the authority is an entity who can take action. The discussion earlier in paragraph 5 about "a regional management approach" and the later mention of "several authorities" that could develop a program to prevent wetland losses both indicate that the author is focusing on organizations that have the ability to take action, which matches **(B)**.

Wrong Answer Explanations

(A) This is a common use of the word "authority," but there is no reference to extensive, specialized knowledge of a subject in paragraph 5.

(C) It is possible to claim to have information "on good authority" when that information is received from a reliable source, but the author does not indicate anything about information sources in paragraph 5.

(D) This is another usage of the word "authority" that is related to the possession of knowledge, but the author never discusses using expertise to influence others in paragraph 5.

Question 10: (D) – Summarize Text

Explanation for Question 10

The author begins paragraph 5 by describing the "currently favored strategy," which protects wetlands with "stringent permit guidelines that do not distinguish by wetland types" and immediately notes that "it has failed to produce meaningful results." The author then pivots to introduce a preferred alternative: "A more promising strategy is to develop a regional management approach focused on valuable wetlands in selected areas." A summary should include both the critique of the current approach and the introduction of the proposed new one. **(D)** is correct.

Wrong Answer Explanations

(A) The paragraph identifies "stringent permit guidelines" as part of the *current* strategy, which the author explicitly states "has failed to produce meaningful results." The author's main point is to propose a new strategy, not to simply continue refining the failing one.

(B) This is an inaccurate distortion of the author's proposal. The author advocates for a "careful review of the trade-offs," which is more nuanced than outright "abandonment." Furthermore, the author's criteria for valuable wetlands is broad ("meet particular local and national needs"), not focused exclusively on ecologic potential.

(C) This is an incomplete summary. While this statement is true according to the paragraph, it only presents the problem and omits the author's proposed solution of a regional management approach, which is the main focus of the paragraph.

Question 11: (C) – Paraphrase Detail

Explanation for Question 11

The author describes multiple "important wetland functions" in the first part of paragraph 2. The specific functions mentioned are the protection of dry land "by inhibiting downstream flooding and preventing erosion along coasts and rivers," protection of the environment "by the removal or assimilation of pollutants," and protection of "endangered species, including birds, mammals, amphibians, plants, and fishes." Items I and III are listed in paragraph 2, whereas renewable forestry options, in Item II, are never mentioned. **(C)** is correct.

Roman Numeral Explanations

(I) True. The author mentions wetlands supporting "endangered species, including birds, mammals, amphibians, plants, and fishes" in paragraph 2.

(II) False. The passage never discusses renewable forestry.

(III) True. Paragraph 2 suggests that wetlands are "inhibiting downstream flooding and preventing erosion along coasts and rivers."

Question 12: (A) – Recognize Opinion

Explanation for Question 12

Asking what the author is a proponent of is another way of asking what the author likes. The author's main purpose is to advocate for effective wetland protection. First, the author critiques existing efforts, pointing out the practical failure of the "currently favored strategy" of stringent permits, which "has failed to produce meaningful results" (paragraph 5). Second, the author proposes a new way forward, calling a regional management approach a "more promising strategy" (paragraph 5). By both critiquing current methods and proposing a new one, the author demonstrates a commitment to a comprehensive approach: finding ways to improve what is already being done while also developing entirely new and better solutions. **(A)** is correct.

Wrong Answer Explanations

(B) The author explicitly argues against this approach in the final paragraph, stating that this "currently favored strategy ... has failed to produce meaningful results." The author is a proponent of replacing this strategy, not maintaining it.

(C) This misinterprets the example in paragraph 4. The author describes businesses that benefit from *protecting* nearby wetlands that serve as visual amenities. This is an argument for preservation, not for the "development of wetlands" themselves.

(D) The author is skeptical about the broad applicability of business involvement, noting that "it is doubtful, however, that these businesses' decisions to save wetlands would have occurred without strong government regulation; the marketplace does not generally recognize the public benefits of wetlands" (paragraph 4). The author attributes the few successful examples to strong regulation, not to government incentives, which are not discussed in the passage.

Question 13: (B) – Recognize Opinion

Explanation for Question 13

The most relevant information about the author's view on how wetland destruction affects humans is in paragraph 2, where the author describes a range of negative effects. First, the author lists tangible benefits of wetlands for the environment, including: "inhibiting downstream flooding and preventing erosion along coasts and rivers, and ... the removal or assimilation of pollutants." Based on the first sentence of paragraph 2, these benefits are lost when wetlands are lost. Later in paragraph 2, the author specifically states that "humans can also mourn the personal loss of aesthetics and pristine natural spaces." Humans would be affected by tangible outcomes like increased flooding and pollution, and here the author specifically mentions additional losses that affect humans in intangible ways. The author believes these intangible results are worth mourning, so **(B)** is correct.

Wrong Answer Explanations

(A) In paragraph 2, the author states "The incalculable loss of these ecosystems is paramount" immediately before mentioning that "humans can also mourn ..." Based on the word "paramount," the author clearly prioritizes the ecological loss above the human-specific losses.

(C) The author does cite a lack of "regional planning, stronger regulation, and greater public understanding" in paragraph 2. However, the tone is one of regret that humans can "mourn" and that benefits have been "sacrificed," not one of moral judgment suggesting the negative effects are deserved.

(D) The entire passage is written to emphasize the seriousness of wetland loss. Phrases from paragraph 2 like "important wetland functions" and citing the sacrifice of "public benefits" show that the author believes the impacts are significant, not low in impact.

UNIT 3

REASONING WITHIN THE TEXT SKILLS

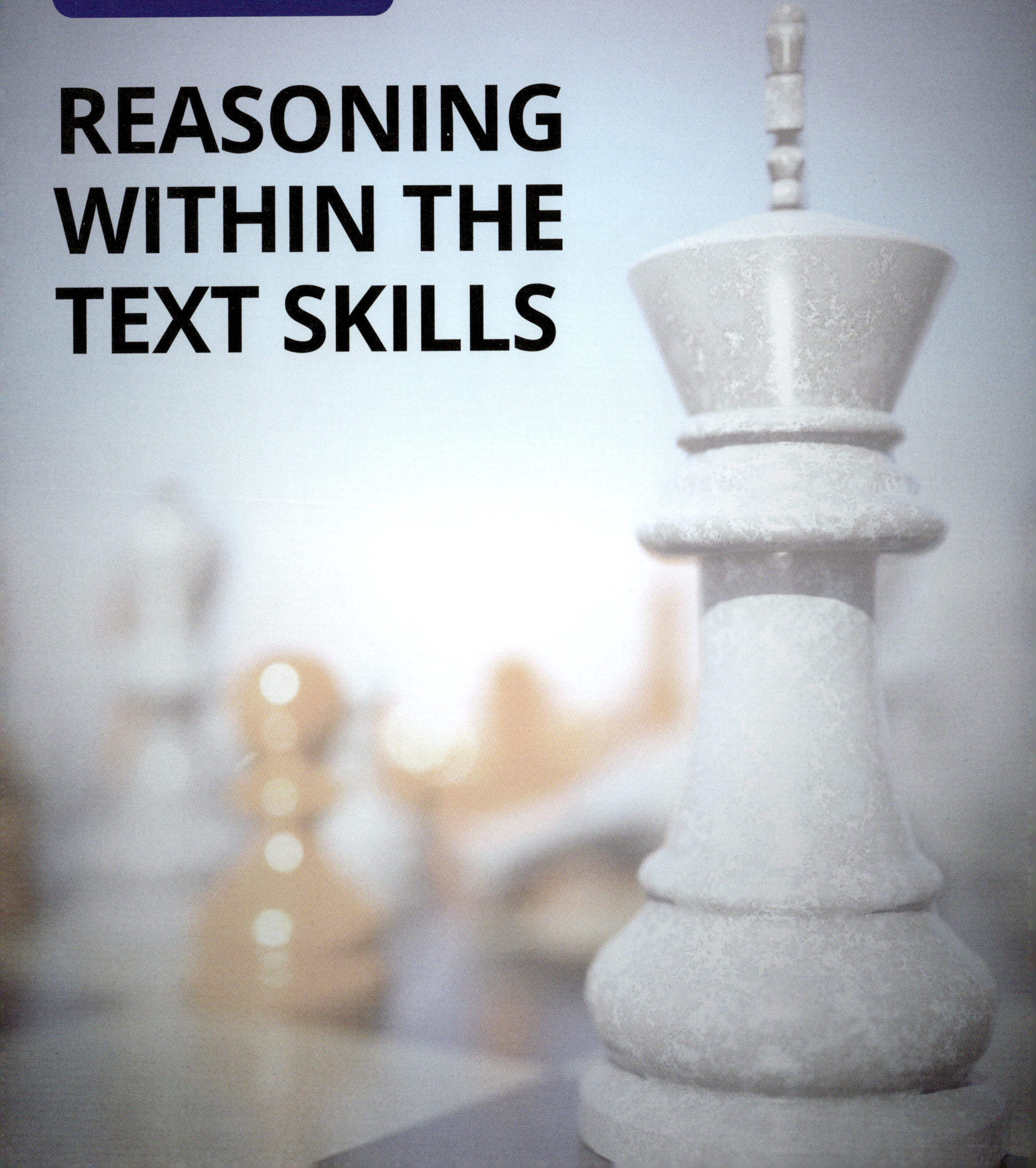

CHAPTER 13

DESCRIBE PURPOSE

In This Chapter

13.1 Skill Description 192

Understanding the Purpose of the Passage as a Whole 193

Understanding the Role of Specific Elements Within a Passage 194

13.2 Question Variations and Examples . . . 194

Passage Element 195

Location Clues 196

Direct Quotation 196

Positive or Negative Phrasing 197

13.3 Applying the Kaplan Method 197

Step 1: Type the Question 197

Step 2: Rephrase the Stem 199

Step 3: Investigate Potential Solutions 200

Step 4: Match Your Prediction to an Answer Choice 200

13.4 Skillbuilder 201

Skill and Strategy Summary 207

LEARNING OBJECTIVES

After Chapter 13, you will be able to:

- Define the Describe Purpose skill
- Discern the author's purpose in writing the passage
- Describe how details within the passage support the author's execution of their purpose
- Identify common wordings for questions that test Describe Purpose
- Apply the Kaplan Method for CARS Questions to Describe Purpose questions
- Evaluate your current proficiency with the Describe Purpose skill

REASONING WITHIN THE TEXT SKILL

Describe Purpose: Identify why the author wrote the passage or a part of it.

Approximate Frequency: 30% of Reasoning Within the Text questions

A company gains first mover advantage when it enters a new market or uses a new technology before its competitors. First movers can capture significant market share, build customer loyalty, secure key resources, and set industry standards, creating powerful barriers for subsequent entrants to the market. For example, by being an early mover in online book sales, Amazon established and maintained a dominant position in e-commerce, which it then leveraged to expand into other product categories and services.

However, pioneers bear the immense costs of initial research and development and must educate the market about the new product, with no guarantee of success. They are also likely to incur technology debt, the eventual cost of investing in an immature technology now instead of more robust, better tested solutions later. Competitors can learn from the first mover's mistakes, entering the market with a superior product and relegating the early entrant to has-been status. Google, for example, entered the search engine market well after competitors and soon dominated it. Countries can also benefit from late-adopter advantages. In Africa and Asia, for instance, many countries that were not able to establish a telecommunications infrastructure in the twentieth century have today leapfrogged to advanced mobile networks and are innovators in areas like mobile money and virtual health services.

What is the author's likely purpose in mentioning "technology debt"?

A. To explain why first movers should not invest in new technologies
B. To highlight a specific risk associated with being a first mover
C. To illustrate how a first mover can secure key resources
D. To show that first movers use technology that can be surpassed

13.1 Skill Description

Employing the **Describe Purpose** skill is much like what a doctor does when they think about the intentions behind a patient's self-assessment. This can be vital: imagine three different patients who, when asked to rate their pain level on a scale of 1 to 10, all smile and say "8." One might be trying to use humor to downplay their pain or make themselves more comfortable, another might be exaggerating in order to obtain opiate painkillers, and a third might actually be grimacing while in excruciating torment. A physician needs to use all available information to decode the deeper meaning behind a patient's words: Things like the patient's underlying condition, personal history, facial expression, and body language could all be relevant.

In a similar way, when an MCAT question asks you for the function of a particular detail in a CARS passage, you should gather all the relevant context from that passage before coming to a conclusion. The author probably won't spell out their motivation explicitly, but there will always be adequate clues. Your job is to find them and assemble them into a coherent picture.

For instance, consider the sample question at the beginning of this chapter. It asks for the author's purpose in mentioning "technology debt," and before looking back at the passage, all the answer choices might seem plausible. Without a systematic approach to this question, it would be easy to simply react to the fact that "technology debt" sounds like something bad, and be attracted to **(A)**, with its focus on the negative aspects of investing in technology.

Instead, however, you must investigate the context surrounding the author's use of this phrase. You should begin with the definition of "technology debt" that appears immediately after the term is introduced in paragraph 2: it is "the eventual cost of investing in an immature technology now instead of more robust, better tested solutions later." And the ones paying this eventual cost are the "pioneers," the "first mover" and "early mover" companies discussed in the first paragraph. Choice **(D)** is also tempting as it closely parallels this definition. However, the question doesn't ask what technology debt is; it asks why the author is talking about technology debt.

Looking at the passage more broadly, paragraph 1 lays out several possible advantages of being a first mover. Paragraph 2, where the term "technology debt" is introduced, is instead devoted to listing possible disadvantages, and in context "technology debt" is clearly one of those disadvantages. This wider view offers the proper perspective into the author's motivations for mentioning the concept. "Technology debt" is introduced as an example of a potential drawback of being a first mover. With this insight in hand, it's clear that **(B)** is the correct answer.

Every time you say something to someone else, you have the intent to communicate something, even if that intent isn't literally reflected in the words of the statement you say. CARS passages are no different: each one has an overall purpose, and every detail has a role to play within that larger context. This chapter will teach you how to reliably discern those purposes. In addition to helping you answer Describe Purpose questions, understanding *why* an author includes various details will also put you in a much better position to utilize other deep and new info question skills, such as Evaluate Reasoning and Strengthen/Weaken Argument.

Understanding the Purpose of the Passage as a Whole

Even when a Describe Purpose question asks about a minor detail, understanding a passage's overall purpose is important, since the detail you are trying to understand must contribute to that purpose in some way. Finding this overall purpose is largely dependent on your ability to successfully distill a passage as you read it.

Chapter 4 discusses how to read actively using the process of elaborative interrogation, while Chapter 5 addresses the Distill step of the **PCRD** Kaplan method. As you read, these techniques lead you to identify important information, either by outlining or highlighting, and your distillation should directly reflect the purpose of each paragraph when possible. Then, when you reach the end of the passage, you should think about how those individual paragraph purposes come together to create a coherent story. A key takeaway from your distillation, if you are doing it this way, should be an understanding of the author's overall intent in writing the passage. That is, you will have reflected on, and likely jotted down, what the author is seeking to accomplish.

While the exact intent of each CARS passage is unique to that passage, authors' goals almost always fall into one of three broad categories:

- To describe or explain something
- To argue for or against something
- To compare and contrast one or more positions on something

If you are having trouble discerning a passage's overall purpose, it can help to think about which of the three categories it fits into, and then move forward from there.

BRIDGE

Questions about a passage's overall purpose are closely related to questions that ask you for the "main point" or "thesis" of a passage, which are covered in detail in Chapter 11, Summarize Text. In essence, if you can build an effective summary of a passage's main idea, you should be able to describe its purpose as well, and vice versa.

Understanding the Role of Specific Elements Within a Passage

Instead of asking about the entire passage, most Describe Purpose questions ask about the author's purpose in including a specific detail or idea, or in mentioning a particular person. Since everything in the passage serves to execute the author's *overall* intention, your understanding of that intention is still important to answering these questions. But your analysis, and the correct answer, will typically center on the specific element the question asks about.

Fortunately, authors of CARS passages don't just randomly scatter information about. Instead, they carefully select the points to include in the passage and arrange them in a way that logically develops their ideas. Each paragraph in the passage has a function. Likewise, every detail within a given paragraph will have some role to play in the development of that paragraph's function.

Keywords that introduce a given detail, as well as the detail's placement within the structure of a paragraph, provide crucial clues as to why the author put it there. Keywords will also connect the detail in question to other details in the same paragraph. If you understand the interrelationships between details, and how the detail you're interested in relates to the paragraph's overall function, you will understand that detail's function as well.

Common functions of details in CARS passages:

- They introduce a new aspect of the topic.
- They provide an example or illustration of something.
- They provide evidence for the author's position.
- They provide evidence for or against a position held by someone other than the author.
- They state a conclusion or opinion of the author or of another person.

Common verbs used to express the functions of details in CARS passages:

- support, justify, establish
- challenge, discredit
- suggest, indicate
- explain, clarify, demonstrate
- emphasize
- provide an example
- illustrate

13.2 Question Variations and Examples

On the MCAT, questions that test the Describe Purpose skill will vary along the following dimensions: the passage element whose purpose must be identified, the presence or absence of location clues, the presence or absence of a direct quotation, and whether they ask for the purpose or for something that is not the purpose.

MCAT EXPERTISE

You've probably been taught to look for topic sentences or thesis statements in short essays. But remember, on the MCAT, every passage you'll see on Test Day is an excerpt from a larger article or book. So, since an MCAT passage isn't a self-contained whole, its overall purpose will probably not be stated directly. If there is an exception to this rule, it concerns passages whose purpose is to *advocate* or *argue*—either for or against something. These passages sometimes do have an explicit statement of purpose. It could be anywhere in the passage, though, so don't waste a lot of time looking for it. Instead, rely on your distillation, and if there happens to be a sentence somewhere in the passage that neatly summarizes its take-home message, so much the better.

BRIDGE

The author's purpose in saying something is often closely related to their *opinion* about that thing. For this reason, the techniques you use to answer Recognize Opinion questions, such as focusing on keywords to understand the author's point of view, are also especially useful for answering Describe Purpose questions. The Recognize Opinion skill is discussed in detail in Chapter 9.

Passage Element

The most significant variation has to do with whether the question asks about the passage as a whole or just a part of the passage.

Entire Passage

A few questions that test the Describe Purpose skill ask you to identify the author's overall purpose in writing. If you identified the author's purpose when outlining, then you will already have a solid prediction of the correct answer with no further research needed.

EXAMPLE QUESTION STEMS

What is most likely the main concern of the passage author?

The primary purpose of the passage is to:

For these questions, it's important to avoid choices that correctly describe the purpose of just one detail or paragraph but do not address the overarching purpose of the passage.

A Detail From the Passage

The vast majority of Describe Purpose questions will test your understanding of how a specific element is used in the passage. The question may be about why the author includes a particular example or chooses to refer to a certain person or event.

EXAMPLE QUESTION STEMS

Why does the author most likely refer to Breton lays (paragraph 4)?

What is the apparent function of the author's description of a WPA poster?

The author most probably mentions Joan Didion in order to:

Research the detail in your distillation or in the passage to understand how it relates to the point the author is making in that paragraph as well as to the purpose of the passage as a whole.

A Segment of the Passage

Occasionally, a Describe Purpose question will test your understanding of the role that an excerpt of several sentences, or even an entire paragraph, plays in the passage as a whole.

EXAMPLE QUESTION STEM

What is the function of the author's discussion of Occam's razor (paragraph 2)?

Location Clues

Paragraph Reference

Many questions about specific elements in the passage include information about which paragraph to go to.

EXAMPLE QUESTION STEMS

What is the author's most likely purpose in emphasizing Japan's legal traditions (paragraph 3)?

Jungian archetypes are most likely mentioned in the first paragraph because they:

No Paragraph Reference

Some questions don't include an explicit location clue. Use your outline and/or highlighting to find the required detail efficiently.

EXAMPLE QUESTION STEMS

What is the function of the author's citation of Peace Corps reports?

The author most likely mentions the trans-Saharan trade network because it:

Direct Quotation

No Quotation

Most Describe Purpose questions about elements in the passage do not quote language from the passage.

EXAMPLE QUESTION STEMS

The author probably mentions Southern Gothic literature because it:

Why does the author most likely cite Leonard Nimoy (paragraph 2)?

Quoted Text

Sometimes the question stem includes a word or phrase from the passage, recognizable because it is within quotation marks.

EXAMPLE QUESTION STEMS

Why does the author most likely use the word "transitional" in the fourth paragraph to describe the Long Depression of the 1870s?

The author describes OpArt as "nauseatingly mind-bending, related in its effects to psychedelic substances" in order to:

Ensure that your analysis focuses on the cited language. In the example question stems, you are not being asked why the author mentions the Long Depression or OpArt in the passage but rather why the author chose specific language to describe them.

Positive or Negative Phrasing

Asks for the Purpose

Nearly all Describe Purpose questions will ask for the purpose of the passage or an element of the passage.

EXAMPLE QUESTION STEM

The passage's main purpose is most likely:

Asks for Something That Is Not the Purpose

You may encounter a question that asks you to identify the one choice out of four that does *not* describe the purpose.

EXAMPLE QUESTION STEM

Which of the following functions does paragraph 3 NOT accomplish in the passage?

Because these questions have three "true" answer choices, they must ask about something that has multiple purposes.

13.3 Applying the Kaplan Method

Step 1: Type the Question

The first step in answering any CARS question, as outlined in Chapter 6, is to read the question stem analytically and glance at the answer choices to determine the skill being tested as well as the apparent difficulty of the question. Start by identifying the broad skill category—Foundations of Comprehension (surface questions), Reasoning Within the Text (deep questions), or Reasoning Beyond the Text (new info questions). You want to tackle the questions you can answer most confidently and efficiently first, saving for later the questions that might take longer or that you are less likely to get right. Whether you can identify the skill with certainty or not, the analysis you do in this step will focus your approach to the subsequent steps and help you answer the question more efficiently.

Identifying the Skill

Describe Purpose questions have fairly predictable wording. Many begin with "Why" and ask directly why the author mentions, cites, or refers to something in the text. Variations on this phrasing include "The author probably mentions [detail] because:" and "the author most likely cites [detail] to:"

Some of these questions actually use the words "purpose," "role," or "function," asking for the "the author's purpose," or "the role of [detail]." They also sometimes include variations on the phrase "in order to," as in "The author includes [detail] in order to:"

A few Describe Purpose questions include atypical phrasing, such as asking what the author is "most concerned with."

In addition, the answer choices of Describe Purpose questions often begin with verbs. If the question stem ends with a question mark, the answer choices might begin with "To."

- To explain ...
- To demonstrate ...
- To argue ...

If the question stem ends with a colon, the choices will often begin with a verb in the form that grammatically continues the sentence.

MCAT EXPERTISE

Like several other MCAT question types, Describe Purpose questions almost always include qualifying language such as "most likely" or "probably." This is most likely because, short of reading an author's mind, there is no way to be absolutely certain about why they said something. Don't let this language fool you into thinking that the question isn't rigorous, though. The correct choice will be unambiguously supported by the passage, and the wrong answers will be unambiguously contraindicated.

EXAMPLE QUESTION

The author most likely cites the work of Jack London to:

A. justify a particular approach to writing fiction.

B. emphasize the difficulty of wilderness survival.

C. compare dogs' behavior to that of wolves.

D. illustrate the variability of animal behavior.

Note that using these and similar verbs in your predictions will help your predictions more closely match what you see in the answer choices.

Deciding When to Attack

Describe Purpose questions involve Reasoning Within the Text and thus dive deeper than Foundations of Comprehension questions. Nonetheless, if you follow the Kaplan Method and read the passage actively, you will (after enough practice) naturally identify the purposes of each paragraph as you distill the passage, and conclude your distillation with the author's overall goal. You'll indicate these purposes either directly in an outline or more indirectly in your choice of highlights. Either way, you should have a solid understanding of why the passage was written and how each paragraph contributes to that goal, which is a good starting point even for questions about the purpose of elements within paragraphs. Consequently, the right strategy for Describe Purpose questions is generally to attack them *now*.

Some exceptions do exist. For example, if a question asks about a detail you don't remember at all and think you will have difficulty finding in the text, then it may be worth tackling other questions first. Similarly, variations that lend themselves to the process of elimination, such as scattered questions that ask for something least likely to be a purpose, should generally be saved for *later* instead.

Step 2: Rephrase the Stem

Having determined that the question is testing the Describe Purpose skill, your next step is to translate the question stem into a concrete task.

First, determine where you will direct your research. If the question asks about the purpose of the passage as a whole, then you'll find your prediction in your distillation. If the question is about an element in the passage, does the question tell you where to find the relevant details? If so, you'll research that paragraph. If not, then your outline or highlighting may help you find the detail efficiently, or you may need to scan the passage for it.

So, for this question stem:

> What is the author's apparent purpose in writing the passage?

The rephrased task would be:

- Consult your distillation for the overall passage goal, or why the author wrote the passage, and use that as a prediction.

For this question stem:

> Why does the author most likely cite the work of Frank Lloyd Wright (paragraph 4)?

Your rephrased tasks need to take into account the detail provided and the paragraph reference:

- Consult your outline or highlights for the author's purpose in writing the fourth paragraph to set initial expectations.
- Scan paragraph 4 for the mention of Frank Lloyd Wright and read the surrounding sentence(s) to understand how that mention relates to neighboring details, and how it functions in the context of the paragraph and passage, then predict its purpose in your own words.

And if the question stem asks about an element of the passage but does not provide a location clue, you will need to add finding the element to your task, such as could occur with this question:

> The function of the author's citation of the Organization for Economic Co-operation and Development (OECD) is most likely to:

Your tasks would be:

- Consult your outline or highlighting for references to the OECD, and look for any information in your distillation about the author's purpose for including that detail.
- Scan the passage for a mention of the OECD, starting with anything revealed in your distillation.
- Read the surrounding text to understand how the citation of the OECD relates to neighboring details, and how it functions in the context of the passage, and use that to make a prediction.

Step 3: Investigate Potential Solutions

To formulate your prediction, just follow the instructions for yourself that you developed in Step 2.

Consult your distillation of the passage and, as needed for questions that direct you to a certain element, review the relevant section of the passage.

When determining the author's reason for including a particular idea or detail, consider how it serves the author's purpose for writing the passage and the particular paragraph. For example:

- If the author is offering an explanation or analysis of a topic, does the detail help make the author's point clearer, or did the author include it to highlight a complication involved in the explanation?
- If the author is comparing two things, does this detail provide evidence of similarity between the things, or does it show that they are different?
- If the passage is making an argument for a point of view or a course of action, is the detail included in support of that argument, or is it included to weaken the position the author is arguing against? Or is it provided simply as background information to help the reader understand the point at issue?

MCAT EXPERTISE

Well over half of all Describe Purpose questions have a correct answer that falls into one of two categories:

- The detail is included to either support or undermine an argument that appears in the passage.
- The detail is included to illustrate or provide an example of something.

If you are having trouble making a prediction for a Describe Purpose question, remember that, all other things being equal, these are your two best candidates!

As noted above, the answer choices for Describe Purpose questions often begin with verbs like *challenge*, *emphasize*, *clarify*, *illustrate*, *identify*, and so on. Even when the verb does not begin the answer choice, it is often in there somewhere, and key to understanding whether the choice is correct or not. Therefore, when phrasing your prediction, be as precise as possible when selecting a verb. Comparing the verb you use to express the author's purpose to the verbs in the answer choices can allow you to more quickly recognize a match, or at least to discard some incorrect answers more efficiently.

Step 4: Match Your Prediction to an Answer Choice

Armed with a clear prediction, you are ready to approach the answer choices.

As mentioned above, a scan of the verbs in the choices can often help you quickly eliminate one or more of them. Is the author providing support for some position? If not, then a choice that talks about "justifying" or "defending" can probably be discarded without closer examination. Is the detail in the question used to explain or show why something is true? Then give serious consideration to choices that talk about "explaining," "clarifying," or "demonstrating."

Finally, as always, be wary of common trap answer choices. For Describe Purpose questions, the most tempting wrong answers are often those that correctly paraphrase something that the author says in the passage. These choices jump out of the list as looking familiar, and a check of the passage shows that, indeed, the author says this very thing—it's true! But these choices are not the correct answers to Describe Purpose questions. Instead, they follow the **Faulty Use of Detail** pattern. This is because, while they accurately convey *content* from the passage, Describe Purpose questions deal with the deeper level of author *per-*

MCAT EXPERTISE

If you do not find a clear match for your prediction in your first review of the choices, you can still identify the correct answer. Using your prediction as a guide, eliminate each choice that you are sure does not express the purpose of the passage or of the detail being asked about. Remember: every wrong answer has something in it that makes it unambiguously wrong, while the correct answer will be unambiguously correct.

spective, the reasons that motivate the author to construct the passage as they do. A rehash of passage details will not necessarily explain the author's purpose for something.

13.4 Skillbuilder

Use the following shortened passage to practice the Describe Purpose skill. The reading is scaffolded to reinforce good active reading habits and to let you devote more of your attention to practicing your critical thinking skills. It includes Active Reading Checks with each paragraph to evaluate how well you're uncovering important passage information at every level. Answer both the Active Reading Check and the CARS question that accompanies each paragraph before continuing. You can check your answers on the next page before you move on to paragraph 2, and the same for paragraph 3.

Paragraph 1

José Saramago's novel Blindness follows an ophthalmologist's wife as she navigates the societal collapse caused by a mysterious epidemic of "white blindness" in an unnamed city, populated by unnamed citizens. Her husband is infected after he treats "Patient Zero," a man who suddenly loses his sight while waiting in his car at a stoplight. As the epidemic spreads, the government responds by quarantining the blind in a derelict asylum, and the protagonist makes the fateful decision to feign blindness and go with her husband. Within the asylum's walls, fear takes over, the powerful are no longer held accountable, established norms of social conduct utterly dissolve, and the community descends into Hobbesian savagery. Eventually, in a violent paroxysm, the starving internees escape, only to discover that the plague has spread throughout the city, where ragged bands wander a ravaged landscape and fight one another for scraps.

Active Reading Check for Paragraph 1

How does the situation inside the asylum relate to the situation in the city?

A. The escape of the internees ends up hastening the city's collapse into chaos.
B. The violence of those inside the asylum was triggered primarily by their isolation.
C. The chaos in the asylum was a preview of what was to happen outside.

1. The author's choice to call the first victim "Patient Zero" primarily serves to:
A. underscore the anonymity of the novel's characters and settings.
B. draw attention to the ways in which "white blindness" was spread.
C. situate the disorder within a familiar epidemiological context.
D. suggest that the man was the subject of a government experiment.

Active Reading Check for Paragraph 1: (C)

(A) The escapees "discover that the plague has [already] spread throughout the city." Since the collapse came *before* the escape, the escape could not have "hastened" the collapse.

(B) The last sentence of the paragraph states that a similar level of violence and chaos was already happening outside of the asylum, where presumably people were not isolated from one another. This directly contradicts the claim that the violence inside the asylum was "triggered primarily by . . . isolation."

(C) The paragraph states that the community within the asylum "descends into . . . savagery." The final sentence reveals that the entire city eventually suffers a similar fate, becoming a "ravaged landscape" populated by "ragged bands" of people who "fight one another for scraps." Thus, the chaos inside the asylum is a small-scale preview of what would later happen to the city as a whole.

Question 1: (A)

Answer Choice Explanations for Question 1

(A) The paragraph opens by establishing a context of anonymity with the phrases "unnamed city" and "unnamed citizens." The author's choice to then use the clinical, impersonal label "Patient Zero" instead of a name for the first victim directly continues and reinforces this theme.

(B) The term "Patient Zero" might help identify the starting point of the epidemic, but it does not do anything to explain the specific manner, or "ways" in which the affliction is supposed to have spread.

(C) While the term "Patient Zero" is commonly used in discussing epidemics, and therefore does have the effect of situating the disorder in a "familiar epidemiological context," this is secondary, since nothing else in the paragraph refers to the medical or epidemiological aspects of "white blindness." Instead, the author merely points out that the affliction is "mysterious" and that it occurs "in an unnamed city, populated by unnamed citizens." The choice, in the very next sentence, to use the impersonal "Patient Zero" rather than a name primarily serves to extend and emphasize this theme of anonymity.

(D) There is nothing in the paragraph to suggest the idea that the man was involved in a government experiment.

Detailed Explanation for Question 1

Skill: This question asks you to identify the author's primary reason for using a specific wording. The task is not simply to understand what the words mean, but to determine what effect the author intended to achieve by selecting them. Therefore, it is testing the Describe Purpose skill.

Question: Since the question asks for the primary purpose of the author's choice to label the first victim "Patient Zero," you need to figure out *why*—within the context of themes introduced in the paragraph—the author selected this specific clinical term instead of giving the man a name or providing a personal description.

Passage: The author introduces the clearly fictional "white blindness," by explaining simply that the epidemic is "mysterious," and that it occurs in an "unnamed city, populated by unnamed citizens." This suggests that *Blindness* may be more a fable or allegory than a realistic story. In the next sentence, the first victim is identified not by a name, but with the clinical designation "Patient Zero" (ironically capitalized as if it *were* a name). The placement of this impersonal label, immediately following the establishment of the setting and characters as nameless, suggests that the two ideas are linked, and that the author is extending and highlighting the themes of anonymity and universality. Check the answer choices one at a time looking for something consistent with this prediction.

Answer: **(A)** fits perfectly. It identifies the term's primary function within the immediate context of the paragraph. The choice to use a label instead of a name "underscore[s] the anonymity of the novel's characters and settings," a theme established in the passage's very first sentence.

Paragraph 2

Although originally pretending to be blind simply to accompany her husband, the doctor's wife quickly discovers that vision would make her a target for the cruel and desperate. And even as she uses her sight to try and help her companions, she must conceal it from them to avoid provoking deadly resentment. Meanwhile, she alone is forced to witness the full spectrum of depravity—the filth, betrayal, and brutality—and the weight of this knowledge becomes almost unbearable. She embodies the plight of anyone who sees the truth in a regime where truth is suppressed. Their clear-sightedness is treated as hostility or unfaithfulness, and simply acknowledging facts becomes a subversive act.

Active Reading Check for Paragraph 2

What is the primary internal conflict the doctor's wife faces in this paragraph?

A. Her loyalty to her husband versus her desire to escape the asylum

B. Her need to use her sight to help others versus her need to hide it to survive

C. Her disgust with the depravity versus her sympathy for the other internees

2. The author says that "simply acknowledging facts becomes a subversive act" (paragraph 2) in order to:

A. argue that the doctor's wife could have incited rebellion inside the asylum.

B. articulate one of the major theses implicit in the plot of Saramago's novel.

C. imply that some internees were aware that the doctor's wife could see.

D. suggest that honesty is less important than the preservation of social order.

Active Reading Check for Paragraph 2: (B)

(A) While loyalty to her husband is the reason the doctor's wife enters the asylum, the paragraph does not suggest any conflict between this loyalty and a desire to escape once she is there.

(B) The doctor's wife "uses her sight to try and help her companions" but at the same time "must conceal it from them to avoid provoking deadly resentment." This opposition between the impulse to help and the need for self-preservation is the central conflict described in paragraph 2.

(C) The paragraph notes that the doctor's wife must witness "filth, betrayal, and brutality," and characterizes this as a great burden, but her internal conflict is never framed as disgust versus sympathy, but rather as a dilemma regarding how to use her vision effectively while simultaneously hiding it.

Question 2: (B)

Answer Choice Explanations for Question 2

(A) The passage never suggests that the doctor's wife could have incited a rebellion by revealing her ability to see—she concealed that ability in order to survive, not to avert rebellion.

(B) The sentence in question continues the transition, begun in the immediately preceding sentence, from describing the protagonist's specific situation to stating a general, universal principle about the relationship between truth, power, and society. In doing so, the author is explicitly articulating one of the main ideas, or theses, that they contend the novel's plot is designed to explore.

(C) This is refuted by the text. The wife must "conceal" her sight precisely because the others are *not* aware of it and would probably react with "deadly resentment" if they found out.

(D) This is contrary to the author's point. The passage speaks of "clear-sightedness" and "facts" in positive terms, referring to "the plight of anyone who sees the truth in a regime where truth is suppressed." These passage clues indicate that the author is prioritizing the value of honesty over the value of preserving a social order based in ignorance.

Detailed Explanation for Question 2

Skill: This question tests the Describe Purpose skill because it asks you to analyze *why* the author included a particular quote. To answer, you must understand how the quote in question serves the author's larger goals.

Question: What is the purpose of the phrase, "simply acknowledging facts becomes a subversive act"? It is a general statement, not a description of a specific event, so your task is to figure out what rhetorical function this generalization serves within the context of the author's overall analysis, and how it connects to the story of the novel's protagonist.

Passage: In paragraph 2, the author describes the personal dilemma of the doctor's wife: she can see the truth, but she must hide her vision to survive. The author then makes a broader point, stating that she "embodies the plight of anyone who sees the truth in a regime where truth is suppressed." Thus, the phrase in the question stem functions to draw a general lesson from the specifics of the novel's plot and directly states one of the novel's primary themes. Evaluate the answer choices looking for a paraphrase of this idea.

Answer: (B) matches this prediction: the generalization contained in the phrase cited by the question stem does indeed seem to "articulate one of the major theses" of the novel, by helping the reader understand a deeper meaning behind an aspect of the book's plot.

Paragraph 3

Unlike the plague's gradual onset, its end is stunningly abrupt. Sight is restored to the population as inexplicably as it had vanished. For most, this marks a return to their previous lives and a deliberate forgetting of the harrowing truths the white darkness revealed. For the doctor's wife, however, vision has become an inescapable moral state. She is left with a final, chilling thought: "I don't think we did go blind, I think we are blind, Blind but seeing, Blind people who can see, but do not see." Writing in 1995, Saramago was surely influenced by the world's response to the HIV/AIDS epidemic, and analogy to the COVID-19 pandemic is inevitable. Ultimately, though, Blindness describes any society swept up in political narratives built on willful ignorance and scoured by delusion. In a world that punishes vision, people learn to hide what they see.

Active Reading Check for Paragraph 3

The passage's final sentence suggests that "to hide what they see" is primarily an act of:

A. survival.
B. rebellion.
C. deception.

3. What is the most likely reason the author explicitly mentions HIV/AIDS and COVID-19 in the final paragraph?

A. To argue that Saramago's novel can be seen as a legitimate foreshadowing of future events
B. To suggest that the epidemic depicted in Saramago's novel is to some extent scientifically plausible
C. To set up a contrast between a more literal reading of *Blindness* and a more metaphorical one
D. To show ways in which *Blindness* can function as a critique of societal responses to real-world pandemics

Active Reading Check for Paragraph 3: (A)

(A) The final sentence, "In a world that punishes vision, people learn to hide what they see," is a straightforward example of operant conditioning—as a matter of survival, people and other animals avoid being punished. Moreover, this directly connects to the experience of the doctor's wife, as described in paragraph 2. She hides her sightedness as a matter of self-preservation because revealing it would make her a "target."

(B) This is the opposite of the point of this sentence. Rebellion would involve showing what one sees despite the punishment, not hiding it.

(C) While concealing one's vision might be a form of deception, the sentence in question (as well as the story of the doctor's wife, as told in the passage) relates it to self-preservation in a world that "punishes vision," not to a desire to deceive.

Question 3: (C)

Answer Choice Explanations for Question 3

(A) The author states that when Saramago wrote *Blindness*, he was likely influenced by past, not future, events (the HIV/AIDS epidemic), and although an analogy is drawn to what, in 1995, were events still to come (the COVID-19 pandemic), no direct similarities are cited between the way society reacted to COVID-19 and the story in *Blindness*.

(B) The passage brings up parallels between the events depicted in *Blindness* and the two real-world epidemics in social and political terms, not medical or scientific terms. In fact there is no real discussion anywhere in the passage of the scientific plausibility of the "white blindness" described by Saramago.

(C) The passage first introduces a more literal reading by linking *Blindness* to the concrete examples of the HIV/AIDS and COVID-19 pandemics. Then, using the phrase "Ultimately, though," the author contrasts this reading with a much broader, metaphorical one: that the novel describes "any society swept up in ... willful ignorance and scoured by delusion." The purpose of mentioning the pandemics, therefore, is to set up a contrast between the first fairly straightforward idea and the second more profound one.

(D) The author points out a relatively evident analogy between the epidemic depicted in *Blindness* and real-world pandemics; it is certainly possible to interpret this as implying that the novel could be understood, at least in part, as a critique of societal responses to those pandemics. However, the passage offers no specifics of this critique, meaning that it cannot be said to "show ways" in which the novel could function as such a critique.

Detailed Explanation for Question 3

Skill: Because it asks why the author included specific references in the passage, this question tests the Describe Purpose skill.

Question: The question asks why the author brings up HIV/AIDS and COVID-19. To answer correctly, you have to go back to the passage and pay close attention to the context within which these real-world epidemics are raised, and particularly to how they relate to the structure of the author's overall argument.

Passage: The author's argument at the end of paragraph 3 has two parts. First, the author mentions that parallels are self-evident between the epidemic depicted in *Blindness* and real-world pandemics like HIV/AIDS and COVID-19. The author then employs the crucial pivot phrase "Ultimately, though ...," which signals a shift to a more important point. The second part of the argument presents this point: the novel is about something even broader, describing "any society swept up in political narratives built on deliberate ignorance and scoured by delusion." The author's purpose in mentioning the real-world pandemics, therefore, is to establish a specific, direct connection that can be used as a springboard and to move toward a more universal interpretation of *Blindness*. Look proactively among the answer choices for something that describes this rhetorical strategy.

Answer: The only answer choice that deals with two different ways to think about the novel is **(C)**, which perfectly captures the rhetorical strategy revealed by research into the passage. The author mentions the pandemics "to set up a contrast" between a more direct, literal reading and a "more metaphorical" one that is broader and more universal.

Skill and Strategy Summary

Skill Description

- The **Describe Purpose** skill involves identifying why the author included something in the passage or why they wrote the passage itself.
  - Describe Purpose accounts for about 30% of Reasoning Within the Text questions.
- Describe Purpose questions do not ask *what* the author says about something but rather *why* they wrote what they did. Thus, this skill involves discerning the author's reasons for writing the passage and for writing the passage in a particular manner.
- The author's purpose is usually not expressed explicitly. However, keywords will unambiguously convey the purpose. Many different types are helpful:
  - Author keywords that indicate the author's attitude toward ideas in the passage
  - Connection keywords that establish relationships between an idea and surrounding ideas
  - Logic keywords, especially those that signal an author's conclusion

Question Variations and Examples

- Describe Purpose questions can vary in the following ways:
  - Passage Element: Questions address the purpose of the entire passage or, more commonly, of a part of the passage, ranging from a single word to an entire paragraph.
  - Location Clues: They either include a paragraph reference or they don't.
  - Direction Quotation: Most lack direct quotations from the passage, but some questions have them.
  - Positive or Negative Phrasing: Questions almost always ask for what the purpose is likely to be but a few ask what it is LEAST likely to be.

Applying the Kaplan Method

- Step 1: Type the Question
  - Identify Describe Purpose questions by their use of "Why" or "purpose" in the question stem, or other question stem variants that can be paraphrased as "Why did the author write this?"
  - Answer most Describe Purpose questions *now*, since your distillation provides a strong guide to answer these questions.
- Step 2: Rephrase the Stem
  - Include the scope of what the question is asking about (i.e., the entire passage or one element of the passage) and the location of the information you will use to answer the question.
- Step 3: Investigate Potential Solutions
  - If asked about the purpose of the passage as a whole, use your distillation to form a prediction.
  - To identify the purpose of specific details, ideas, or language, locate the relevant section of the passage and check the surrounding text for keywords to use in forming a prediction.
- Step 4: Match Your Prediction to an Answer Choice
  - Compare the verbs in the choices (e.g., to argue, to explain, to illustrate) with your prediction.
  - Avoid the **Faulty Use of Detail** trap, where an incorrect choice accurately reflects something said in the passage but does not address the question, which is about *why* the author said it.

CHAPTER 14

EVALUATE REASONING

In This Chapter

14.1 Skill Description 210

Analyzing Components of Arguments. 211

Analyzing Other Logical Connections. 216

14.2 Question Variations and Examples . . 216

Find the Requested Role. 216

Determine the Connection 217

Assess Support 218

Identify a Problem. 219

Describe the Passage's Structure 219

14.3 Applying the Kaplan Method. 219

Step 1: Type the Question. 219

Step 2: Rephrase the Stem 220

Step 3: Investigate Potential Solutions 221

Step 4: Match Your Prediction to an Answer Choice. 221

14.4 Skillbuilder. 222

Skill and Strategy Summary 230

LEARNING OBJECTIVES

After Chapter 14, you will be able to:

- Define the Evaluate Reasoning skill
- Identify ways that the author relates ideas
- Analyze the components and validity of arguments
- Recognize common wordings for questions that test Evaluate Reasoning
- Apply the Kaplan Method for CARS Questions to Evaluate Reasoning questions
- Evaluate your current proficiency with the Evaluate Reasoning skill

REASONING WITHIN THE TEXT SKILL

Evaluate Reasoning: Characterize logical connections between ideas in the passage.

Approximate Frequency: 40% of Reasoning Within the Text questions

The Nazca (or Nasca) Lines of Peru, a collection of colossal geoglyphs etched into the arid plains, have long puzzled archaeologists and captivated the public imagination. Consisting of hundreds of geometric shapes and stylized animal figures visible in their entirety only from the air, their purpose has been the subject of intense speculation. For decades, the dominant scholarly theory proposed that the lines functioned as a vast astronomical calendar, meant to track the movement of celestial bodies. Support for this idea is drawn from figures like the iconic spider geoglyph, whose legs appear to align with the rising of the Orion constellation. This interpretation, however, struggles to account for many of the figures, particularly the winding, labyrinthine paths that seem to have no astronomical correlation. Additional theories propose uses tied to religious rituals or pilgrimage.

While debates about the lines' purpose continue, the physical method of their creation is well understood and surprisingly straightforward. The Nazca people created these massive figures by carefully removing the reddish-brown, iron oxide-coated pebbles that form the desert's surface. This exposed the lighter, sandy soil underneath, creating a stark color contrast that defines the lines. Archaeologists have found ancient wooden stakes at the endpoints of many long, straight lines that form vast geometric shapes. Such discoveries point to the use of simple surveying techniques, likely involving stretched ropes to achieve precision. Executing the more complex animal figures would have required scaling up a smaller model or grid-based drawing onto the desert floor, an act of meticulous planning and engineering.

The assertion that the Nazca people used simple surveying techniques in creating the geoglyphs is supported in the passage by:

A. the color contrast between different soil layers.
B. ropes discovered near the spider geoglyph.
C. wooden stakes found at the ends of straight lines.
D. small-scale models of the geometric shapes.

14.1 Skill Description

Applying the **Evaluate Reasoning** skill is like the process of examining and judging a proposed treatment plan for a patient. A resident might propose an aggressive therapy for a specific ailment, presenting evidence that it is highly effective. This is a simple argument: the evidence supports the conclusion. An experienced physician, however, immediately evaluates this reasoning by considering the patient's complete health profile. They might find a conflicting factor, a strong counterpoint that makes the proposed therapy too risky. This critical step—assessing what evidence supports a claim, but also what other arguments are given—is precisely what Evaluate Reasoning tests. You must analyze an author's logical connections, identify which points are supported and which are not, and sometimes judge the validity of their argument in whole or in part.

This is, of course, not an everyday use of the word "argument," in which two people disagree about something and express that disagreement, sometimes loudly. In CARS, **arguments** refer to claims that have justification provided for them. **Conclusions** are the claims that are the primary focus of the argument: what the author (or someone else) believes to be true. **Evidence** is the reason or reasons given to support the conclusion. (See the discussion of Logic keywords in Chapter 3 for additional details on how these terms are used.)

The passage that accompanies the sample question provided evidence for multiple distinct claims. When answering questions that test the Evaluate Reasoning skill, it is important to move beyond simply noticing *what* the author says and instead to analyze *how* the author builds their case. Which piece is actually given as evidence for a specific conclusion?

The sample question above helps demonstrate the need to pay attention to specific connections in the author's reasoning. The question asks for support regarding the techniques used in creating the geoglyphs, and these were discussed in the second paragraph. A reader who located the term "simple surveying techniques" and sees that these techniques were described as "likely involving stretched ropes" might select **(B)** because it mentions ropes. However, the author never relates the ropes to the spider geoglyph from paragraph 1, so this is a faulty connection. The passage also never states that ropes were discovered, merely that they were likely involved.

Instead, the sentence about surveying techniques begins with the phrase "such discoveries point to the use of simple surveying techniques," which indicates that you need to read earlier in the passage to see what these discoveries were. The preceding sentence mentions that archeologists have *found* wooden stakes, so these stakes are the discoveries that support the use of surveying techniques.

Alternatively, it might be tempting to go back even farther in the paragraph to the different colors of soil that are mentioned in **(A)**. However, the color contrast is mentioned to describe the *method* that the Nazca used to create the physical lines, which was removing the top layer of earth. The question asks for support for the assertion that the Nazca used simple surveying techniques, which is a question about the *plotting* of the lines rather than the method for etching them in the earth. The wooden stakes cited in **(C)** could be used with stretched ropes to serve this purpose. **(C)** is correct because it creates the right kind of connection with the right claim in the passage.

Ultimately, the most common way that Evaluate Reasoning is tested in CARS is based on the relationship between evidence and conclusion, and so recognizing those components is the foundation of this skill.

Analyzing Components of Arguments

Use of Keywords

A good place to start to recognize the parts of an argument is by looking for Evidence and Conclusion keywords. Many examples of keywords are summarized in Chapter 3 of this book. Recall from that chapter that CARS authors often use keywords to reveal relationships. We start with keywords because, when they are present, they clearly identify the evidence or conclusion without any need to understand the context or the relationships that constitute the argument. Evidence keywords are always directly followed by evidence, and Conclusion keywords are always directly followed by a conclusion. However, both of these types of keywords can indirectly indicate where other parts of the argument are located, based on the sentence structure.

For example, if we only used letters to present the argument "X because Y," you can still identify that X is the conclusion based on the keyword "because," which indicates that Y is the evidence. You use this structure often in conversation:

"I was late because my alarm didn't go off."

"I don't drive a car often because we have good public transportation where I live."

"You need to study for the MCAT because the MCAT is challenging."

In each of the above, the first part of the sentence is the conclusion and the second part is the evidence for that conclusion, and we identify that based on the word "because." Using keywords that authors put in passages is the most direct way to identify argument components.

Review Chapter 3 on keywords if necessary and practice identifying the evidence and conclusion in the simple examples below:

> The novel should be understood as a political allegory, since its main characters clearly represent competing contemporary ideologies.

In this example, "since" is used as an Evidence keyword. The full argument is contained in one sentence, and the comma functions to separate the two parts. The "since" indicates that the fact about the main characters representing ideologies serves as evidence to support the conclusion that the novel should be understood as a political allegory.

Now consider how you might identify parts of the argument in this next example:

> The Impressionist painters focused on capturing fleeting moments and the transient effects of light. Thus, their work often appears less detailed and more spontaneous than that of their predecessors.

This example consists of two sentences, and this time a Conclusion keyword, "thus," is included. That allows you to identify the second sentence as the conclusion: the Impressionist painters' work appears less detailed and more spontaneous than their predecessors. When a sentence begins with a Conclusion keyword, it indicates that evidence has already been given. Check the sentence that immediately precedes the Conclusion keyword to find that evidence. In this case, the "fleeting moments" and "transient effects of light" serve the role of evidence, creating an argument.

This fits with the way you use words that indicate logic in everyday life. You would never tell a story by *beginning* with "Thus, I was late to class," and follow that up with *why* you were late. Instead, you would tell your friend something like "Ugh, the line for coffee was so long and then they messed up my order and had to redo it. So, I was late to class." In this case, that last "so" is the Conclusion keyword.

The above examples demonstrate that an individual Logic keyword can point to both the evidence and conclusion. Sometimes multiple keywords need to be untangled instead to interpret the argument. Consider the following example:

> The policy was ultimately a failure, not because its goals were misguided, but because it was implemented without sufficient funding.

In this sentence, the word "because" appears twice, which *could* indicate two pieces of evidence. However, each "because" is also paired with a contrast keyword, so you need to consider which part of the sentence is truly playing the role of evidence. The claim that needs support is the first clause in the sentence: that the policy was ultimately a failure. If someone walked up to you and told you that a policy was a failure, you would want to know why they think that. If that same person replied to you "it's not because they had bad goals," you might start to get a little frustrated and insist that they tell you why they do think it's a failure, not why they don't.

That response helps you recognize that the role of the second clause is to rule out possible evidence. The third clause finally gives the author's reason: the policy was implemented without enough funding. Now you have a reason for their claim that the policy was a failure, so now you have enough to identify the parts of the argument. The implementation without sufficient funding is the evidence, and it supports the conclusion that the policy was ultimately a failure.

BRIDGE

Chatting with the author while reading a CARS passage includes asking questions like "Why do you believe that?" This is an important part of interrogating the passage and helps to uncover the architecture of a passage, including arguments. For more on interrogating passages, see Chapter 4.

Of course, most CARS paragraphs are noticeably longer than a single sentence. The next skill to practice is recognizing an argument contained within a larger block of text.

> The term "food desert," coined in the early 1990s, describes urban neighborhoods with limited access to affordable and nutritious food. These areas are typically saturated with fast-food restaurants and convenience stores that primarily stock processed, high-calorie items. Residents of food deserts exhibit higher rates of diet-related diseases compared to other communities. Therefore, the scarcity of supermarkets offering fresh produce is a major public health issue. In recent years, community gardens have emerged as one popular grassroots effort to combat this problem.

The author provides multiple facts within this paragraph, including the definition of food deserts and the possible solution of community gardens. It might be easy to focus on the facts, but the argument is embedded in the middle of the paragraph, and the keyword "therefore" is a red light signal to stop and recognize that argument. The keyword indicates a bold conclusion: the lack of stores with fresh produce is a major public health issue. When a sentence begins with a Conclusion keyword, then you know, first, that this sentence includes a conclusion. Second, it also means that sentences before it include the evidence. This is the same structure that was used earlier in the example sentences about the Impressionist painters.

However, the Conclusion keyword does not mean that *every* sentence that comes before the conclusion must serve the role of evidence. The information immediately before the conclusion in this paragraph is clearly related to health: diet-related disease rates are higher in food deserts than in other places, and so this sentence serves as evidence. The first two sentences in the paragraph describe food deserts and provide context, but they don't truly serve as support for the claim that there is a major public health issue. Only the higher rate of disease clearly serves as evidence for the conclusion.

The sentence after the conclusion turns to a new idea: the possibility of community gardens as a solution. If this were part of a full CARS passage, it's quite likely that the author would explore this solution in the next paragraph, but the community gardens cannot be taken as a reason to believe that the lack of produce is a major health issue. This sentence is not part of the argument.

Focus on Relationships

The previous examples focused on the use of keywords to identify the conclusion and evidence, but Logic keywords are not always given in a passage. Identifying the core relationship of which part *needs* support and which part *provides* support can be used to identify conclusion and evidence regardless of the presence or absence of Logic keywords. For example, suppose someone pokes their head into the room you're in and says:

> "We should leave the building. The sprinklers in the ceiling just turned on!"

Even without keywords, you know that the sprinklers are the reason you should leave the building, and not the other way around. The spraying sprinklers are the evidence for the conclusion that it's time to leave the building.

Identify the conclusion and evidence in the following paragraph:

> Public policies, even those with noble intentions, can fail spectacularly by creating perverse incentives that encourage the very behavior they seek to prevent. A classic historical illustration of this phenomenon occurred in colonial India when British officials in Delhi, hoping to reduce the city's

MCAT EXPERTISE

Some arguments in CARS passages may not include clear keywords for either the evidence or conclusion. In these situations, focus on the relationship between passage statements. Which is given to provide support for another? That's evidence. Which statement needs support? That's the conclusion, when support is given. (A claim with no support is just a claim. An argument needs both evidence and conclusion.)

> venomous cobra population, offered a cash bounty for every dead snake. Citizens responded to this incentive by breeding cobras in large numbers to be killed for the reward. When the government eventually scrapped the program, the breeders released their now-worthless snakes, drastically increasing the wild cobra population and worsening the original problem.

The first sentence includes an assertion that would greatly benefit from supporting evidence. You may have read it and wondered how a policy would end up encouraging something that it's trying to prevent. Alternatively, you may have read that first sentence and immediately thought of a time when you have seen this outcome. If that is your response, then you just thought of an example, which is a popular type of support for passage assertions.

Next, the sample paragraph provides details about a historical event in Delhi. It would be easy to read this as a simple accounting of facts. However, keep in mind that CARS authors build their ideas very deliberately. After noticing that the first sentence in the paragraph could use some support, you might pause and ask yourself: what is the relationship between this story about cobras in Delhi and that first claim? Then you might notice that the example is introduced with the phrase "historical illustration of *this* phenomenon." The use of the Continuity keyword "this" indicates that the situation in Delhi is an example of the claim from the preceding sentence: that public policies can lead to the opposite outcome. Clearly, that happened in Delhi. Using the clues and thinking about the relationships is how you identify that the claim in the first sentence is a conclusion, the supporting example is evidence, and together they form an argument.

MCAT EXPERTISE

Opinionated-sounding statements are more likely to be conclusions, and neutral and factual-sounding statements are more likely to be evidence, but there are many exceptions to both trends. So while these tonal clues can point us in the right direction, we always need something a bit more definitive (either keywords or a clear relationship between ideas) to be sure.

Counterarguments

There will also be occasions when a passage includes a counterargument. Recall from Chapter 3 that when an author presents an argument *against* some idea in the passage, this negative argument is called a **counterargument**; the claim that is called into question is the **target**, and any reason given for doubting the target is called a **counterpoint**.

Locate the counterargument in the following paragraph:

> Proponents of global free trade agreements argue that such policies are unequivocally beneficial, leading to lower prices for consumers and greater economic efficiency. However, this perspective is undermined by the localized but significant economic disruption that can result from globalization. Often, domestic industries unable to compete with cheaper foreign imports are forced to downsize or close, leading to widespread job losses in specific sectors.

MCAT EXPERTISE

When a sentence includes a reference to "this phenomenon" or "that situation," don't just read passively through that phrase. Instead, pause and think about what specific idea in the passage the author is referring to with that phrase, even if you have to check the preceding paragraph. Making this a habit will help you locate logical connections.

The author uses the Contrast keyword "however" to indicate a point of difference but then adds the Counterpoint keyword "is undermined by" to signal that, more than mere contrast, this is a challenge to what was just discussed. The target claim is in the first sentence: the global free trade agreements are "unequivocally beneficial." The amplifier "unequivocally" makes this a very strong claim, which means it will be easier for the author to counter this assertion. The author does so by providing the counterpoint that "significant economic disruption" can be a result, and follows this with additional information about industries closing and job losses. Such outcomes certainly would not be "unequivocally beneficial."

A common pattern in CARS is that authors set up claims that they intend to counter. Watch for Contrast keywords paired with Counterpoint keywords to locate these counterarguments.

Incomplete Arguments

Another aspect of evaluating CARS arguments is determining whether the passage provides *any* support for a claim.

> The rise of citizen science has democratized data collection, as volunteers can gather vast amounts of environmental information that would be impossible for professional researchers to collect alone. This approach, however, will never fully replace the work of trained scientists. The rigorous, hypothesis-driven methodology central to formal scientific inquiry requires a level of expertise that volunteer programs cannot replicate.

Which assertions in this paragraph are supported by evidence and which are not? The first assertion is that the "rise of citizen science has democratized data collection." Whether or not you know exactly what the author means by "democratized," they elaborate on it in what follows. Volunteers are able to collect far more information than researchers working on their own. The first sentence introduces and defines a situation.

Next, the author makes a prediction (a claim about the future), which is a type of assertion that needs supporting evidence in order to be accepted as valid. In this case, the author predicts that the "citizen science" approach will never completely replace research done by trained scientists. The final sentence explains why the author thinks they can make that prediction: volunteer programs cannot reproduce the rigorous methods needed for scientific research.

While the last sentence provides a reason for the author's prediction in the previous sentence, where is the support for why the author thinks that volunteer programs *cannot* reliably follow the scientific methodology? You might think to yourself that the level of training for scientists takes years, and that's true. However, it's important not to rely on your own reasoning when you're looking for support in a passage. This final sentence is a claim that the author makes, and they undoubtedly consider it to be a reasonable claim, but they never give you a reason to believe it.

This leads to a related aspect of the skill of evaluating the reasoning in arguments: recognizing problems in arguments. Often this happens when an argument fails to account for something or the claim in the conclusion is too strong for the evidence provided. Consider the following example:

> Gentrification profoundly reshapes a neighborhood's economic character and erases its authentic cultural identity. The initial phase of this process is visibly marked by a shift in the local business landscape, as longtime businesses aimed at the lower-to-middle class residents are systematically replaced by upscale establishments like artisan coffee shops and boutique fitness studios. This commercial turnover is a direct reflection of rising property values and the new consumer demands of wealthier residents.

This paragraph opens with two claims about gentrification: it reshapes the economic character of the neighborhood and erases the cultural identity. The evidence that follows this claim addresses the changing economic conditions. It would be easy to focus on this as a complete argument, but something has not been addressed! Where does the author provide evidence or explanation regarding the loss of cultural identity? Nowhere! If the author never addresses cultural erasure elsewhere in the passage, then this part of the claim is completely unsupported and the argument is incomplete.

Analyzing Other Logical Connections

You will also sometimes be asked to characterize other kinds of relationships between ideas besides that of evidence and conclusion. One such relationship is a **paradox**, which is created when two parts of the passage seem to conflict with each other, such that they cannot both be true at once. For example, suppose a passage on economics addresses factors in the job market. This discussion could include both the fact that hiring managers want to hire people with experience at any level of employment and also the fact that, in order to gain experience, an individual must first be successful in obtaining employment. This sets up a paradox for inexperienced job seekers, who can't get a job without experience but also can't get experience without a job.

Another key relationship CARS authors establish is **cause** and **effect**, found when explaining why events occur or when examining the consequences of events. Consider the following paragraph:

> Many early twentieth-century skyscrapers are still admired for their ornate, art-deco facades. The interior design of these historic buildings was primarily driven by the need to maximize rentable floor space on a limited urban footprint. Consequently, their layouts often consist of dense, repetitive floor plans with minimal regard for communal areas or natural light. This architectural approach stands in stark contrast to the modern focus on open, collaborative workspaces.

The first sentence is an assertion of fact that introduces the subject, early 20th-century skyscrapers. In the next sentence, the Cause keyword "driven by" indicates a cause-and-effect relationship: the need to make the most of limited space in an urban setting caused a particular trend in the interior design. The Effect keyword "consequently" at the start of the next sentence indicates what this resulting trend is: the floor plans are dense and repetitive.

To identify cause-and-effect relationships, look for Cause keywords or Effect keywords like "as a result of," "caused by," "leading to," or "consequently." Identify the direction of the relationship in terms of which event caused the other. You can establish the order either by paying attention to the type of keyword (Cause keywords precede causes, and Effect keywords precede effects) or by using your common sense about which is capable of causing the other. It would make no sense to try to say that the dense floor plans caused the need to maximize rentable space, but it does make sense for that need to cause the design of dense floor plans. For more on Cause and Effect keywords and the chain of causality, see Chapter 3.

14.2 Question Variations and Examples

The MCAT tests the Evaluate Reasoning skill in a variety of ways because authors can create the passage architecture in a variety of ways. Most of these questions take one of four general approaches in asking about the reasoning in the passage. Questions can ask how the author connects ideas in the passage, which ideas are connected in a particular way, whether support for an assertion is or is not given, or for any problems with the passage's reasoning. Rarely, Evaluate Reasoning might be tested in a more general way when a question asks you to describe passage architecture as a whole or in part.

Find the Requested Role

These questions specify a type of logical role—most often evidence or conclusion, but sometimes others like counterpoint, target, cause, or effect—and ask you to identify the *specific element that performs that role* in the passage.

Locate Evidence

You are asked to find the evidence that supports a conclusion mentioned in the question stem.

EXAMPLE QUESTION STEMS

The assertion that poetry rarely aims to convey a single, limited meaning is supported in the passage by:

The claim that Kingsley Amis had a favorable view of science fiction novels is supported by the author's reference to:

Locate Conclusion

In the reverse of the previous variant, this one involves locating the conclusion that is supported by the evidence mentioned in the question stem.

EXAMPLE QUESTION STEMS

The author mentions the invention of portable paint tubes that allowed artists to work outdoors in order to support the conclusion that:

The author's discussion of the widespread adoption of social media serves primarily as evidence that:

Locate Another Connected Idea

These questions ask you to identify an idea that is connected to a statement in the question stem in a way that does not reflect an evidence/conclusion relationship. This is uncommon compared to the others, and most often involves cause and effect.

EXAMPLE QUESTION STEM

Which of the following is presented in the passage as a cause of the economic shift described in paragraph 4?

Determine the Connection

This variant asks for a description of the connection between specific ideas in the passage.

EXAMPLE QUESTION STEMS

The passage implies which of the following relationships between an author's personal letters and the themes in their published novels?

In what way is the author's discussion of the artist's early life (paragraph 3) most directly relevant to the main argument of the passage?

Based on the passage, which of the following best describes the relationship between the goals of archeologists and the goals of historians?

A variety of types of connections are possible here, but some common ones include evidence-conclusion, cause-effect, counterpoint-target, and conflict (either an apparent paradox or an actual contradiction). Many of the Connection and Logic keywords from Chapter 3 will be found in the answers to these questions, so return there if you need a refresher.

Assess Support

These questions focus on the *presence* or *absence* of support for a claim made in the passage. As a result, they focus on the role of evidence in supporting a claim and on whether or not such evidence has been given. Some questions include a yes-or-no component in the answer.

Absence of Support

This is the most common variant, but it can take quite a bit of time to search in the passage for all of the claims from the choices. Occasionally, the choices include paragraph references, which makes locating the claims more efficient.

EXAMPLE QUESTION STEMS

Which of the following claims from the passage is NOT supported by evidence or reasoning?

The passage provides NO information that would be useful in verifying:

Presence of Support

Less frequently, a question may ask for the assertion that is supported by evidence, and sometimes the question will specify the type of support, such as an explanation or examples.

EXAMPLE QUESTION STEMS

For which of the following assertions does the author provide an explanation?

Which of the following claims regarding political polarization is most directly supported by evidence in the passage?

Determining the Presence or Absence of Support

The least common variant poses a yes-or-no question. The first part of the answer will be either yes or no, followed by elaboration on the nature of the presence or absence of support.

EXAMPLE QUESTION STEMS

Is evidence given in the passage for the claim that gentrification erases cultural identity?

Is the critics' assertion about the rise of abstract painting supported in the passage by examples?

Sometimes an Evaluate Reasoning question will ask whether evidence is verifiable or whether an idea can be confirmed. In this case, check not only for the presence of evidence, but also for whether it can be authenticated. A claim that is highly subjective is difficult to verify.

BRIDGE

Chapter 9 discusses the skill of distinguishing opinions from facts. Facts are objective and therefore are more straightforward to verify than opinions, which are subjective. If a question asks to identify verifiable evidence, be wary of choices that include subjective language.

Identify a Problem

This variant requires you to act as a critic, identifying weaknesses, paradoxes, or gaps in the author's reasoning.

EXAMPLE QUESTION STEMS

Which of the following best describes a weakness in the author's argument regarding the significance of the printing press?

The author's description of the politician's behavior appears to contrast with the passage claim that:

The passage description of the decline of the Mayan civilization does NOT account for the role of:

Describe the Passage's Structure

This rare variant asks for the author's approach to the passage as a whole or a specific part of it.

EXAMPLE QUESTION STEMS

In the final paragraph, what method does the author use in presenting the solution?

The author's overall approach to the subject matter of the passage can best be described as:

Answer choices for these questions often describe the passage architecture in general terms. They may also list specific rhetorical devices like analogies or mention particular arguments or causal claims.

BRIDGE

A question that uses some of the same argument-related terminology but also includes new information is most likely testing the Strengthen/Weaken Argument skill. For more on applying your analysis of arguments in the context of new information, see Chapter 19 on the Strengthen/Weaken Argument skill.

14.3 Applying the Kaplan Method

Step 1: Type the Question

As described in Chapter 6, the first step of the Kaplan method is to read the question stem, glance at the choices, and use what you notice to determine the question type and decide whether to attempt the question now or triage it for later. Always try to identify the broad skill category of the question: Foundations of Comprehension (surface questions), Reasoning Within the Text (deep questions), or Reasoning Beyond the Text (new info questions).

As previously mentioned, this will help guide your approach to the question and answer choices, even if you cannot precisely identify the specific skill.

Identifying the Skill

Questions testing the Evaluate Reasoning skill often ask about what "supports," "explains," or "is supported" in the passage. Questions also frequently include a reference to "evidence," "conclusion," "examples," or "relevance." These questions will only include ideas from the passage, whether in the question, the answer choices, or both. Even when a question does not include some of these common terms, you can recognize the Evaluate Reasoning skill when a question asks about relationships between ideas in the passage.

Deciding When to Attack

Evaluate Reasoning is a Reasoning Within the Text skill, meaning these are deep questions that require you to analyze the passage's architecture. Your decision to attack the question now or save it for later often depends on the specific variant of the question and on how comfortable you are with your interrogation of the passage, along with your confidence at applying this skill.

If a question asks about the reasoning in a specific part of the passage and you feel that you have a solid understanding of the passage architecture in that part, you may choose to go ahead and do the question *now*. This is more likely to be the case with questions that ask how specific ideas are related or which passage claim plays a specific role.

On the other hand, if you are less confident in your grasp of the passage architecture or if the question is more open-ended, then you will likely benefit from saving the question for *later*. Sometimes answering other questions helps solidify your understanding of the passage's reasoning, allowing you to use your time more effectively when you return to the question. In particular, it is nearly always a good plan to wait until later to answer questions that ask you to evaluate four different claims from the passage to identify which is or is NOT supported by some form of evidence. These are some of the most time-consuming—and potentially frustrating—variations of Evaluate Reasoning questions.

Step 2: Rephrase the Stem

After you recognize that you are being tested on the Evaluate Reasoning skill, the next step is to rephrase the question stem in a way that focuses your thought process. In particular, you need to identify two pieces: the concepts from the passage and the kind of relationship between them.

The concepts are the specific claims or examples from the passage, or they could be a broad reference to the passage argument as a whole. The most commonly tested relationship is that of evidence and conclusion, but cause-and-effect or counterpoint-and-target connections could show up as well.

Rephrase the question such that you clearly state which of these pieces the question provides—a concept, a type of relationship, or perhaps one of each—and which piece(s) you need to identify in the choices. This allows you to be specific about your task in answering the question.

For example, consider this question stem:

> The passage implies which of the following relationships between an author's personal letters and the themes in their published novels?

This question refers to two specific concepts: an author's personal letters and themes in their published novels. Your rephrased task is:

- Locate the discussion of personal letters and themes in published novels within the passage and look for any keywords that connect them, especially any Logic or Connection keywords, to determine their relationship.

On the other hand, a different rephrase is needed for this question stem:

> The author mentions the invention of portable paint tubes that allowed artists to work outdoors in order to support the conclusion that:

In this case, one concept and the type of relationship are specified in the question stem. Your task in answering this question is:

- Locate the invention of portable paint tubes in the passage and determine what conclusion is supported by this claim.

Regardless of the variant, with the Evaluate Reasoning skill you want to try to spell out the specific connections between ideas as clearly as possible to facilitate your investigation.

Step 3: Investigate Potential Solutions

Once you have identified the task(s) required to answer the question, it's time to go back to the passage to check the relevant architecture. Sometimes a question stem will include a paragraph reference, which will help you locate claims in the passage, and sometimes it will not. When you do not have a paragraph reference, use your outline or highlights from your distillation of the passage to locate the parts of the passage that you need.

When a question asks about a specific paragraph, or about a concept that is only covered in one paragraph, start there. Your primary goal is to identify the logical structure of the relevant section. Look for Logic keywords that signal evidence (*because, since, as*) or a conclusion (*therefore, thus, consequently*). If there are no Logic keywords, look for Connection keywords. Ask yourself how the author built relationships between ideas in this part of the passage. Then predict what you can about the kind of connection or the claim that the correct answer should include. Some Evaluate Reasoning questions allow you to make a very specific prediction, especially questions that ask for the conclusion supported by a specific piece of evidence or vice versa.

When a question asks which of four claims does or does NOT have support in the passage, it is best to save this question for later, and possibly for last in the question set. Then, when you return to it, check the claims in the choices to see which you encountered while answering other questions. If you can clearly eliminate any of those choices, do so. Otherwise, your task will be to locate the claims in the passage as efficiently as possible and quickly scan for any sentence or phrase that provides direct evidence for that specific claim. Check each choice until you find the one that matches the question's criteria.

MCAT EXPERTISE

If it is time to move on from a passage and question set, make a strategic guess on questions that ask you to determine which claim is or is not supported rather than spending a lot of time tracking down those claims in the passage. It's not worth devoting too much time to these questions when you could conceivably answer two or more questions in the same amount of time with the next passage.

Step 4: Match Your Prediction to an Answer Choice

When you have a specific prediction in hand for the concept or relationship that the correct answer needs to include, conduct a targeted search for that idea in the choices. Before selecting the choice, check the reasoning to be sure it reflects the kind of relationship that you predicted, even if it uses slightly different wording.

If you only have a vague idea of the relationship that you are looking for or encounter multiple claims from the passage that play a role like evidence, then eliminate any choices that clearly do not fit your general prediction. If you have time, compare any remaining choices to the passage, not to each other. The passage is the source of the reasoning that the question asks you to evaluate.

When you have to approach the choices by process of elimination, especially for questions that ask you which claim is NOT supported in the passage, be strategic in the way you check choices. Sometimes the MCAT provides paragraph references with the claims in the choices. Start by checking shorter paragraphs or parts of the passage that you understood better. When looking for an unsupported claim, check whether any of the claims from the choices appear at the end of a paragraph. Such claims are easier to locate and often lack support, but remember to check the following paragraph to see if support is given there.

The most common wrong answer trap for Evaluate Reasoning questions is the **Faulty Use of Detail** trap, where a choice includes a detail or claim that was mentioned in the passage but that is wrong because it doesn't answer the question that was asked. These wrong answers often contradict the passage architecture by connecting the wrong pair of claims or by connecting the right claims in the wrong way.

You can also characterize some of the wrong answer choices as the **Opposite** of what you are looking for, especially on questions that ask about the presence or absence of support. For questions that ask what was NOT supported in the passage, for example, the choices all tend to be claims from the passage, and the wrong choices all fit the Opposite wrong answer pathology because they *do* have support in the passage.

14.4 Skillbuilder

Use the following shortened passage to practice the Evaluate Reasoning skill. The reading is scaffolded to reinforce good active reading habits and to let you devote more of your attention to practicing your critical thinking skills. It includes Active Reading Checks with each paragraph to evaluate how well you're uncovering important passage information at every level. Answer both the Active Reading Check and the CARS question that accompanies each paragraph before continuing. You can check your answers on the next page before you move on to paragraph 2, and the same for paragraph 3.

Paragraph 1

The so-called "paradox of fiction" presents a significant philosophical quandary. At its core, the paradox arises from a set of three intuitively plausible, yet seemingly contradictory, propositions. First, individuals experience genuine emotional responses—pity for Anna Karenina or fear of Dracula—towards fictional characters and situations. Second, for an emotion to be considered genuine, one must believe that its object actually exists. Third, readers and viewers are fully aware that such fictional characters and situations do not, in fact, exist. This triad of propositions creates a logical inconsistency that demands resolution. Consequently, any coherent theory of readers' emotional response must involve the rejection or substantial reinterpretation of at least one of these foundational claims.

Active Reading Check for Paragraph 1

Based on the final sentence of paragraph 1, what will likely come next in the passage?

A. An explanation of why it is impossible to solve the paradox of fiction

B. At least one way that one of these claims can be changed or set aside

C. A summary of several books and emotions experienced while reading them

1. The author's basic approach in presenting the "paradox of fiction" is to:

A. present the claims and dispute each individually.

B. appeal to the emotions of passage readers.

C. summarize the claims and take their contradictions to be evident.

D. describe the ways in which the claims are logically inconsistent.

Active Reading Check for Paragraph 1: (B)

(A) The passage states that the logical inconsistency "demands resolution." This language clearly claims that a resolution is needed for a coherent theory, which means the author must believe that resolution is possible in the first place. This is the opposite of saying the paradox is impossible to solve.

(B) The final sentence of the paragraph explicitly sets up something that the author believes is necessary: to build a coherent theory by either rejecting or reinterpreting at least one of the foundational claims. Therefore, the most logical next step for this author is to explore one of these attempts to change or set aside a claim.

(C) While the paragraph does mention book characters and emotions, they are mentioned in the context of the paradox created by the three propositions that are described in paragraph 1. The last sentence calls for rejection or reinterpretation of one of these propositions, so the focus is on the paradox and not on specific books.

Question 1: (C)

Answer Choice Explanations for Question 1

(A) The passage describes the three claims as "intuitively plausible" and states that the "triad of propositions creates a logical inconsistency" when they are considered together. The author does not present a case against any individual claim.

(B) The author's tone is academic and analytical, using phrases like "philosophical quandary," "propositions," and "logical inconsistency." The author writes *about* emotions experienced by readers, but they do so by presenting a logical argument rather than by making an appeal to emotion.

(C) The author lists the three propositions, providing a summary of each. Then the author states that together they form a "logical inconsistency." The passage treats the contradiction as a clear and obvious result of trying to hold all three beliefs at once.

(D) While the author states that the claims are logically inconsistent, the author does not go on to describe the inconsistencies in detail. The passage simply presents the inconsistency as a fact, which is a subtle but important difference from providing a detailed description of the logic.

Detailed Explanation for Question 1

Skill: This question asks you to look beyond the content of the passage to analyze how the author writes. To answer correctly, you must assess the logical and rhetorical structure of the author's presentation of the paradox in the first paragraph. This level of analysis means that the question is testing the Evaluate Reasoning skill.

Question: The question stem asks you to identify the author's "basic approach" in the first paragraph. Your task is to select the answer choice that best describes the method the author uses to introduce the paradox of fiction to the reader.

Passage: The author begins by introducing "a set of three intuitively plausible, yet seemingly contradictory, propositions." After listing these three propositions, the author claims "This triad of propositions creates a logical inconsistency that demands resolution." The author does not provide a detailed description of *how* they are inconsistent, and this lack of explanation shows that the author thinks the reason for the inconsistency should be obvious to a reader of the passage. This suggests that the basic approach is to present the claims and assume the contradiction is clear.

Answer: Based on the passage, the author's method is to list the three plausible ideas and then simply state that they result in a "logical inconsistency." The author presents the contradiction as self-evident, so this approach is described perfectly by **(C)**.

Paragraph 2

One prominent resolution, championed by philosopher Colin Radford, targets the first proposition—that readers experience genuine emotional responses—for reinterpretation. Radford concedes that the emotions felt are phenomenologically real; the pity for Anna Karenina feels like actual pity. However, he argues that this entire emotional response is fundamentally irrational. If one believed that something terrible had happened to a real person but then discovered that event had not truly happened, it would no longer be rational to feel pity for that person. An emotional engagement with fiction is, therefore, a testament to a curious flaw in human psychology. People are, in his view, sentimental creatures who indulge in emotional responses that lack a proper rational foundation, a conclusion many find both compelling in its honesty and unsatisfying in its implications.

Active Reading Check for Paragraph 2

How do the ideas in paragraph 2 relate to those in paragraph 1?

- **A.** Paragraph 2 presents one of the new interpretations requested at the end of paragraph 1.
- **B.** Paragraph 2 explains why the "paradox" presented in paragraph 1 isn't actually a paradox.
- **C.** Paragraph 2 changes direction from paragraph 1 to discuss a new aspect of fiction.

2. Which of the following ideas from the passage best serves to support Radford's view that people embrace irrational emotional responses?

- **A.** The emotion felt for a fictional character feels real to the individual.
- **B.** The reasonableness of an emotion is affected by knowledge of whether something is true.
- **C.** Many people appreciate the honesty of Radford's conclusions.
- **D.** Books about highly flawed characters are more likely to prompt emotional responses.

Active Reading Check for Paragraph 2: (A)

(A) Paragraph 1 ends by stating that any resolution to the paradox must involve the "rejection or substantial reinterpretation" of one of its core claims. Paragraph 2 then introduces Radford's theory, which "targets the first proposition ... for reinterpretation." Therefore, paragraph 2 provides one of the reinterpretations requested in paragraph 1.

(B) This paragraph does not attempt to explain away the paradox of fiction from paragraph 1. Rather, it presents a "reinterpretation" of one of the claims, which is a way of resolving the paradox instead of trying to claim that it isn't one.

(C) Paragraph 2 does not change the subject to a new aspect of fiction. Instead, it takes the next logical step of examining a specific philosophical resolution to the problem from paragraph 1.

Question 2: (B)

Answer Choice Explanations for Question 2

(A) The passage identifies this idea as a point that Radford "concedes" is true before making his main argument. A concession usually refers to an idea from an opposing point of view that one accepts as true while arguing against that opposing point of view as a whole. Because it lends greater support to the opposing paradox-of-fiction view than to Radford's view, this choice does not provide strong support for Radford's view.

(B) Radford's argument for the irrationality of these emotions rests on a hypothetical example given in the passage: the feeling of pity for someone would no longer be rational if someone discovered that a bad event never really happened. This example directly illustrates the principle that an emotion's rationality (paraphrased here as "reasonableness") depends on knowing whether its object is real, so it is used to support Radford's view.

(C) his phrase from the passage describes how Radford's argument is received by an audience. A description of how an argument is received does not function as support for the argument itself.

(D) Paragraph 2 describes Radford's view that emotional responses are due to a flaw in human psychology. The passage never claims that emotional responses are more likely when the characters are highly flawed. This claim distorts the argument.

Detailed Explanation for Question 2

Skill: This question requires you to move beyond simply understanding the details of the passage and instead analyze the logical structure of an argument. To find the correct answer, you must identify an argument's central claim and then determine which piece of passage information is the best evidence or support for that claim. Because you must identify specific support used in an argument, this question tests the skill Evaluate Reasoning.

Question: The question asks you to find the idea that best supports Radford's view that people embrace irrational emotional responses to fiction. Your task is to locate Radford's conclusion and then identify the specific reason or explanation that is provided in the passage to justify that conclusion.

Passage: Paragraph 2 begins by stating that Radford reinterpreted the first proposition of the paradox: that readers have genuine emotional responses. After admitting that the emotions feel real, the keyword "However" introduces Radford's true argument: that the emotional response to fiction is "fundamentally irrational." This is the view that is addressed in the question and for which you need to find support.

The passage immediately offers Radford's reasoning for the claim with a hypothetical situation: "If one believed that something terrible had happened to a real person but then discovered that event had not truly happened, it would no longer be rational to feel pity for that person" (paragraph 2). This thought experiment is the key piece of support for Radford's view that people "indulge in emotional responses that lack a proper rational foundation." This hypothetical situation needs to be included in the correct answer.

Answer: The question requires you to identify the best support for Radford's view that people's emotional responses to fiction are irrational. The passage explains his reasoning with a hypothetical thought experiment. This idea is used to demonstrate that the rationality of an emotion depends on someone's knowledge of the truth. This reasoning is accurately paraphrased as a claim that the reasonableness of emotion is affected by knowledge of truth in **(B)**.

Paragraph 3

Kendall Walton's influential "make-believe" theory, on the other hand, offers a resolution by directly rejecting the first proposition. Walton posits that what readers experience are not genuine emotions but "quasi-emotions." These affective responses are generated as prescribed parts of a game of make-believe, authorized by the fictional work. When a reader claims to feel "quasi-fear" from a horror novel such as Dracula, they are not actually afraid for their safety. Rather, their physiological arousal is part of their imaginative participation in Dracula's story. In this framework, the response is not an irrational mistake but a sophisticated engagement with a fictional world according to its rules. This approach elegantly sidesteps the paradox by asserting that because the emotions are not genuine, they do not need to be validated by a belief in the object's existence.

Active Reading Check for Paragraph 3

Which of the following words from paragraph 3 most clearly reveals the author's personal opinion of Walton's theory?

A. genuine
B. imaginative
C. elegantly

3. Which of the following claims is best supported in the passage by an accompanying explanation or example?

A. Radford's conclusion about human psychology is found by many to be unsatisfying.
B. Readers are aware that fictional characters do not actually exist.
C. A reader experiencing "quasi-fear" is not truly afraid for their safety.
D. Walton's "make-believe" theory is an influential one in philosophy.

Active Reading Check for Paragraph 3: (C)

(A) The word "genuine" is used within the passage to describe a type of emotion ("not genuine emotions"). It is a term that is part of the philosophical debate over whether the emotions themselves are real, not a word that reveals the author's own judgment of Walton's theory.

(B) The word "imaginative" is used to describe the type of participation a reader has in a story according to Walton's theory. The author uses this word while summarizing Walton's view, not to express their own personal opinion about Walton's theory.

(C) The author uses the word "elegantly" to characterize how Walton's theory solves the paradox of fiction. "Elegantly" is a word of praise, suggesting the author finds the solution to be clever and well-crafted. This word choice directly reflects the author's own positive assessment of Walton's theory.

Question 3: (C)

Answer Choice Explanations for Question 3

(A) The author asserts this claim at the end of paragraph 2 but offers no further evidence or explanation to describe who finds the conclusion unsatisfying or why they do so.

(B) This statement is one of the foundational premises of the paradox presented in paragraph 1. The passage describes it as one of three "intuitively plausible" ideas but does not provide any supporting evidence.

(C) **(C)** The passage makes this specific claim in paragraph 3 and immediately provides a supporting explanation in the next sentence: "Rather, their physiological arousal is part of their imaginative participation in Dracula's story." This explanation serves as direct support for the claim.

(D) The author introduces Walton's theory as "influential," but this is presented as a simple fact. The passage does not provide any specific evidence to support this assertion, such as describing the theory's impact or citing other philosophers who have adopted it.

Detailed Explanation for Question 3

Skill: This question tests your ability to Evaluate Reasoning. Specifically, it asks you to differentiate between claims that the author simply states and claims that the author substantiates with evidence. This requires analysis of the passage's structure around a claim to see if a statement stands alone or is supported by an example, a thought experiment, or a direct explanation.

Question: The question asks you to identify which of the listed claims is "best supported" by an accompanying explanation or example in the passage. Your task is to locate each claim, look for examples or explanations for the claim, and determine which claim is clearly supported by the most information in the passage.

Passage: This is a question that needs to be addressed by process of elimination, likely involving multiple paragraphs. The mention of Radford in **(A)** directs you to paragraph 2. The claim that many people find Radford's theory to be "both compelling in its honesty and unsatisfying in its implications" is made in the last sentence of the paragraph. There is no further explanation of these responses to Radford and no example of specific people who had that response, so **(A)** can be eliminated.

The claim in **(B)** is the last of the three propositions mentioned in paragraph 1 as "intuitively plausible, yet seemingly contradictory, propositions." After mentioning the claim that readers know that fictional characters do not exist, the author did not spend any time explaining or giving examples. Instead, the author moved on to their point that the inconsistency among the three claims needs resolution. Therefore, **(B)** has no explanation or example and can be eliminated.

The mention of "quasi-fear" in **(C)** directs you to Walton's theory in paragraph 3. The passage author gives the example of "'quasi-fear' from a horror novel such as Dracula" in making the claim that the reader is "not actually afraid for their safety." The very next sentence provides the explanation that the physical feelings are instead a part of the reader's "imaginative participation in Dracula's story." This is a clear case of a claim that is presented with an example and a supporting explanation. The claim from **(D)** that

Walton's theory is influential is stated in the first sentence of paragraph 3 without any further explanation or examples of people who were influenced by it.

Answer: To answer this question, you must find the claim that is most directly backed by evidence. The claim in (A) is made at the end of paragraph 2 with no further explanation. The claim in **(B)** is one of the propositions that are introduced in paragraph 1 without any explanation. The claim in **(D)** is made at the beginning of paragraph 3 without any explanations or examples of people influenced. The passage makes the claim in paragraph 3 that a person feeling "quasi-fear" is not genuinely afraid. This claim is made in the context of the example of the novel *Dracula* and is also immediately followed by an explanation clarifying what that feeling is instead: a form of "imaginative participation." This direct pairing of a claim with its supporting explanation makes **(C)** the best-supported idea among the options.

Skill and Strategy Summary

Skill Description

- The **Evaluate Reasoning** skill is your ability to recognize how the author creates relationships between ideas and to identify the components of those relationships, including arguments.
  - Evaluate Reasoning accounts for about 40% of Reasoning Within the Text questions.
- When using this skill, start by looking for keywords that indicate relationships, especially Logic and Connection keywords.
- As you read passages, look for claims that need support (conclusions) and reasons that are given to provide support (evidence). A complete argument needs both parts.

Question Variations and Examples

- Evaluate Reasoning questions can vary in the following ways:
  - **Find the Requested Role**: Many questions ask for a specific statement that performs a particular type of logical role: evidence, conclusion, or (rarely) others like cause or effect.
  - **Determine the Connection**: Other questions ask for a description of the connection between specific ideas in the passage.
  - **Assess Support**: Some questions request a statement that is (or is not) supported by evidence in the passage.
  - **Identify a Problem**: Sometimes, questions ask for a weakness, paradox, or gap in the author's reasoning.
  - **Describe the Passage's Structure**: Rarely, a question may ask for the author's approach to the passage as a whole or a specific part of it.

Applying the Kaplan Method

- Step 1: Type the Question
  - Recognize the Evaluate Reasoning skill by a reference to relationships between ideas in the passage, especially arguments.
  - As deep (Reasoning Within the Text) questions, triage depends on your comfort with the passage architecture, the specificity of the question, and personal preference.
- Step 2: Rephrase the Stem
  - State the task in terms of the kind of relationship you need to identify in the passage and the concepts that need to be a part of that relationship.
- Step 3: Investigate Potential Solutions
  - When the question asks about a specific relationship in the passage, locate the relevant part of the passage and look for Logic and Connection keywords.
  - When a question asks you to locate a claim that is or is NOT supported, check the claims one at a time and look for Logic keywords. Consider making a strategic guess to save time.
  - Predict the concept or relationship (or combination of the two) that you expect to find in the correct answer.
- Step 4: Match Your Prediction to an Answer Choice
  - Assess the answer choices using your prediction to locate the best fit. Compare the question and answer to the reasoning in the passage if necessary.
  - Watch out for the **Faulty Use of Detail** traps that make inaccurate connections between passage claims.

CHAPTER 15

MAKE DEDUCTION

In This Chapter

15.1 Skill Description 232
Combining Claims 234
Uncovering Assumptions 235
15.2 Question Variations and Examples . . 236
Nature of the Deduction 236
Location Clues 237
15.3 Applying the Kaplan Method 238
Step 1: Type the Question 238
Step 2: Rephrase the Stem 239
Step 3: Investigate Potential Solutions 240
Step 4: Match Your Prediction to an Answer Choice 241
15.4 Skillbuilder 241
Skill and Strategy Summary 249

LEARNING OBJECTIVES

After Chapter 15, you will be able to:

- Define the Make Deduction skill
- Draw inferences by combining multiple claims from the passage
- Uncover assumptions implicit to passage arguments
- Recognize common wordings for questions that test Make Deduction
- Apply the Kaplan Method for CARS Questions to Make Deduction questions
- Evaluate your current proficiency with the Make Deduction skill

REASONING WITHIN THE TEXT SKILL

Make Deduction: Infer a claim that follows from multiple parts of the passage, such as an assumption in an argument.

Approximate Frequency: 30% of Reasoning Within the Text questions

The sociologist Pierre Bourdieu proposed the concept of "cultural capital" to explain how power and social status are transferred across generations outside of direct economic inheritance. Cultural capital comprises the non-financial social assets—such as education, intellect, style of speech, and manner of dress—that signal membership in a particular social class. According to Bourdieu, these assets function as a kind of social currency. Educational systems and elite professions, while ostensibly meritocratic, often implicitly reward the possession of cultural capital. Because this capital is typically acquired through upbringing and socialization, this process allows social stratification to persist, as the markers of a high-status background are often misrecognized as signs of innate talent or intelligence.

The world of classical music has provided a compelling case study of this phenomenon. For decades, auditions for positions in major symphony orchestras were conducted face-to-face. Studies of this era revealed that a musician's likelihood of being selected was strongly correlated with the prestige of the conservatory they attended and their history of studying with renowned masters. In the 1970s and '80s, however, orchestras began adopting "blind" auditions, in which aspiring musicians perform behind a screen to conceal their identity from the jury. The results were dramatic. The implementation of the screen significantly increased the probability that women would be hired and opened doors for musicians from less prestigious educational backgrounds who had previously been overlooked.

The passage suggests that the success of blind auditions in diversifying orchestras is best explained by their ability to:

A. reduce the impact of explicit gender bias among judging panels.
B. increase the economic value of a musician's formal training.
C. isolate assessment of musical skill from a musician's social and educational background.
D. encourage judges to be more open-minded about unconventional musical styles.

15.1 Skill Description

Making deductions is classically the talent of the skilled diagnostician. It's no coincidence that the famous fictional detective Sherlock Holmes, renowned for joining seemingly unrelated facts together to make impressive deductions that can solve murders, has been used as inspiration for characters in medical dramas such as *House, M.D.* The recognition that a high iron level in a blood test isn't a coincidence for a patient presenting with swollen joints, but in fact both are symptoms of hemochromatosis, is a deduction that depends upon knowledge gained from medical training.

A **deduction**, also known as an **inference** or **implication**, is a statement that must be true (or is most likely to be true) given that other claims are accepted as true. On the CARS section, the **Make Deduction** skill is your ability to make more complex inferences, connecting the dots between distant paragraphs in a passage or unpacking arguments to uncover necessary assumptions.

Unlike the Paraphrase Detail skill, which sometimes involves simple inferences based on a single part of the passage, Make Deduction delves more deeply into the architecture of the passage, requiring inferences that depend on understanding logical arguments or other conceptual connections that span multiple parts of the text.

One of the most important things to remember about deductions or inferences is that they aren't just statements that could be true. In the sample question at the beginning of the chapter, **(A)** presents a plausible explanation for "the success of blind auditions in diversifying orchestras" because the passage notes that this type of audition "significantly increased the probability that women would be hired." The problem with this conclusion is that "explicit gender bias" is not the only possible explanation, and there's nothing in the passage that suggests this possibility is better than any other. In fact, the discussion in the first paragraph mentions how cultural capital is "implicitly reward[ed]" by giving people who possess more of it an advantage in education and professional life. The passage would be more supportive if the bias mentioned in **(A)** were implicit, but it's in fact the opposite, "explicit."

The question mentions "the success of blind auditions in diversifying orchestras," which refers to a claim in the second paragraph: "The implementation of the screen [used in blind auditions] significantly increased the probability that women would be hired and opened doors for musicians from less prestigious educational backgrounds who had previously been overlooked." There are actually two results mentioned here that could be interpreted as "diversifying orchestras." **(A)** focused on the first of these, gender, but having more musicians from a broader array of educational backgrounds would increase diversity in a different way. Does the passage help us know which success the author is focusing on?

This is a place where keywords come in, helping you to uncover connections between different ideas in the passage. The question references ideas from paragraph 2, so think about that paragraph's purpose or function, which you should aim to uncover when reading actively. Paragraph 2 is introduced as offering "a compelling case study of this phenomenon." The Continuity keyword "this" points us back to the discussion in paragraph 1, which ends with the statement that "markers of a high-status background are often misrecognized as signs of innate talent or intelligence." Because it immediately precedes the keyword, that is what "this phenomenon" probably refers to.

An example of the phenomenon as described in that last sentence of P1 is actually given in P2: before blind auditions, "a musician's likelihood of being selected was strongly correlated with the prestige of the conservatory they attended and their history of studying with renowned masters." That's to be expected if those status markers are taken as signs of musical talent.

Putting the pieces together, it makes sense that blind auditions would counteract this process by rendering it impossible to know any characteristics of the person who's playing music behind the screen. Only the music is left to judge, and it carries no information about a person's cultural capital. That's precisely what **(C)** suggests: greater educational diversity was a result of assessing only the music and not also personal characteristics like "social and educational background." This might even explain the success in diversifying gender, at least in part, if it were true that women were less likely to attend prestigious conservatories or study with renowned masters in the 1970s and 1980s.

Thus, **(C)** is the best explanation because it follows a chain of reasoning that begins with clues in the stem. Based on the passage, it is more likely to be true than any other answer choice. This is the minimum requirement for an inference, that it be significantly more likely than any alternative. Often, such as when a question asks you for an assumption that is necessary for an argument, the correct answer *must* be true, given what the passage states.

Not all Make Deduction questions require such elaborate chains of reasoning, but as deep (Reasoning Within the Text) questions, they almost always involve more cognitive effort than Paraphrase Detail or other surface questions. Let's break down this process into its parts and understand the most common ways this skill is tested in CARS.

Combining Claims

The single most common way Make Deduction is tested is by having you find connections between different parts of the passage to draw inferences that the author never states. Doing this requires that you find the relevant points of connection and reason through them to the appropriate inference.

When putting statements together to draw inferences, limit yourself to claims that are absolutely certain, or extremely close to it. This will help you to avoid falling for trap answer choices on questions that test the Make Deduction skill. For example, consider the following text:

> Lucas said that he never eats pizza because he doesn't like cheese and that he always prefers to cook with olive oil over butter. No one has ever seen him have ice cream or a milkshake or even a glass of milk.

Many students see an example like this and naturally jump to an explanation like "he must be lactose intolerant!" That's definitely a possibility, but it's making an extra leap that wouldn't be justified on the CARS section. The better-supported inference is that Lucas doesn't consume dairy products: that's the common thread linking cheese, butter, ice cream, and milk. But no hints are suggested about why he dislikes or avoids these products.

MCAT EXPERTISE

In CARS, all correct answers will be based only on the passage, not any real-life information you happen to have about the topic. It can be especially tempting to apply your personal knowledge when making deductions, so be careful.

Finding points of connection can sometimes be challenging, as in the sample question, which required moving along a chain of reasoning through multiple sentences. In other cases, the connection may be easier to make because the question gives you the common thread. For example, if the question asks for a statement that is "probably true" about a person who is described in the first two paragraphs of the passage, you'll likely just look at what is said about that person in those paragraphs and see if anything follows that the author didn't spell out.

Once you've found claims in the passage that you believe could be relevant for a Make Deduction question, combine them logically. For example, suppose the following excerpts appear in a passage:

> **Paragraph 1:** "... historians generally agree that there are only two plausible explanations for the court's decision to ban the serialized publication of James Joyce's *Ulysses* in *The Little Review*. Either the panel of judges genuinely feared for the corrupting influence of the novel's "Nausicaa" episode on young minds, or the ruling was a paternal attempt to weaponize obscenity law against a politically radical magazine run by women."

> **Paragraph 4:** "... thus it stretches the bounds of credulity that even the 1921 judicial panel could have seriously believed that any American youth were reading such an avant-garde publication, or would have been capable of interpreting Joyce's oblique stream-of-consciousness prose if they had read it."

In paragraph 1, the author asserts that there are only two possible explanations for the court's ruling: genuine fear of corrupting youth, or an attack against the magazine. In paragraph 4, the author conclusively refutes the first explanation, saying that it couldn't have been fear for the youth. The passage might never say

MCAT EXPERTISE

In rare cases, a Make Deduction question might ask you to resolve a paradox or reconcile an apparent contradiction. A **paradox** in CARS is usually just a pair of claims that seem to conflict at the surface but don't actually clash if you fully understand what the author means. In these cases, identify the two claims in the passage that seem to conflict, and then consider what else would have to be true so that both of them could be true at the same time. Resolving paradoxes is just a special type of deduction.

explicitly that the second explanation is true and the obscenity ruling was an attack on the magazine *The Little Review*, but we can deduce that this is the case based on the language of the passage.

Uncovering Assumptions

One of the toughest deductions to make is uncovering an assumption in a logical argument. Assumptions are a special kind of inference: to understand how they work, let's review and expand upon some important concepts introduced earlier in this book.

As explained in the discussion of Logic keywords in Chapter 3 and further addressed in Chapter 14 on the Evaluate Reasoning skill, an **argument** is made up of a claim or **conclusion** that is supported by one or more pieces of **evidence**. In a strong argument, the evidence does a good job of convincing the reader that the conclusion is true. But often, authors don't present every single piece of evidence that would be needed to prove the conclusion.

An **assumption** is a statement that isn't written in the argument, but that *needs* to be true in order for the logic of the argument to work. It's a missing piece of evidence, often one that connects the existing evidence more strongly to the conclusion and clarifies why that evidence suggests that the conclusion is true.

However, accurate assumptions don't have to *guarantee* that the conclusion is true or that the argument works; they're just something that the argument needs. It's comparable to the way that a supply of oxygen to the bloodstream doesn't guarantee good health, even though it's definitely *necessary* for good health.

> **MCAT EXPERTISE**
>
> In CARS passages, it's rare for arguments to be absolutely "perfect" and prove the conclusion beyond a shadow of a doubt: that's a very high standard to meet. Authors more commonly make arguments in which the evidence makes it very likely that the conclusion is true but stops short of absolute certainty.

Consider the following simple argument and ask yourself what it assumes:

> The patient is presenting with a fever and a sore throat, so he should be prescribed the antibiotic amoxicillin.

Since this argument draws a conclusion (antibiotic prescription) based on the presence of certain symptoms (fever and sore throat), it assumes that the cause of these symptoms can be effectively treated by antibiotics. In other words, it assumes the symptoms are caused by a bacterial infection (because that's the only condition antibiotics effectively treat).

That is not the only assumption in the argument, of course. Others include:

- Amoxicillin does not have dangerous side effects that outweigh its benefits.
- The patient is not taking any other drugs that have seriously harmful interactions with amoxicillin.
- There is no antibiotic superior to amoxicillin in every way (effectiveness, availability, cost, safety, etc.).

Fortunately for Test Day, you'll only ever need to identify one assumption for any particular question. But it's important to remain open-minded and recognize that even if you predict a genuine assumption, the correct answer might match a different, equally valid assumption.

Assumptions are claims that the argument absolutely needs, not statements that *could* help the argument or that *might* be true according to the argument's logic. Consider another simple argument and try to identify any assumptions it makes.

> There is a swim meet at the high school tomorrow morning, so Amina can't go out dancing at the club tonight.

It might be tempting to say that this argument assumes Amina is one of the swimmers competing at tomorrow's meet. You might ask, "Why else would the swim meet affect what she can or can't do the night before?" But in this case, there could be multiple other explanations.

Perhaps Amina is a coach of one of the teams or a maintenance person responsible for setting up the pool before the swim meet. Any of these facts could *potentially* connect the evidence to the conclusion, but none of them *need* to be true for the argument to work, so none of them are valid assumptions. Instead of being more specific than what the argument needs, consider what all these possibilities have in common. They all try to connect Amina to the swim meet.

In addition to that, the argument needs a connection between the swim meet and dancing at the club. Even if we know Amina's connection to the swim meet, why does this mean she can't go to the club the night before? Again, it's important not to be too specific.

So this argument is assuming a couple of things:

- Amina has some obligation related to the swim meet.
- This obligation prevents her from going out to the club the night before.

Unlike the possibilities discussed before, denying either of these points completely ruins the argument, so they are both valid assumptions.

15.2 Question Variations and Examples

Make Deduction questions vary in two basic dimensions: the type of deduction required and whether they have location clues.

Nature of the Deduction

There are two main kinds of inferences that questions testing the Make Deduction skill ask for. As discussed in Section 15.1, they require somewhat different approaches.

Indirect Inference

Some questions that test the Make Deduction skill require you to identify that two or more pieces of information from different parts of the passage are logically related to one another, then combine them to draw a new conclusion that must be true.

MCAT EXPERTISE

Because assumptions have to be true for an argument to work, one way to test out a potential assumption is to evaluate what would happen to the argument if the potential assumption were *false*. If a valid assumption is false, it should make the argument fall apart. Consider how this might apply to the amoxicillin argument: if the sore throat and fever were caused by a viral infection that is not treatable with antibiotics, then there's *no reason* to prescribe amoxicillin. The conclusion is no longer true, so pretending that this potential assumption is false ruins the argument. This means that the potential assumption is valid, and the argument indeed assumes a bacterial infection that can be treated effectively with antibiotics.

MCAT EXPERTISE

Phrases such as "based on the passage" and "according to the passage/author" each appear in both Make Deduction questions and Paraphrase Detail questions, as well as others. So these words are not a reliable guide to the skill being tested.

EXAMPLE QUESTION STEMS

The passage argument implies that the Etruscan language:

In referring to the "hegemony" of mass media (paragraph 1), the author implies that advertising functions as:

Based on the passage, the author most likely believes that urban renewal and gentrification may be:

According to the author, a key difference between folk tales and myths is:

What statement about Velasquez can reconcile the claim that he was always generous with his friends (paragraph 3) with his cruelty toward his stepchildren (paragraph 6)?

Necessary Assumption

Less commonly, Make Deduction questions ask for a different kind of unstated idea that must be true: something that a passage argument must be assuming in order for that argument to make sense.

EXAMPLE QUESTION STEMS

Implicit in the author's argument that the fall of the Roman Empire was caused primarily by economic factors is the assumption that:

Whittington's argument about the Cambrian explosion (paragraph 2) necessarily requires which of the following?

Location Clues

Make Deduction questions can also be subdivided based on whether they provide a paragraph reference pointing you toward a particular part of the passage.

No Paragraph Reference

In this most common format, the question stem does not directly state where the author discusses the topic or concept that you must make a deduction about, so you must use context and your distillation of the passage to locate it.

EXAMPLE QUESTION STEMS

Based on the passage, it can be reasonably inferred that academics widely adopted post-structuralist literary theory because it:

Which of the following is implied, but not stated, in the passage?

In arguing that early photography is not properly considered a fine art, the author implicitly disputes the idea that:

Passage context suggests that when Erik Satie disassociated himself from Les Six, he intended to:

Paragraph Reference

Less often, the question stem directly states which paragraph mentions the concept that the question is asking about, narrowing your search for the relevant information.

EXAMPLE QUESTION STEMS

The author's critique of traditional economic models (paragraph 3) implies a belief that:

What relationship between the "aesthetic of the sublime" (paragraph 1) and the "aesthetic of the beautiful" (paragraph 4) is implicit in the passage argument?

Since the Make Deduction skill involves more complex logic, however, question stems that mention a particular paragraph will regularly require you to locate information in other paragraphs as well.

15.3 Applying the Kaplan Method

Step 1: Type the Question

See Chapter 6 for more information on how to identify the broad AAMC question type: Foundations of Comprehension (surface questions), Reasoning Within the Text (deep questions), or Reasoning Beyond the Text (new info questions). Identify this type along with the relative difficulty of the question as the basis for your triage decision: attack the question *now* or *later*. Optionally, after you've learned the question skills, you can try to identify the specific skill and factor that into your triaging decision.

MCAT EXPERTISE

Very rarely, Make Deduction questions reverse the usual line of thinking by asking for a statement that *cannot* be deduced from the text. In other rare cases, they ask about multiple potential inferences in a Roman numeral format. These questions are very similar to comparable variants of the Paraphrase Detail skill discussed in Chapter 10, as well as other skills.

Identifying the Skill

Make Deduction questions are not always easy to identify. Words like "implicit," "implied," "inferred," "inference," "necessary," "assume," and "assumption" are common, along with phrases like "must be true" or "most likely to be true." However, these words can also appear when other skills are being tested, such as Paraphrase Detail, which usually involves a much less elaborate solution process. As a Reasoning Within the Text skill, Make Deduction questions will not include new information, although answers almost always include information that is only implied in the passage and not explicitly stated.

Deciding When to Attack

Because Make Deduction questions can be some of the most time-consuming to track down an answer, you should usually save them for *later*, as long as you can recognize them. If you start on one of these questions because you initially misidentified it as surface rather than deep, continue working through it if you see a path forward to an answer. Otherwise, consider changing your triage decision and finishing the investigation later, or even making an educated guess if you're running low on time or significantly behind on your pacing for the section.

The only exception to saving these for later would be if the question asks about a connection or assumption that you happened to uncover during your active reading of the passage. This is relatively rare but can become more frequent as you gain additional experience with CARS and establish more grounded expectations about what questions ask. If you have a good sense of how to answer the question before even starting your investigation, you should definitely attempt the question *now*.

Step 2: Rephrase the Stem

With a Make Deduction question, try to specify the exact piece of information that the question is looking for, as well as any clues about where to start looking in the passage. Location clues can include: paragraph numbers, names or technical terminology used in the passage, direct quotations, paraphrases of important concepts or claims from the passage. The less direct the clues, the more you'll need to rely on your distillation (your outline or highlights) to isolate the relevant text from the passage.

With Make Deduction questions, expect that you'll probably also need to rely on other information from the passage, often from different paragraphs than anything that appears in the question stem. You may need to find a mention from a distant paragraph of an idea that appears in a quotation in the question. Or you may need to follow a less direct chain, as was the case with the sample question at the beginning of the chapter.

For most students, the easiest way to follow these chains is to start at the end point and see if you can make a connection back to the question stem. In other words, default to a process of elimination, especially on Make Deduction questions with few context clues.

For example, for a question like the following:

> The passage argument implies that the Etruscan language:

One thorough rephrase would be:

- Using your distillation (highlights or outline), find information from the passage on the Etruscan language to set initial expectations.
- Review each answer choice. If any match the information about the Etruscan language already uncovered, select it and move on.
- Otherwise, evaluate each choice based on how well the passage connects it to the Etruscan language. The choice with the strongest textual support that doesn't otherwise contradict the passage is correct.

It's possible that your investigation might end with the second step, as typically occurs when a question that appeared to test Make Deduction is actually testing Paraphrase Detail. But if not, you're ready with a backup plan for how exactly to deploy the process of elimination.

When the question contains language like "assume," "assumption," or "must necessarily be true," your rephrase will look a little different, and it's less likely that you'll need to jump to other parts of the passage for a solution. Instead, you'll need to delve more deeply into the logic of the argument and uncover what it has to assume in order to function.

BRIDGE

The skill that you're most likely to confuse with Make Deduction is Paraphrase Detail. Sometimes you won't identify something as Make Deduction right away: you may not discover until the Investigate step whether a question has a relatively quick answer that can be extracted from a single part of the passage, or whether you'll need to interconnect ideas from multiple paragraphs to find a solution. If you're expecting the skill is Paraphrase Detail but then discover there isn't an obvious answer where you thought, it's okay to pivot, putting that revealed Make Deduction on pause until you've earned some points tackling other questions. See Chapter 10 for more on Paraphrase Detail.

KEY CONCEPT

If a lot of information is provided in the stem without specific paragraph references, consider starting with the **rarest concept**, as explained in Chapter 10. Briefly, this is the piece of information least likely to appear in the passage, making it easier to isolate. For example, given a question about "Schopenhauer's philosophy of art," look for "Schopenhauer" or "philosophy" in a passage on the arts, but for "art" and similar ideas in a passage on Schopenhauer's thought.

Because any argument consists of evidence and conclusion, your first task will be to identify exactly what each piece is, as presented in the passage. There may be only one piece of evidence or there may be multiple, but try to be comprehensive. An assumption could affect any or all evidence included in an argument.

The second task for any assumption is finding a missing piece of the argument. The passage could hint at this missing piece elsewhere, but often it is just something that the test maker believes a reasonable student will naturally recognize. Ask yourself: what does this argument take for granted, or what must be true for this evidence to actually make the conclusion more likely? Your backup plan, in case nothing jumps out at you as the missing piece, will be the process of elimination, as is often needed for this skill.

For example, with a question like this:

> Whittington's argument about the Cambrian explosion (paragraph 2) necessarily requires which of the following?

A strong rephrase would be:

- Go to paragraph 2 and identify the evidence and conclusion of the argument.
- Identify any missing piece of evidence as a prediction.
- If no match (or no prediction), evaluate each answer choice by negating it: the choice that most weakens the argument after being negated is correct.

In this case, "weaken" could mean that denying the choice makes the conclusion false. Alternatively, denying it might just sever the connection between evidence and conclusion, removing any reason there may have been for accepting the evidence as evidence. For more on weakening arguments, see Chapter 19 on the Strengthen/Weaken Argument skill.

Step 3: Investigate Potential Solutions

When you investigate most Make Deduction questions, you should be strategic and flexible. It's worthwhile to spend some time investigating the passage, but (as was clear from the start of this chapter with the sample question) sometimes chains of reasoning can be intricate and time-consuming to unpack.

If a modest investment of time looking over your distillation and rereading select parts of the passage gives you a clear prediction, then approach the answer choices with that. Otherwise, don't force it and be willing to jump into process-of-elimination mode as soon as the trail goes cold.

During the process of elimination, your investigation is centered around the answer choices. See if you can follow clues in the choices to specific parts of the passage that support them, or that give a possible exit point from the chain of reasoning that started with the question. If you can find a clear connection from question to answer choice through different pieces of the text, you'll have your correct answer.

When dealing with assumptions and sometimes with the other types of inferences requested in Make Deduction questions, you can use the denial test strategy mentioned above to guide your process of elimination: choose the choice that, when negated, most weakens the author's argument.

Step 4: Match Your Prediction to an Answer Choice

This question skill is more likely to require a process of elimination, but if you do find yourself able to make a good prediction with a solid match, don't hesitate to choose it and get the point.

More likely, this step will involve selecting the one choice you weren't able to eliminate. However, you should keep in mind the option of making an educated guess or even a wild guess when time is low. Because they're more likely to be time-consuming and difficult, but they aren't worth any additional points, these are good questions to strategically guess on.

A common trap with Make Deduction is an answer choice that *could* be true, but is not the most likely to be true. More than being a mere possibility, the correct answer to a Make Deduction question must be highly likely, and sometimes it's even an absolute certainty.

15.4 Skillbuilder

Use the following shortened passage to practice the Make Deduction skill. The reading is scaffolded to reinforce good active reading habits and to let you devote more of your attention to practicing your critical thinking skills. It includes Active Reading Checks with each paragraph to evaluate how well you're uncovering important passage information at every level. Answer both the Active Reading Check and the CARS question that accompanies each paragraph before continuing. You can check your answers on the next page before you move on to paragraph 2, and the same for paragraph 3.

This page is intentionally blank. Chapter continues on the next page. ▶ ▶ ▶

Paragraph 1

Before World War II had ended, delegates from all 44 allied nations, including the Soviet Union, met in Bretton Woods, New Hampshire, to plan post-war reconstruction and stabilization of the global economy. What became the World Bank was established to provide loans for specific reconstruction and development projects while the International Monetary Fund (IMF) would monitor exchange rates and make short-term balance-of-payment loans. However, the Soviet Union later declined to ratify the agreement, rejecting the U.S. Treasury Department's sway as the largest shareholder and exchange rates pegged to the dollar. This rift expanded into competing development ideologies between Western capitalistic democracies (the so-called "First World") and communist bloc countries ("Second World") for influence over the remaining "Third World" nations. Throughout the Cold War, loans frequently arrived with economic restructuring conditionalities. Notably, the 1980s "Washington Consensus" mandated market liberalization, private takeover of government services, and fiscal austerity in exchange for Western development assistance.

Active Reading Check for Paragraph 1

The passage author's use of the term "so-called" and the quotation marks they place around "First World," "Second World," and "Third World" serve to:

A. suggest that these classifications were universally accepted and accurate in their time.
B. merely cite historical terminology without any implied judgment or critical distance.
C. indicate such hierarchy is potentially outdated and biased to a particular ideology.

1. The passage implies that during the Cold War nations borrowing development funds for state-run enterprises would be:

A. more likely to secure a loan from the International Monetary Fund than the World Bank.
B. less likely to achieve economic growth or prevent economic collapse than nations pursuing privatization.
C. more likely to qualify for a lower interest rate by joining a specific military alliance.
D. less likely to meet the conditions for economic restructuring stipulated by "First World" lenders.

Active Reading Check for Paragraph 1: (C)

(A) While signals that these terms are not the author's own way of referring to parts of the world could suggest that is how they were commonly designated at that point in history, paragraph 1 describes a world separated by "competing development ideologies." A development framework that ranked some nations above others would therefore not have been "universally accepted," especially by the nations subordinated within it.

(B) These rhetorical tools create a "critical distance" between the author and the terminology that suggests the author finds them problematic, not just old-fashioned. The author's "implied judgment" that they don't necessarily agree with the fairness of the historical framing of Western nations as "first" is evident in their scrutiny of positioning the U.S. dollar as the world's reserve currency and the "U.S. Treasury Department's sway as the largest shareholder."

(C) That the author is trying to distance themself from the terminology, suggesting they don't fully endorse it or want to be associated with its use, is reflected by the core argument of paragraph 1: the First, Second, and Third World framework is not an objective ranking but instead a biased product of the "competing development ideologies" that defined the Cold War.

Question 1: (D)

Answer Choice Explanations for Question 1

(A) Since the question stem asks about an "enterprise," the World Bank, which provides "loans for specific reconstruction and development projects," would be the more appropriate lender than the IMF that provides "short-term balance-of-payment loans." Furthermore, both institutions were part of the Bretton Woods system that conditioned loans on restructuring away from "state-run" organization, making neither a likely lender for such an enterprise.

(B) Paragraph 1 describes the "Washington Consensus" mandate for "private takeover of government services" but does not provide details on the relative economic "growth" or "collapse" that resulted from pursuing or rejecting these policies during the Cold War.

(C) Paragraph 1 discusses loan "conditionalities" and "competing development ideologies" between Western and communist blocs for "influence over the remaining 'Third World' nations," but contains no information about "military alliance[s]" or their impact on "lower interest rate[s]" for securing funds.

(D) Loans from "First World" lenders came with "economic restructuring conditionalities." For example, the "Washington Consensus" explicitly "mandated ... private takeover of government services," meaning nations with "state-run enterprises" would be "less likely to meet" these terms for "Western development assistance."

Detailed Explanation for Question 1

Skill: This question tests the Make Deduction skill since it requires you to use logical reasoning to infer a claim that is not explicitly stated but is justified by connecting multiple ideas within the passage.

Question: The question asks for a logical consequence regarding nations pursuing development loans for "state-run enterprises" during the Cold War, based on implications from the passage. Locate information in the passage about these nations and the "Cold War" era to deduce what must be true.

Passage: Paragraph 1 explains that Cold War loans from "First World" lenders (Western capitalistic democracies) frequently included "economic restructuring conditionalities." Specifically, the "Washington Consensus" "mandated ... private takeover of government services ... in exchange for Western development assistance." Since this requirement directly opposes the concept of "state-run enterprises," it is reasonable to predict such entities would not meet the terms set by these lenders.

Answer: **(D)** aligns with the prediction that "state-run enterprises" would not meet the terms set by "First World" lenders. The other choices make unsupported claims about economic outcomes and lending terms or present an inaccurate comparison based on the passage.

Paragraph 2

Polarization gave way to globalization with the fall of the Berlin Wall and the apparent triumph of market capitalism. However, optimism for the potential to reallocate resources from geopolitical competition and military buildup to poverty reduction amounted to little more than a superficial reclassification of the world into two strata: "developed countries" and "developing countries." Anthropologist James Ferguson's 1990 book dismantled this false dichotomy that premised development agency priorities on conflating two different definitions of "development": "(1) poor countries are (by definition) 'less developed'; (2) less developed countries are (by another definition) those which have not yet been fully brought into the modern economy." Yet, the Millennium Development Goals (MDGs), endorsed by the UN in 2000, formalized the two-tier hierarchy with externally defined targets for developing countries to achieve by 2015 in exchange for official development assistance and technical expertise within the established finance paradigm.

Active Reading Check for Paragraph 2

When the author describes the "optimism for the potential" of the era following the Cold War, their tone suggests in hindsight it was:

A. tempered by the persistence of perceived superiority.
B. discredited as misguided anti-communist posturing.
C. vindicated by the radical reordering of global power structures.

2. The passage author suggests that the Millennium Development Goals:

A. set aspirational rather than measurable objectives.
B. assumed economic globalization would reduce poverty.
C. created equitable partnerships for mutual benefit.
D. circumvented lending contingent on economic restructuring.

Active Reading Check for Paragraph 2: (A)

(A) Describing the optimism as having "amounted to little more than a superficial reclassification of the world into two strata" suggests a lost opportunity to mitigate underlying power imbalances. This allowed the "perceived superiority" to continue under the name "developed" rather than "First World," despite the hopes for change.

(B) While paragraph 2 mentions the "apparent triumph of market capitalism" after the Cold War context of paragraph 1, the author's discouragement focuses on the persistence of hierarchical relations, not discrediting opposition to communism as misguided.

(C) The author implies the optimism was not vindicated, describing the post-Cold War reclassification as "superficial," stating that the "established finance paradigm" remained, and directly contradicting any characterization of "radical reordering."

Question 2: (B)

Answer Choice Explanations for Question 2

(A) According to paragraph 2, the Millennium Development Goals set "targets for developing countries to achieve by 2015 in exchange for official development assistance," suggesting they were intended to be measurable objectives, not merely aspirational.

(B) Paragraph 2 states that the Millennium Development Goals "formalized the two-tier hierarchy" that categorized countries as either "developed" or "developing." The passage author calls this a "false dichotomy" that set priorities by "conflating two different definitions of 'development.'" To treat "integrating into the modern economy" (i.e., economic globalization) and "alleviating poverty" as interchangeable, the MDGs must take for granted that the former inherently causes the latter.

(C) Paragraph 2 presents the Millennium Development Goals as part of a "two-tier hierarchy" with "developed countries" providing "official development assistance and technical expertise" and determining "externally defined targets" for "developing countries," which does not suggest a power balance of "equitable partnerships for mutual benefit."

(D) Paragraph 2 indicates that the Millennium Development Goals were formalized "within the established finance paradigm" that, as described in paragraph 1, involved "economic restructuring conditionalities," indicating they did not "circumvent[] lending contingent on economic restructuring."

Detailed Explanation for Question 2

Skill: Because this question requires you to infer an unstated claim by logically connecting details provided in the passage, it assesses the Make Deduction skill.

Question: The question asks for a claim the passage author implicitly makes about the Millennium Development Goals. To answer, review the author's description and treatment of the MDGs within the passage and infer their suggested characteristic or consequence.

Passage: Paragraph 2 introduces the Millennium Development Goals as formalizing a "two-tier hierarchy with externally defined targets." Such "priorities" are "premised ... on conflating two different definitions of 'development'" during an era when countries were sorted as either "developed" or "developing," which effectively suggests that any poor "developing" country was insufficiently integrated into the global economy. The author characterizes this two-tier hierarchy as a "false dichotomy" and simply a "superficial reclassification" of the prior three-world model, which served to maintain "the established finance paradigm." Look for an answer choice that reflects the passage author's criticism of the MDGs, perhaps their perpetuation of power imbalances that they purported to combat or their faulty rationale.

Answer: **(B)** is correct because it points to a consequence of conflating poverty and lack of global integration. If "developing" means both poorer and less globalized "by definition," it stands to reason that increasing globalization would decrease poverty as a nation shifted from "developing" to "developed." The author views this assumption as a weakness in the MDGs.

Paragraph 3

The MDG deadline arrived with mixed success, as the "development" binary ceded to quantitative classification of countries across a spectrum of income levels. The post-2015 UN Development Agenda set 17 interconnected Sustainable Development Goals (SDGs), which still prioritized poverty reduction but applied universally to all countries, recognizing development was not a static or evenly distributed outcome within (let alone between) countries. At the same time, the BRICS (Brazil, Russia, India, China, South Africa) group of emerging economies had already begun to forge an alternative to the Bretton Woods system, culminating in the 2014 establishment of the New Development Bank (NDB). The NDB's core philosophy purportedly emphasizes mutual benefit and non-interference. With the SDG 2030 horizon approaching and the United States contracting its foreign assistance, the future of global development finance is increasingly multipolar and less reliant on traditional models.

Active Reading Check for Paragraph 3

According to paragraph 3, which of the following labels is most consistent with country classifications during the SDGs era?

A. "Third World Country"

B. "Developing Country"

C. "Lower-Middle-Income Country"

3. The author indicates belief in each of the following EXCEPT:

A. every country has an internal range of development and no country stops developing.

B. the Millennium Development Goals relied on the Bretton Woods system.

C. shareholders' national security interests do not influence NDB lending.

D. the world is moving away from a unipolar order where one superpower dominates.

Active Reading Check for Paragraph 3: (C)

(A) This term was used during the Cold War era (paragraph 1) to refer to countries that were not allied with either the "Western capitalistic democracies" or the "communist bloc countries." So, it is inconsistent with the "post-2015" SDG era.

(B) This is a classification associated with the MDG era (paragraph 2). While still used colloquially, the passage emphasizes this "'development' binary ceded" to a more nuanced system in the SDG era (paragraph 3).

(C) Paragraph 3 explains that the SDG era moved to "quantitative classification of countries across a spectrum of income levels," which is consistent with a label such as "Lower-Middle-Income Country."

Question 3: (C)

Answer Choice Explanations for Question 3

(A) Paragraph 3 indicates this belief by stating the Sustainable Development Goals (SDGs) applied universally to all countries, "recognizing development was not a static or evenly distributed outcome within (let alone between) countries." This implies that every country has an internal range of development and that development isn't a process that simply comes to an end.

(B) This claim can be inferred when paragraph 2 states the Millennium Development Goals (MDGs) emerged "within the established finance paradigm" because paragraph 1 set up the reliance of that paradigm on the existing Bretton Woods system.

(C) The author does not support this claim. As paragraph 3 explains, while the New Development Bank's declared guiding principle is "mutual benefit and non-interference," the author's use of "purportedly" casts doubt on this assertion. Even assuming "non-interference" implies an absence of economic restructuring conditionalities like those from the Bretton Woods system, it does not necessarily mean shareholders forego national security advantages in their lending; indeed, the concept of "mutual benefit" within the philosophy suggests some form of advantage to all parties.

(D) Paragraph 3 explicitly states "the future of global development finance is increasingly multipolar and less reliant on traditional models," suggesting a move away from a unipolar order where one superpower dominates.

Detailed Explanation for Question 3

Skill: This question tests the Make Deduction skill by requiring you to logically connect information from across the passage to infer which claim goes unsupported.

Question: The question asks you to identify a claim that the passage author does not support, either implicitly or explicitly. Thus, three wrong answer choices will be stated or at least suggested, and the correct answer will be unsupported. To answer, evaluate each statement against the passage to determine if the author indicates a belief in it.

Passage: Without any indication in the question stem about what implicit or explicit claims from the passage will appear as wrong answers and an infinite number of possible claims that the author would NOT endorse, it is impossible to evaluate the answer choices with a prediction in mind. Instead, eliminate each answer choice that is supported in the passage. Unless you remember the author explicitly making a claim paraphrased by an answer choice, which can be eliminated immediately, revisit the part(s) of the passage related to each choice, and determine if the author implies that they believe this answer choice to be true. Repeat the process until you locate the correct choice that the author expresses disagreement with or takes no position about.

Answer: **(A)** makes a claim consistent with the author's assertion that "development was not a static or evenly distributed outcome within (let alone between) countries" in paragraph 3. **(B)** is supported by logically concluding that the "established finance paradigm" that paragraph 2 indicates the MDGs emerged within was based on the Bretton Woods system. **(C)** is the claim that lacks support in the passage. Paragraph 3 states the NDB's core philosophy "purportedly emphasizes mutual benefit and non-interference." The author's use of "purportedly" suggests that they don't believe this claim. But even if granted, there's no reason given in the passage to suppose that "mutual benefit" would exclude national security considerations entirely. **(D)** is supported as paragraph 3 concludes: "the future of global development finance is increasingly multipolar and less reliant on traditional models."

Skill and Strategy Summary

Skill Description

- The **Make Deduction** skill is your ability to derive complex inferences from the passage, either by combining distant claims or uncovering assumptions in passage arguments.
  - Make Deduction accounts for about 30% of Reasoning Within the Text questions.
- Many **inferences** are found by combining claims from different parts of the passage, which are interconnected through shared terminology or concepts.
- An **assumption** in an argument is something that must be true for the conclusion to follow from the evidence.

Question Variations and Examples

- Make Deduction questions can vary in the following ways:
  - **Nature of the Deduction**: They can ask for an indirect inference combining information in a complex way (or from multiple parts of the text) or, less commonly, for an assumption required by a passage argument.
  - **Location Clues**: Stems usually do not provide a paragraph reference with this skill, but sometimes.

Applying the Kaplan Method

- Step 1: Type the Question
  - Recognize Make Deduction by language like "infer," "imply," "assume," and "necessarily true." They usually ask for a specific piece of information that can be deduced from the passage.
  - Save these questions for *later* but watch out for ones that look more like Paraphrase Detail.
- Step 2: Rephrase the Stem
  - Be clear on the precise piece of information you need, as well as any clues about where to start looking in the passage.
  - If you need to combine information from multiple paragraphs or uncover an unclear assumption, plan to use the process of elimination.
- Step 3: Investigate Potential Solutions
  - These can be harder to predict but try your best to follow the chain of reasoning in the passage efficiently.
  - If no prediction is forthcoming, use the process of elimination, letting answer choices potentially guide you to text in the passage that can confirm or eliminate them.
  - For assumptions and sometimes other inferences, deny the answer choices and see what effect it has on the author's argument. The greatest weakener after negation is correct.
- Step 4: Match Your Prediction to an Answer Choice
  - Process of elimination is common with these questions but also be willing to guess when timing demands it.
  - Common trap answers are choices that only *could* be true instead of being the most likely to be true.

CHAPTER 16

REASONING WITHIN THE TEXT PRACTICE

How to Use This Chapter

This practice chapter contains two full MCAT passages and question sets, designed to help you practice answering Reasoning Within the Text (RWT) questions using the skills discussed in Chapters 13–15. While RWT questions make up only 30% of the questions you will see on Test Day, the passage sets within this chapter contain *only* RWT questions. Use the strategies discussed in Chapters 1–6 to Read and Distill the passages and answer the associated questions. Then, use the answer explanations at the end of the chapter to review your practice (information on how to review your practice can be found in Chapter 7).

Passage 1 (Questions 1–6)

Yugoslav folk dances have always played a central role, not only within Yugoslavia as an expression of core ideologies, but also internationally, as a medium for achieving diplomacy and cultural branding. Framed as folklore—that is, the cultural production of the people transmitted through generations, in which individual authors are unknown and authorship is collective—social participatory dances practiced in the villages of Yugoslavia gained momentum in the 1930s. However, it was during the 1940s that a profound transformation took place. This change was catalyzed by the establishment of cultural and artistic associations, which assumed the role of embodying socialist principles of leisure as work through the execution of folklore.

These organizations, often encompassing folk dance ensembles, choirs, drama, and sports divisions, were primarily designed to propagate the concept of amateurism, meaning the transformation of leisure into a productive endeavor. By highlighting amateurism as a spontaneous collective expression, Yugoslav officials extolled the cultural contributions of the entire working populace. They regarded amateurism as a fundamental requirement for every individual seeking to become an integral part of the broader social community. Popular culture, encompassing music and dance, assumed a central role in cultural propaganda due to its association with populism. Consequently, cultural and artistic associations served as platforms that not only united the working class but also attracted the working intelligentsia, providing opportunities for the public presentations of staged music and dance. The social chain dances eventually evolved into symbolic representations of national culture.

These social dances are locally known as *kolo* or *oro*, which are often translated into English as "circle dance" or "chain dance." They represent a prevalent dance genre in the region, present in all Yugoslav republics and neighboring Balkan nations. While the *kolo/oro* dances exhibit variations in names, rhythms, and tempos, a common characteristic is the facilitation of mass participation within circular formations, either open or closed. Participants, joined by their hands, execute synchronized steps, thus fostering a sense of equality and collective spirit. These dances offered an avenue for an unrestricted number of participants to come together, forge bonds, and engage in collective interaction, all while immersed in the rhythms of the dance.

Notably, no formal training is required to partake in these dances as proficiency is acquired solely through immersion. These dances are performed at all types of events, including religious holidays, weddings, and social gatherings. The participatory nature of the dance fosters inclusivity, allowing every community member to take part, and results in a tangible sense of egalitarianism irrespective of individual skill levels. All of these mentioned values held particular significance for Yugoslav ideologues, who adeptly incorporated them into their propaganda efforts, accentuating themes of unity, equality, and collective solidarity.

The popularization of cultural and artistic associations gave birth to the idea of forming the first national and professional dance ensembles. The ensembles' mandate was to gather, adapt, and preserve the folk dances and songs of their respective regions. Cognizant of the potential for folk dance performances to catalyze separatism and nationalism, Yugoslav authorities advocated for the creation of a pan-Yugoslav repertoire, encompassing dances and music from all of the diverse ethnic groups and republics within the country. This strategic decision, rooted in the principle of brotherhood and unity, served as a proactive measure aimed at averting ethnic, religious, and political discord. Within their music and dance ensembles, Yugoslav dancers and musicians were required to acquaint themselves with the music and dance cultures from other republics. Meanwhile, local village performing groups were exempted from the pan-Yugoslav program because they were regarded as the authentic custodians of folklore traditions.

Adapted from F. Petkovski, "How to Choreograph a Socialist Society?" *Arts*. ©2024. Petkovski et al.

1. The author implies that Yugoslav cultural and artistic associations served to:
   A. preserve the cultural heritage of village dances for future generations.
   B. encourage financial support of working-class artistic performances by the intelligentsia class.
   C. professionalize folk dancing to showcase Yugoslav culture for international audiences.
   D. promote certain political values across multiple social classes.

2. Why does the author most likely mention folklore in the first paragraph?
   A. To imply that Yugoslav officials were incorrect in applying the label of folklore to their dance ensembles
   B. To emphasize the continuity of dance traditions, suggesting they were resistant to the changes initiated in the 1940s
   C. To provide context for the history of social dances and introduce their later ideological transformation
   D. To introduce the concept of collective cultural production as a theme that runs throughout Yugoslav history

3. What is the primary purpose of the author's discussion of the *kolo* and *oro* dances (paragraph 3)?
   A. It attributes the dances' popularity to the lack of a formal training requirement.
   B. It evaluates the rationale for the creation of a pan-Yugoslav repertoire for the dance ensembles.
   C. It establishes the authenticity of *kolo* and *oro* by their prevalence across all Yugoslav republics.
   D. It exemplifies a dance genre whose features were well-suited to the state's promotion of solidarity.

4. Which of the following claims does the author support with an explanation in the passage?
   A. "... social participatory dances practiced in the villages of Yugoslavia gained momentum in the 1930s."
   B. "Meanwhile, local village performing groups ... were regarded as the authentic custodians of folklore traditions."
   C. "Notably, no formal training is required to partake in these dances ..."
   D. "These dances are performed at all types of events, including religious holidays, weddings, and social gatherings."

5. What assumption best explains the Yugoslav authorities' decision to exempt local village performing groups from the pan-Yugoslav program?
   A. That these groups were a more powerful tool for propaganda than the national ensembles
   B. That the small-scale nature of these groups made them an unlikely vehicle for political separatism
   C. That these groups would eventually adopt the pan-Yugoslav repertoire without official enforcement
   D. That these groups lacked the skill required to perform the complex choreographies of the pan-Yugoslav repertoire

6. The author's primary purpose for discussing amateurism (paragraph 2) is most likely to:
   A. explain the core ideological concept that officials used to redefine folk traditions as a form of state-building.
   B. suggest that the transformation of leisure into work was the most significant cultural policy in socialist Yugoslavia.
   C. argue that the state failed to appreciate the intrinsic artistic merit of the social dances that they appropriated.
   D. describe the process by which amateur performers were later recruited into the professional dance ensembles.

Passage 2 (Questions 7–12)

Victor Moscoso's psychedelic posters have captivated collectors, musicians, and historians alike for decades. Moscoso's freeform innovation brought forth a new type of print that blurred the line between static image and moving picture—now coined as his "moving posters," or his kinetic lithographs. These posters, though few in number, present a broader question for museum curators who must contend with the quandary of installing a shapeshifting medium that refutes standards for works on paper and media art alike.

It is important to note that these posters do not actually have moving parts in the literal sense, like flaps or spinning dials. Instead, they appear to move. When viewed in stable white light, the imagery in kinetic lithographs appears as double (or triple) exposure photography. Dizzying at first glance, the composition is only clarified by flashing lights of the same hues as the inks used in the poster, whether the poster is witness to a psychedelic light show at a dance hall for which it was designed or staged in a museum context. Different portions of the print dissolve one by one as light of the same hue washes out the ink on the page. Red ink vanishes in red light, only to reappear as blue light strikes the poster's surface seconds later. In effect, the dance hall becomes the organizing mechanism, but only for a moment or two. The legibility of the poster is entirely dependent on its environment, destabilized in conventional viewing settings.

In 2021, an exhibition in Moscoso's hometown—A Coruña, Spain—featured his kinetic lithographs in an isolated context within the broader exhibition, further underlining their eccentricity as a medium. As visitors moved through the exhibition, they happened upon a small, glowing room with a cartoonish opening. Curator David Carballal designed the room to house the kinetic lithographs, creating a semi-enclosed space to better experience them. Tube lights hung around the ceiling's perimeter and radiated varying hues, including red and green. Visitors could enter the dynamic room and shift under the colorful hues alongside the posters' cast of characters, including a hovering set of lips and floating butterflies. Looking down at one's hands, glancing across the room at someone else's face, staring at one's shoes—the impact was universal.

The shifting lights above stood in the way of a museum's conventional aims. Changing constantly and skewed by their environment, the lights eliminated visual stability. As the posters oscillated between the categories of print and animation, beholden to the lights' steady flash, the ritual of the museum's concentrated gaze was substituted with the ritual of the psychedelic dance hall, one centered on communal engagement and embodied participation. As Carol Duncan explained in her seminal 1995 essay, the sacredness of the modern museum is deeply tied to its uncluttered and individually lit displays that isolate objects, subsequently elevating them to an otherworldly level through aesthetic choices.

However, although Carballal's installation of the kinetic lithographs could not be further from the white cube world Duncan refers to, I argue it functioned in a similar manner and created a ritual of its own: still an entirely different mode of being but one without the baggage of poised expectations and revelatory observations—one could simply be. In its original context, the light show emphasized a collective experience above an individual one, and the same is true of the communal experience of museumgoers. Regardless of identity, the lights cast a uniform glow onto everyone in the room, projecting a new, heavily saturated existence that allowed visitors to step outside of themselves.

Adapted from A. Barton, "Contemplating Light: Experiencing Victor Moscoso's Psychedelic Lithographs in the Museum." *Arts*. ©2023. Barton et al.

7. Why does the author most likely mention Carol Duncan (paragraph 4)?
   A. To criticize the degree to which Carballal departed from the methods of other curators
   B. To underscore the difference between traditional museum settings and the exhibit of Moscoso's posters
   C. To argue that the experience of viewing art should be elevated to the level of religious ritual
   D. To describe the type of display that the author finds aesthetically pleasing to view

8. The author provides details about the posters' behavior under varying colors of light primarily to support the assertion that they:
   A. embrace a higher standard for works of communal art.
   B. fascinate viewers who are mystified by the way they were created.
   C. create optical illusions that can be disorienting for viewers.
   D. are fundamentally reliant on their surroundings for proper display.

9. What relationship between museums and dance halls is implied in the passage?
   A. Their pursuit of different purposes prevents meaningful evaluation of their relationship.
   B. They are alike in their ability to promote robust physical movement while appreciating art.
   C. They have a common potential to create a powerful joint experience for the people.
   D. They are typically distinct and should imitate each other when displaying unusual items.

10. The primary purpose of the passage is to:
   A. examine the challenges that unconventional media pose to traditional museum curation.
   B. illustrate that communal engagement is a more valuable museum experience than solitary contemplation.
   C. explain the technical process used to create Moscoso's innovative kinetic lithographs.
   D. describe a particular exhibition to explore how a museum can create a meaningful viewer experience.

11. Given the information in the passage, it can reasonably be inferred that the displays in traditional museums:
   A. fail to engage visitors who prefer interactive experiences.
   B. create pressure on viewers to properly respond to these displays.
   C. are more concerned with historical accuracy than with visitor enjoyment.
   D. rely on complex lighting systems to isolate and protect valuable objects.

12. The details of the exhibit room designed by Carballal (paragraph 3) provide support for the idea that:
   A. the display affected the appearance of other items in addition to the posters.
   B. Moscoso's "moving posters" have long attracted the attention of viewers.
   C. under white light, the posters appear to have multiple exposures.
   D. a museum can only display a unique medium in a customized setting.

Answers and Explanations

Passage 1 (Questions 1–6)

Question 1: (D) – Make Deduction

Explanation for Question 1

The passage states that the cultural and artistic associations "assumed the role of embodying socialist principles" (paragraph 1), the desired political values of Yugoslav officials. It also notes that the associations' staged performances served as platforms that "united the working class but also attracted the working intelligentsia" (paragraph 2), thereby promoting a state-endorsed ideology across different social strata. **(D)** is correct because it accurately paraphrases this result in slightly different wording, with "certain political values" as a reference to the socialist principles and "multiple social classes" including both the working class and the intelligentsia.

Wrong Answer Explanations

(A) The passage states these associations were established to "embody socialist principles," which is an explicitly political purpose rather than a cultural one. Paragraph 5 clarifies that local village groups, not these associations, were regarded as the "authentic custodians" of tradition.

(B) Paragraph 2 explicitly states that these associations "not only united the working class but also attracted the working intelligentsia," indicating their purpose was to promote the nation's values across class lines, not to encourage one class to financially support the other.

(C) While the passage mentions international branding (paragraph 1) and the later formation of professional ensembles (paragraph 5), the primary domestic function of the associations described in paragraph 2 was based on "amateurism," not professionalization for international performance.

Question 2: (C) – Describe Purpose

Explanation for Question 2

The author defines folklore as "the cultural production of the people transmitted through generations" (paragraph 1) and identifies Yugoslav dance as an example that "gained momentum in the 1930s." The author then pivots to discuss the "profound transformation" that occurred in the 1940s, when associations were formed that promoted "socialist principles of leisure as work through the execution of folklore." This suggests that the dances were adapted from fulfilling cultural roles to political roles when they were tied to socialist ideology. **(C)** is correct because it explains how the concept of folklore is context for the author's account of Yugoslav dance's transformation.

Wrong Answer Explanations

(A) The author's tone is descriptive, not critical. The passage mentions folklore to establish the past history of the social dances and not to criticize the use of the label by Yugoslav officials in the 1940s.

(B) This choice contradicts the main point of the paragraph, which states that a "profound transformation took place" in the 1940s, altering the function and meaning of these dances.

(D) This choice is too broad. While the passage discusses collective production, its focus is on a specific period beginning in the 1930s and its effect on folk dance, not on a theme spanning all of "Yugoslav history."

Question 3: (D) – Describe Purpose

Explanation for Question 3

The author's primary purpose for a specific part of the passage will be related to how the discussion fits into the author's overall purpose for the passage. The passage as a whole explores the way that Yugoslav officials of the 1940s used social dances to promote socialist ideals, especially "amateurism as a spontaneous collective expression," as described in paragraph 2. The *kolo* and *oro* dances were introduced in paragraph 3, where the author described them as "fostering a sense of equality and collective spirit." In paragraph 4, the author claims that these values "held particular significance for Yugoslav ideologues, who adeptly incorporated them into their propaganda efforts, accentuating themes of unity, equality, and collective solidarity." **(D)** is correct because it connects the details of the dances to their use by the Yugoslav state, which is the author's primary purpose in mentioning them.

Wrong Answer Explanations

(A) The fact that formal training was not required is mentioned in paragraph 4, but the primary reason that the author mentions these dances is not to focus on how they were learned or why they were popular. Instead, the purpose is to introduce the collective nature of the dance, which establishes why Yugoslav officials used them to promote their ideals.

(B) These specific dances are examples of some of the dances that were popular in the Yugoslav republics. However, the author does not use the discussion of these specific dances to evaluate the rationale behind the creation of a pan-Yugoslav repertoire, which is discussed in the final paragraph but never judged by the author.

(C) While the prevalence of the dances might contribute to a sense of their authenticity, the primary purpose of this paragraph within the author's argument is to describe the *specific qualities* of the dance that made it useful for propaganda, not simply to establish its credentials as authentic folklore.

Question 4: (C) – Evaluate Reasoning

Explanation for Question 4

Paragraph 4 describes the inclusive nature of the dance for all participants. The first sentence of paragraph 4 includes the claim from **(C)**, that no formal training is required to partake in these dances. The author proceeds to explain that "proficiency is acquired solely through immersion" and that these dances were performed at a wide variety of events, which would give opportunities for that immersion. Therefore, **(C)** is correct.

Wrong Answer Explanations

(A) This claim is from the middle of paragraph 1. After the author states that the social dances gained momentum in the 1930s, they change the subject to the role of artistic associations in the 1940s. No more details are given about dance in the 1930s, so this claim is not supported with an explanation.

(B) This claim is in the last sentence of the passage, and it is also the first time that local village performing groups are described as the authentic custodians of folklore traditions. Because there is no other mention of these groups and specifically why they were regarded as the authentic custodians of folklore traditions, this claim is not supported with an explanation.

(D) The passage states that the dances are performed at these events but doesn't explain anything about these different kinds of "social gatherings" or how they're able to incorporate dance.

Question 5: (B) – Make Deduction

Explanation for Question 5

According to paragraph 5, the Yugoslav authorities were "cognizant of the potential for folk dance performances to catalyze separatism and nationalism." Their response was to create the pan-Yugoslav program with dances from all regions. Paragraph 5 also states that this decision was "rooted in the principle of brotherhood and unity" and "served as a proactive measure aimed at averting ethnic, religious, and political discord." However, at the end of the paragraph, the author mentions that "local village performing groups were exempted from the pan-Yugoslav program." The authorities must have assumed that these village groups were not likely to promote the separatism or discord that they were trying to prevent with the pan-Yugoslav program. **(B)** attributes this lack of risk to the small size of the village groups and is correct.

Wrong Answer Explanations

(A) This misinterprets the state's strategy. While the groups were seen as "authentic custodians," the passage shows the authorities used the *national ensembles* as their primary tool for propagating the pan-Yugoslav ideology, suggesting they saw those as the more powerful vehicle for their specific political project.

(C) This is unlikely, as the passage presents the pan-Yugoslav program as a deliberate and necessary state intervention to *counteract* regionalism, implying it would not happen naturally.

(D) The passage provides no information to support this assumption. The decision is presented as a political and ideological one, not one based on an assessment of the villagers' abilities. The passage emphasizes their role as "authentic custodians," which suggests respect for their skill, not a dismissal of it.

Question 6: (A) – Describe Purpose

Explanation for Question 6

The author uses paragraph 1 to introduce "a profound transformation" in the performance of social dances in Yugoslavia in the 1940s, noting that this change involved using "cultural and artistic associations" to embody "socialist principles of leisure as work through the execution of folklore." In paragraph 2, the author defines amateurism as "the transformation of leisure into a productive endeavor." Paragraph 2 also states that the officials "regarded amateurism as a fundamental requirement" for people to be a "part of the broader social community." Therefore, the author's purpose in discussing amateurism in paragraph 2 is to explain how Yugoslav officials used the amateurism of cultural and artistic associations to promote their desired values in society. **(A)** is correct.

Wrong Answer Explanations

(B) This is an extreme claim that the author does not make. While the passage details the policy of amateurism, it never claims it was the "most significant" one in the country, which is an unsupported overstatement.

(C) The author's purpose in discussing amateurism is to describe the officials' ideas about "leisure as work" and their appropriation of the dances to promote socialist principles. However, the author never criticizes the Yugoslav officials for failing to appreciate the artistic merit of the dances.

(D) This choice incorrectly links two distinct concepts. The passage discusses amateurism as a principle for the entire populace, while the professional ensembles were a separate development. The author does not present amateurism as a recruitment pipeline.

Passage 2 (Questions 7–12)

Question 7: (B) – Describe Purpose

Explanation for Question 7

The first two sentences of paragraph 4 describe how the shifting light of the poster exhibit "eliminated visual stability" and ran counter to traditional museum displays. The author referred to Carol Duncan's essay to introduce her description of a modern museum. The "uncluttered and individually lit displays that isolate objects" mentioned by the author sound very different from the changing lights and the impact of the poster display described in paragraph 3. Duncan's description therefore emphasizes the difference between the poster exhibit and a traditional museum. **(B)** states that the purpose of mentioning Carol is "to underscore the difference" between the two and is correct.

Wrong Answer Explanations

(A) The author's tone in describing Carballal's exhibit in the passage is positive, so "to criticize" is too negative to match the author's purpose in mentioning Duncan.

(C) While the author's reference to Duncan includes a mention of elevating objects to an otherworldly level, the author gives no reason to connect that idea with religious ritual. And the passage does not argue how art should be experienced, but merely describes different environments for it.

(D) The author does not use the reference to Duncan to introduce a personal preference, and in fact does not express any personal preferences at all in this paragraph.

Question 8: (D) – Evaluate Reasoning

Explanation for Question 8

In paragraph 2, the author states that the "moving posters" do not have parts that literally move, but that they instead "appear to move." The author proceeds to describe how the posters look like "double (or triple) exposure photography" in steady white light and then claims that "the composition is only clarified by flashing lights of the same hues as the inks used in the poster." After elaborating on how "red ink vanishes in red light, only to reappear as blue light strikes the poster's surface," the author uses these details to conclude that the appearance of the poster "is entirely dependent on its environment, destabilized in conventional viewing settings." This is summarized in **(D)**.

Wrong Answer Explanations

(A) The passage states that the posters *refute* standards and create a "quandary" for curators (paragraph 1). It also never claims that the unique features of the posters lead to the creation of a higher standard.

(B) While the passage does say that the posters have "captivated collectors, musicians, and historians alike for decades," it never suggests that these people are mystified by the posters' creation.

(C) The passage does mention that the posters are "dizzying at first glance," but that is before the poster is "clarified" by the use of the varying colors of light. The purpose of describing the light mechanism is to explain *how* the illusion of movement is created, and the central conclusion of that explanation is about the posters' relationship to their environment.

Question 9: (C) – Make Deduction

Explanation for Question 9

The passage first sets up a contrast between traditional museums and dance halls. In paragraph 4, it describes how Carballal's exhibit replaced the "ritual of the museum's concentrated gaze," substituting it with "the ritual of the psychedelic dance hall, one centered on communal engagement and embodied participation." However, the author's main argument in paragraph 5 is that the Carballal exhibition of Moscoso's work actually "functioned in a similar manner" to a dance hall. The author explains this claim by stating that in "its original context," which is the dance hall, "the light show emphasized a collective experience, and the same is true of the communal experience of museumgoers" in this special room. This shows that despite their typical differences, the author believes both venues have the capacity to create a shared experience as stated in **(C)**.

Wrong Answer Explanations

(A) This choice overlooks the author's ultimate argument in the final paragraph: that the special museum installation for the kinetic lithographs successfully created a communal experience, much like that of a dance hall.

(B) The description in paragraph 3 that visitors could enter the Moscoso exhibit "and shift under the colorful hues alongside the posters' cast of characters" refers to shifting appearances under the changing lights, not to the bodily motions of museumgoers. The last sentence of P3 makes this clear by only describing changes in what people see: "looking down at one's hands, glancing across the room at someone else's face, staring at one's shoes." Nothing in the passage suggests "robust physical movement" in museums, so that could not be a common point of connection with dance halls.

(C) **(D)** The author acknowledges differences in their traditional environments but does not make a universal recommendation that museums and dance halls should imitate each other when displaying something unusual.

Question 10: (D) – Describe Purpose

Explanation for Question 10

The passage first introduces Moscoso's kinetic lithographs and describes the way they need to be viewed under shifting lights to be properly viewed. The author then discusses the special exhibit designed by David Carballal to creatively display the posters, emphasizing how people could enter the room to be immersed in the experience of the shifting lights. In the last two paragraphs, the author contrasts this display with traditional museum displays before concluding in paragraph 5 that the special exhibit designed by Caraballal "functioned in a similar manner and created a ritual of its own." Therefore, the author's primary purpose is to describe this display and the special experience that it created for visitors. **(D)** is correct.

Wrong Answer Explanations

(A) While the passage does begin by framing the kinetic lithographs as a "quandary" for curators, its primary focus is not simply to examine this challenge. Instead, it analyzes a specific, successful *solution* to the challenge—the 2021 exhibition—and explores the unique viewer experience that resulted.

(B) The author does not make this value judgment. The passage analyzes the communal experience created by the exhibition and contrasts it with the individual ritual of traditional museums, but it never claims one is "more valuable" than the other.

(C) This choice is too narrow and somewhat out of scope. The technical process of displaying the lithographs is explained in paragraph 2, but the process of creating them is not.

Question 11: (B) – Make Deduction

Explanation for Question 11

In paragraph 4, the author cites Carol Duncan's description of a modern museum as made up of "uncluttered and individually lit displays that isolate objects, subsequently elevating them to an otherworldly level through aesthetic choices." In describing Carballal's exhibit of the kinetic lithographs in paragraph 5, the author claims that this special display was "one without the baggage of poised expectations and revelatory observations." The use of the term "baggage" in particular indicates that the author thinks the traditional displays that elevate objects also create a burden or pressure on viewers to respond according to "poised expectations," which lines up with **(B)**.

Wrong Answer Explanations

(A) While it is a plausible consequence that some visitors *might* be disengaged by traditional displays, the passage never suggests the stronger claim that the displays definitely *will fail* to engage visitors who have this preference.

(C) The passage never discusses the concept of historical accuracy. The author frames the purpose of traditional museum displays in terms of ritual and aesthetics, not education or accuracy.

(D) This choice introduces concepts not supported by the text. The passage mentions "individually lit displays" but never describes their lighting as "complex" or states that their purpose is "protection." The stated purpose of traditional lighting is only to "isolate objects" for aesthetic elevation.

Question 12: (A) – Evaluate Reasoning

Explanation for Question 12

In paragraph 3, the author describes the exhibit location as "a small, glowing room with a cartoonish opening" and adds that Carballal created a "semi-enclosed space" for the exhibit to better experience the posters. The author also describes the changing colors of lights in the room and the way that visitors who entered the room could "shift under the colorful hues alongside the posters' cast of characters." The author concludes the paragraph by writing, "Looking down at one's hands, glancing across the room at someone else's face, staring at one's shoes—the impact was universal." Based on this last sentence, the author described the enclosed space and changing lights to support the idea that the exhibit affected the appearance of everything in that room, like hands, faces, and shoes. **(A)** is correct.

Wrong Answer Explanations

(B) While the first paragraph does state that Moscoso's posters are captivating to many, the specific details of Carballal's exhibition in paragraph 3 are used to illustrate the *nature and effect of that specific display*, not to prove the posters' general popularity.

(C) The fact that the posters look like double exposures under white light is mentioned in paragraph 2. The details of Carballal's exhibit, which used colored, flashing lights rather than stable white light, serve to explain the dynamic experience of the installation, not to support a point about how the posters appear in a different lighting context.

(D) This choice presents an overly strong and unsupported conclusion. The passage uses the Carballal exhibit as a successful case study, but it never claims that a customized setting is the *only* way a museum can display a unique medium. This is a generalization that the author does not make.

UNIT 4

REASONING BEYOND THE TEXT SKILLS

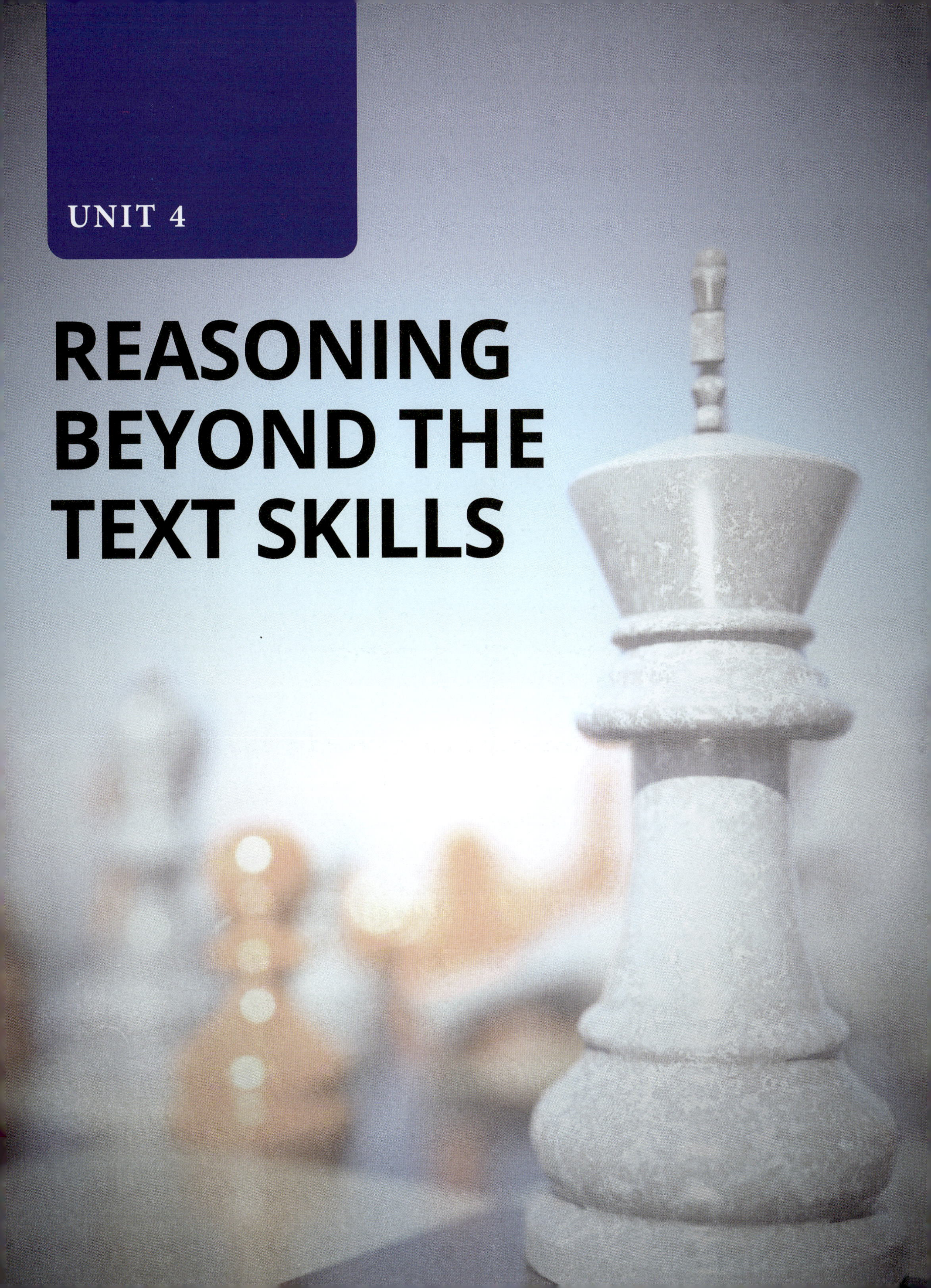

CHAPTER 17

ANTICIPATE RESPONSE

In This Chapter

17.1 Skill Description 264

Finding Clues about the Responder 265

Finding Clues about the Situation and the Response 266

17.2 Question Variations and Examples. . . 267

Identity of the Responder 268

Element Requested 268

Justification in the Answer 269

17.3 Applying the Kaplan Method. 270

Step 1: Type the Question. 270

Step 2: Rephrase the Stem 271

Step 3: Investigate Potential Solutions 272

Step 4: Match Your Prediction. 274

17.4 Skillbuilder. 274

Skill and Strategy Summary 281

LEARNING OBJECTIVES

After Chapter 17, you will be able to:

- Define the Anticipate Response skill
- Recognize who the responder is and what new situation requires a response
- Use passage clues about the responder or other elements of the question to predict a likely response
- Identify common wordings for questions that test Anticipate Response
- Apply the Kaplan Method for CARS Questions to Anticipate Response questions
- Evaluate your current proficiency with the Anticipate Response skill

REASONING BEYOND THE TEXT SKILL

Anticipate Response: Identify what the author or someone else would feel/say/do about a new situation based on its similarities to passage ideas.

Approximate Frequency: 15% of Reasoning Beyond the Text questions

The sociological theories of Max Weber are animated by a profound pessimism regarding the trajectory of modern society. Weber described a process of "rationalization," an inexorable shift toward a social order based on efficiency, calculability, and bureaucratic control. He argued that this process traps humanity in an "iron cage"—a system so dominated by impersonal rules and specialized expertise that it stifles individual spontaneity and human values. In this "disenchanted" world, the charismatic hero is replaced by the technical expert and the career politician. For Weber, this bureaucratic order was our inescapable fate, a vast, self-perpetuating mechanism from which there was no easy exit.

Yet, Weber was no passive fatalist. He believed that even within the iron cage, meaningful political action is not only possible but morally necessary, and advocated for an "ethic of responsibility." He argued that the worth of a political act is not found in its ultimate success, but in the courage of the attempt itself. For Weber, the heroic struggle against the overwhelming forces of the bureaucratic order was the highest expression of human dignity. While he insisted that people must soberly understand the real-world consequences of their actions, he believed that asserting one's values and fighting for a cause was a profound act of human will, and was what gave meaning to political life.

Suppose a political reform movement sought to dismantle a nation's entrenched bureaucratic state and replace it with a system based on direct, community-level democracy. How would Max Weber most likely have viewed the actions of the leaders of this movement?

A. With dismay, because his theories predicted that the movement would ultimately fail

B. With admiration, because of the movement's brave struggle against inexorable historical forces

C. With optimism, because the movement provided a probable counterexample to his more pessimistic theories

D. With suspicion, because he believed that charismatic leaders are ultimately driven by self-interest

17.1 Skill Description

Using the **Anticipate Response** skill is like evaluating how a patient is likely to react to a set of diagnostic test results. Some news might be fine to deliver by email, while other news will clearly merit a personal conversation. Likewise, a patient who might respond to a possibly unwelcome diagnosis with initial denial will need a very different kind of support than one who wants to begin discussing treatment options right away. To achieve the best possible outcome, a physician needs to think in advance about how that individual patient is likely to react, and plan accordingly. They should consider everything they know about the patient's personality and history, as well as about the diagnosis involved.

Successfully answering Anticipate Response MCAT questions requires the same kind of proactive thinking: you have to consider the new information introduced in the question stem within the context of everything the passage tells you about the person whose response you are anticipating, and decide which of four answer choices best represents their most likely reaction.

All Anticipate Response questions share three characteristics:

1. A **situation**: a phenomenon or circumstance (usually something new, but sometimes something dealt with to a varying extent in the passage) that someone is responding to

2. A **responder**: a person or group of people whose reaction is being asked about; approximately half the time it's the author, but the rest of the time it's some other person or group of people mentioned in the passage
3. A **response**: how the responder will probably react to the situation

The passage will always make a connection between the responder and the situation, and that connection is what will allow you to identify the correct answer. To see how this approach works in action, consider the sample question at the beginning of this chapter: Max Weber is the *responder*, the actions of the reform movement's leaders are the *situation*, and Weber's likely view of those actions is the *response* you are looking for among the answer choices.

In dealing with this question, you might be attracted at first to **(A)** because it correctly notes that Weber's "theories predicted that the movement would ultimately fail," and surely Weber would have been dismayed by this fact. However, this interpretation focuses on the wrong part of the passage, because it misidentifies the situation in the question stem. The question doesn't ask about Weber's response to the reforms' *ultimate fate*, or even to the reforms themselves, but about his response to *"the actions of the leaders* of [the reform] movement."

The second paragraph of the passage addresses this issue: Weber believed that "the heroic struggle against the overwhelming forces of the bureaucratic order was the highest expression of human dignity," and that "the worth of a political act is not found in its ultimate success, but in the courage of the attempt itself." So, surely, Weber would not have viewed the leaders of the reform movement and their actions "with dismay," as stated in **(A)**. Instead, Weber would admire and respect them and their "heroic struggle." **(B)** is the correct answer.

As is true for Anticipate Response questions in general, finding the right answer to this sample question depended on gathering information about the responder, properly identifying the situation, and using the links between the responder and situation that were presented in the passage to predict the likely response. This chapter will teach you about clues and strategies you can use to reliably do all of these things, and approach Anticipate Response questions like a seasoned CARS expert.

Finding Clues about the Responder

The more you know about the responder, the more effectively you can attack an Anticipate Response question. Thus, gathering relevant clues about the responder is a crucial component of the Anticipate Response skill.

If the responder is someone other than the author, they may well make only limited appearances in the passage; in this case, there will probably be just one or two major clues associated with them. For example, consider this question stem:

> Based on the passage, which of the following artistic movements would the critics mentioned in paragraph 3 most likely condemn?

Information concerning the responder (the "critics" cited in the stem) will be found in paragraph 3, and will almost surely be restricted to one or two sentences. So it should be pretty easy to find this information, and once you've done so, you will possess a huge clue as to what sort of things the critics mentioned in the stem would "most likely condemn."

Even if the stem doesn't give a paragraph reference, information about a responder who is not the author will often be fairly localized. Consider this stem:

> How would the "consequentialist philosophers" described in the passage most likely view a public policy designed to keep people from harming themselves?

Although no paragraph reference is given, the passage probably mentions more than one group of people—probably even more than one kind of philosopher—so discussion of the "consequentialist philosophers" will probably be confined to only a portion of the passage. Moreover, this stem also provides the additional clue that the relevant information regarding these philosophers will in some way be related to a policy "designed to keep people from harming themselves."

If, on the other hand, most of the passage is devoted to talking about the responder, or if the responder is actually the passage author, the whole passage is in play, and there will probably be a number of potential clues about the responder to choose from. Nevertheless, there will also undoubtedly be other information in the question stem itself, or in the way the answer choices are written, that can help you narrow things down.

BRIDGE

Because Anticipate Response questions always ask you to think about what the passage tells you about the responder, they will often require some of the same types of thinking you will use to answer Recognize Opinion questions (covered in detail in Chapter 9). But this is only part of what you need to do with Anticipate Response, and that's one of the reasons that Reasoning Beyond the Text questions in general can be challenging—because you have to take several steps, each one of which might be enough to find the answer to a Foundations of Comprehension question. On the other hand, it's comforting to realize that the same fundamental skills are involved with even the most challenging questions.

Finding Clues about the Situation and the Response

Consider the following stem:

> Suppose a new scientific study proves the standard belief regarding the use of organic pigments in ancient Roman frescos to be incorrect. The author would most likely react to this news with:

The responder here is the author, so it may seem unclear as to just where in the passage you should look for clues. But notice that a lot of information about the situation is also provided in this stem. Somewhere in the passage, the author must discuss something relevant to "the standard belief" about "organic pigments in ancient Roman frescos," and that's where the best clues for this question will undoubtedly be found. In general, when the responder is the author (or anyone else who appears repeatedly throughout the passage), the most useful clues will relate to the parts of the question stem that talk about the situation or the response. If you can find those clues, you are halfway to finding the correct answer choice.

In addition to identifying the responder, an Anticipate Response question stem will also always include either the situation or the response. If the stem includes the situation (about three-quarters of the time), the answer choices will all be potential responses. If the stem instead includes the response (about a quarter of the time), the answer choices will all be potential situations. Either way, it is important to be able to locate anything in the passage that relates to that hypothetical information. In the question above, for example, the stem outlined a situation—what people believe about the use of organic pigments in ancient Roman frescos—so there must be something in the passage that relates to that situation and tells you how the responder (the author) will likely react.

Sometimes the connection between the responder and the situation will be obvious, but not always. In most of the cases where it's less visible, the hard part will be connecting the situation described in the question to some similar idea from the passage. For instance, the situation in the question stem will often *fit into a broader category* discussed in the passage. Suppose you encounter this question:

> A study of the geographic distribution of cultural resources prompts a billionaire's charitable foundation to donate a new wing to a city's art museum. How would the author most likely view this donation?

In the passage, you find that the author harshly criticizes "large, impersonal philanthropic organizations" for "funding projects based on abstract metrics rather than genuine community needs." Since the situation in the question stem is a perfect example of such an impersonal donation, the author's response is clear—they would disapprove!

Sometimes, on the other hand, the situation will simply be *similar* to something discussed in the passage. Consider this question stem:

> Amos Tutuola's novel *The Palm Wine Drinkard*, which is largely written in a dialect of English sometimes termed "Pidgin," has been criticized for being ungrammatical. How would the author most likely view this critique?

Looking into the passage, you find a sentence in which the author praises Mark Twain's *Huckleberry Finn* as "giving its narrator an authentic voice rather than subjugating him to some artificial standard of so-called 'correct' speech." The aspect of Tutuola's work that is being *criticized* in the question stem is plainly analogous to the aspect of Twain's work that the author praises in the passage. Therefore, you can confidently predict that the author would view the criticism of Tutuola's book as "unfair," "unwarranted," or "unjustified."

Generally, once you have found the link between the situation in the stem and its counterpart in the passage, the passage will usually tell you pretty straightforwardly what the response will be.

Answer choices can provide additional clues about what *kind* of response you're looking for (e.g., approval or disapproval, recommended action, emotional reaction, agreement or disagreement, etc.). For example, consider this question along with its answer choices:

> Based on the passage, the author's reaction to a proposal to fund the arts through a national lottery would likely be one of:
>
> **A.** strong endorsement.
> **B.** cautious optimism.
> **C.** mild disapproval.
> **D.** outright condemnation.

Without a peek at the answer choices, it would be hard to tell what aspect of the author's opinions you should focus on, and how much detail you are going to be asked to provide. A quick scan, though, lets you know that the issue at hand is simply whether—and to what extent—the author would approve or disapprove of the new proposal. Nothing else is really relevant.

BRIDGE

When you find links that relate a situation in the question stem to something in the passage, you are doing some of the same things you do when dealing with Imagine Example/Analogy questions (discussed in detail in Chapter 20), but with Anticipate Response you just have to take an extra step, and think about how the situation will affect the responder. In general, the more you engage in active reading (discussed in detail in Chapter 4), the better you will get at finding such connections and at predicting how a responder will react, since anticipating what comes next and seeing relationships is what active reading is all about!

17.2 Question Variations and Examples

Anticipate Response questions vary in three primary ways: who the responder is, whether the question asks for a response or a situation, and the presence or absence of justification in the answer.

Identity of the Responder

About half or more of the time the responder is the author, but the rest of the time it is some perspective described in the passage.

The Responder Is the Author

In this common format, the passage author responds to the situation.

EXAMPLE QUESTION STEMS

How would the author of the passage most likely view a social media platform designed to maximize engagement by intentionally fragmenting user communities into ideologically isolated "bubbles"?

The author would most likely characterize a government's decision to replace public parks with privately-owned, commercially operated green spaces as:

When the responder is the author, the question stem will usually include the situation as well, and the answer choices will be various possible responses.

The Responder Is Someone Else

It is also common for the responder to be a different person or group whose attitudes are discussed in the passage.

EXAMPLE QUESTION STEMS

The "language poets" described in paragraph 2 would most likely praise a poem that:

How would the consequentialist philosophers discussed in the passage most likely view a public policy designed to keep people from harming themselves?

In the example question stems above, the responder is the language poets and the consequentialist philosophers, respectively.

Element Requested

Questions testing the Anticipate Response skill also vary based on whether they request a response for a given situation or a situation for a given response.

The Answer is a Response

For this variant, your task is to determine the appropriate response to a particular situation.

EXAMPLE QUESTION STEMS

A composer of the Viennese school (paragraph 3) would most likely have reacted to the introduction of polytonality by:

A new biography of Willa Cather focuses on her personal life and largely ignores her work. With which of the following statements about this biography would the author most probably agree?

This is a common variant and includes questions where the responder is the author as well as cases where the responder is another person.

The Answer is a Situation

This less common variant is the reverse of the previous one. The goal is to determine the situation that would have led to the response described in the question stem.

EXAMPLE QUESTION STEMS

According to the passage, which of the following scenarios would be most likely to elicit a feeling of "deep unease" in the Romantics?

One can infer from the discussion that Longinus would have considered an argument sublime if it:

Based on the passage, which of the following narrative structures would the critic Janet Maslin be most likely to dislike?

For this variant, the responder is typically a person other than the author. And a response described in the question stem is usually briefer and simpler, commonly addressing a simple emotional reaction like the "deep unease," "sublime" feeling, and "dislike" in the example stems above.

Justification in the Answer

The answers to Anticipate Response questions can also involve varying degrees of justification. Consider the following question stem:

EXAMPLE QUESTION STEM

Suppose a city decides to replace its historic public library with a modern, multi-use commercial complex. Based on the passage, the author would most likely view this decision as:

The variants below include examples of different potential responses to this stem.

Response Is Not Justified

There is no context or reasoning provided to indicate why the responder would provide the response that the question discusses.

EXAMPLE ANSWER CHOICES

a welcome change.

a regrettable loss.

Response is Justified

These responses are more detailed and include some reasoning along with the reaction or value judgment.

EXAMPLE ANSWER CHOICES

justifiable, because economic development should be prioritized over historical preservation.

misguided, because cultural resources play a crucial role in fostering community identity.

For these questions, the justifications will often reflect the same part of the passage that you would use to predict the nature of the response. There's just an extra step beyond determining the response: first weed out choices with the wrong kind of response, then look for agreement in the remaining justifications with the relevant text you just reread.

17.3 Applying the Kaplan Method

Step 1: Type the Question

As described in Chapter 6, your first step is to read the question stem and glance at the answer choices to assess the question type and difficulty, which will inform your decision to attack it now or save it for later. Always try to identify the broad skill category of the question as Foundations of Comprehension (surface questions), Reasoning Within the Text (deep questions), or Reasoning Beyond the Text (new info questions). Anticipate Response questions, like other RBT questions, can be recognized first by their use of new information.

Identifying the Skill

Whenever a question asks how the author, or someone else from the passage, would react to a new situation, or asks which new situation would most probably provoke a particular reaction, it is an Anticipate Response question.

Sometimes it can be hard to distinguish between Anticipate Response questions and Predict Outcome/Explanation questions (covered in detail in Chapter 18). The key difference is that even though a Predict Outcome/Explanation question may *seem* to ask what someone might do or think, its focus is not really on the responder, but on some other content from the passage.

So, for example, imagine this question stem:

> Which of the following claims would someone who believes Artificial General Intelligence (AGI) systems require a "world model," as described in paragraph 2, most probably make?

BRIDGE

Questions testing the Anticipate Response skill very occasionally have "scattered" variants that involve considering combinations of Roman Numeral statements or ask for reactions/situations that would *not* align with the passage. These variants are very similar regardless of which skill they test, and there is a broader discussion of them in Chapter 10 on the Paraphrase Detail skill, in Section 10.2, defined as the variations "Number of Details Requested" and "Present or Absent Details."

Notice that the "someone" in the question stem is just a prop—they aren't actually someone mentioned in the passage. All you're being told about them is that they have a particular belief, and the focus is on the belief, not the person. Consequently, this would be a Predict Outcome/Explanation question, not an Anticipate Response question. Anticipate Response focuses on a subjective, personal reaction, while Predict Outcome/Explanation focuses on an objective connection of some kind, such as cause and effect.

When you're in the middle of taking the MCAT, the difference between these two question types can sometimes be hard to discern. There's no reason to sweat that fact, though, since you should be able to successfully attack any question that lies close to the dividing line using the strategies and analysis discussed in *either* this chapter or in Chapter 18.

Deciding When to Attack

Anticipate Response questions are Reading Beyond the Text (RBT) or new info questions. This makes them good candidates to triage for later. But just because a question is RBT doesn't mean you *have* to triage it. Make a quick judgment call along the following lines.

If the question gives you the situation and wants you to identify the response, ask yourself if you already feel comfortable about how the situation fits in with what you know about the responder. Do you just need to dip into the passage for a short refresher? Make a prediction and do the question *now*. Are you unsure where in the passage to find the relevant information instead? Save it for *later*.

Likewise, if the question gives you the response and asks you to identify the situation, ask if you feel comfortable with how much you know about the responder and the response (for example, do you know what the passage author would disapprove of?), and whether you already have a sense of what situation might make them react in that particular way.

MCAT EXPERTISE

All this analysis of the triaging step might seem a bit abstract and complicated, but in the end, it's a combination of training, intuition, and practice that will lead to success. The more familiar you become with what the MCAT can throw at you, the better you will be at making these triaging judgment calls. Basically, if you feel you'll be able to make a prediction, and you know where to look in the passage for any information you might need, do the question *now*. Otherwise, triage it for *later*—after you've finished the more straightforward questions on the same passage.

Step 2: Rephrase the Stem

After figuring out that a question is testing the Anticipate Response skill, you have to translate the stem into a specific task. Your first step should be determining whether the responder is the author or someone else. This should be relatively straightforward, as the responder is always called out explicitly in the stem.

If, as in a slight majority of Anticipate Response questions, the responder turns out to be the author, the stem often describes the situation too. If the stem includes a paragraph reference as well, that's where you are going to look in the passage for clues. If there isn't a paragraph reference, your next task is to locate, in the passage, something that is directly linked to the situation described in the stem, and then investigate the surrounding text to see how the author responds to that thing. For example, consider the stem:

> What would the author most likely think of a library policy designed to deter loitering by playing high-frequency sounds that only teenagers can hear?

The author is the responder, so your rephrased tasks become:

- Find something in the passage that relates to a library policy meant to stop teenagers from loitering by playing high-pitched sounds only they can hear.
- Once you find the counterpart to that situation, focus on the same general area in the passage, using Author keywords and other clues to identify the author's probable opinion about such a policy.

If the responder is someone else besides the author, you need to evaluate whether the stem also includes the situation, and the answer choices are potential responses or, alternatively, whether the stem includes the response, and the answer choices are potential situations. Either way, your first job is to locate the responder in the passage.

Then, if the answer choices are responses, and there are many scattered references to the responder in the passage, treat the question much as you would if the author were the responder: find something in the passage that is linked to the situation in the stem, and look for clues about how the responder would react. However, if references to the responder are relatively localized, as they usually are, zero in on that section of the passage (where the responder is discussed) and your clues about the response should be in the same neighborhood. For example, imagine the following stem:

> How would a "Socratic designer," as described in the passage, most likely judge a new software program that is praised for its powerful features but criticized for its steep learning curve?

Your rephrased tasks are:

- First, search the passage for references to "Socratic designer[s]," focus on the portion of the passage that talks about them, and note what opinions and beliefs the author attributes to them.
- Evaluate which of these opinions seems relevant to a software program that's powerful but difficult to learn. This opinion should lead directly to their likely response.

If the responder is not the author, but the answer choices are potential situations, your approach should be very similar. The stem will supply you with a response, which will typically be simple and expressed in one or two words. Your job is to focus on the portion of the passage that discusses the responder, and look for language that describes a reaction consistent with the response mentioned in the stem. Anything in the passage that matches up with that response will be a crucial clue. Consider this example from earlier in the chapter:

> Based on the passage, which of the following narrative structures would the critic Janet Maslin most probably dislike?

Your rephrased task is:

- Check all the references to Janet Maslin in the passage, and look for any that talk about her disliking or disapproving of something. Whatever sort of things the passage says she disapproves of or criticizes will be important clues.

Anticipate Response questions can be intimidating, because every one of them comes with several moving parts. When you rephrase the question stem and transform it into an action plan, however, you simplify it. Here, you can use your active reading skills in much the same way that you simplify a passage when you distill it.

Step 3: Investigate Potential Solutions

After you've rephrased the question stem, it's time to investigate the passage text and make a prediction about the correct answer. The scope of this investigation can vary widely. If your understanding of the responder named in the stem is already very strong, you may not need to do much investigating, but you should at least briefly revisit the relevant parts of the passage anyway to double-check your understanding—sometimes memory plays tricks on us! Then, assuming everything looks okay, use your relevant knowledge of the responder to make a prediction.

If, as is more likely, your understanding of the responder is less comprehensive, use the instructions in your rephrased task and your outline or highlighting from the Distill step of the Kaplan method (discussed in detail in Chapter 5) to guide your investigation.

If the responder is the author, find something in the passage connected to the situation (or, more rarely, the response) specified in the stem. Usually, this will be a *broader category* that includes the situation in the stem, or alternatively, it will be something *similar* to the situation in the stem, and they will *both* fit into the *same* broader category. Your rephrased task is to find that related material in the passage and use it to make a prediction. For example, consider this question:

> How would the author of the passage most likely view the rise of "fast fashion," a trend in which clothing is produced inexpensively to be worn for a single season and then discarded?

Look for anything in the passage related to the description of "fast fashion"— things that are cheap, or things that are disposable—and follow that lead to find out how the author feels about such things. That will be your prediction!

If the responder is *not* the author, your task is to first note what other information the stem gives you. Then look in the passage for references to the responder, and read the surrounding text carefully, searching for anything that links the responder to the other stem information. Finally, use what you discover to make a prediction. For example, consider this question:

> The "19th-century positivists," as described in the passage, would consider an argument valid if it:

In this case, the response (considering the argument valid) is contained in the stem, and the answer choices are situations. Your task is to find the "19th-century positivists" in the passage and understand their core principles. In particular, you want to look for anything that tells you what kind of arguments they would consider "valid." Once you find that, it will be your prediction. Note that predictions for this subset of Anticipate Response questions will typically be broad categories rather than specific situations. So, for the above question, your prediction might be something like "The argument's conclusion follows from its premises, even if the premises aren't true."

Now, imagine a very similar-appearing question:

> The "19th-century positivists," as described in the passage, would most likely have viewed the emergence of abstract art with:

Here, the situation (the emergence of abstract art) is contained in the stem, and the answer choices are responses. Just as with the first example, your task is to find the responder, the "19th-century positivists," in the passage, and understand their beliefs. The passage will undoubtedly also say something about "abstract art" (remember, outside knowledge should never be needed to answer CARS questions—everything necessary will be in the passage). Once you've found that, think about the connection between the positiv-

KEY CONCEPT

As mentioned before, most Anticipate Response questions that ask about somebody other than the author are easier to do passage research on, since you will, in all probability, either know in advance exactly where in the passage to look for information or be able to discover it quickly from your distillation. But even if you don't know where to go, there should be something in the question stem that points to very specific information within the passage. Find that information, and you are well on your way to making a prediction and identifying the correct answer.

ists' beliefs and abstract art's qualities. Your prediction will be the logical extension of that connection, and it should be fairly specific.

Step 4: Match Your Prediction

Anticipate Response questions should always allow you to make some kind of prediction, so you shouldn't examine the answer choices too closely until you have done so. If the answer choices are responses, you should have been able to make a fairly targeted prediction. In this case, simply evaluate the answer choices by comparing them to that prediction.

If, on the other hand, the answer choices are situations, they may well be pretty specific, and your prediction will probably be rather broad. Look for an answer choice that fits within the broader category of your prediction. For example, if the question asks what the responder would be frightened by, and you notice that the passage says the responder is particularly scared of being poisoned by animals, you can scan the answer choices looking for a situation involving some type of venomous spider or snake.

If you can't find a match, or for some reason were not able to make a clear prediction in the first place, you may have to engage in a process of elimination. When doing so, be especially attuned to any answer choice that refers to something in the stem, or something your investigation has revealed as possibly relevant.

Be wary of **Faulty Use of Detail** traps that are based on a misidentification of the situation or the responder mentioned in the stem. These can even be **Opposite** traps, especially if there are people in the passage that disagree with each other—make sure you are thinking about the right responder! Another trap to be on the lookout for is an **Out of Scope** that superficially seems like plausible response, but is not supported anywhere in the passage as a reaction that the responder would have.

REAL WORLD

When you boil things down to their essentials, answering Anticipate Response questions is really no different than figuring out how a friend might react to something you're thinking of saying or doing, or figuring out what to say or do to get your friend to react in a particular way. The key lies in connecting your proposed action to what you know about your friend. It's the same kind of thinking we engage in on an everyday level all the time.

17.4 Skillbuilder

Use the following shortened passage to practice the Anticipate Response skill. The reading is scaffolded to reinforce good active reading habits and to let you devote more of your attention to practicing your critical thinking skills. It includes Active Reading Checks with each paragraph to evaluate how well you're uncovering important passage information at every level. Answer both the Active Reading Check and the CARS question that accompanies each paragraph before continuing. You can check your answers on the next page before you move on to paragraph 2, and the same for paragraph 3.

Paragraph 1

The genesis of a truly new idea remains one of the most mysterious of human experiences. In his landmark work, The Act of Creation, author Arthur Koestler posits that this phenomenon is not divine inspiration; it "does not create something out of nothing." Instead, it "uncovers, selects, re-shuffles, combines, synthesizes already existing facts, ideas, faculties, skills" in a confluence he termed "bisociation." Far from being a simple association, bisociation is a revolutionary spark that connects two self-consistent but previously unrelated conceptual matrices. "The more familiar the parts, the more striking the new whole." Koestler argued this single mechanism underpins all forms of human creativity: in scientific discovery, where new theories or technologies emerge from the synthesis of seemingly unrelated principles; in artistic expression, where juxtaposition forges a new aesthetic experience; and even in a simple joke, where the punchline forces an abrupt and ludicrous shift from one frame of reference to another.

Active Reading Check for Paragraph 1

The examples of "scientific discovery," "artistic expression," and "a simple joke" are mentioned in the first paragraph primarily to:

A. illustrate the wide-ranging applicability of the concept of bisociation.
B. suggest that creativity in the arts and sciences is more significant than the creativity found in humor.
C. provide readers with a practical guide for inducing their own creative revelations.

1. According to the passage, how would Koestler most likely respond to an artist who studied paintings of old masters in order to meticulously recreate their techniques using only historically accurate materials and subjects?

A. He would have praised the artist's technical achievement for scientific rather than artistic creativity.
B. He would have argued that a creative spark is ultimately lacking from the artist's craftsmanship.
C. He would have identified the artist's connection with a conceptual matrix from the past as "bisociation."
D. He would have attributed the artist's ability to a higher power rather than their own imagination.

Active Reading Check for Paragraph 1: (A)

(A) Paragraph 1 presents Koestler's view that a "single mechanism underpins all forms of human creativity" and then lists these diverse examples after a colon to demonstrate this wide-ranging applicability.

(B) While paragraph 1 calls making a joke "simple," this word serves to emphasize the broad applicability of Koestler's "single mechanism" for creativity, not to compare the significance or complexity of humor to the other examples.

(C) Paragraph 1 introduces Koestler's theoretical explanation for "the genesis of a truly new idea," rather than how to implement it in practice.

Question 1: (B)

Answer Choice Explanations for Question 1

(A) While the artist's technical approach might sound more like the "technologies" and "principles" mentioned in the explanation of scientific creativity, paragraph 1 states that Koestler's theory applies to "all forms of human creativity," including science and art, through a "single mechanism," so he would not have separated them in this way.

(B) Painstakingly replicating traditional techniques might involve "uncover[ing and] select[ing] … already existing … faculties [and] skills" within "one frame of reference" but lacks the revelatory "synthesis" of bisociation, which, according to paragraph 1, requires "connect[ing] two … previously unrelated conceptual matrices," not just skillfully working within one.

(C) Paragraph 1 says bisociation involves "connect[ing] two … previously unrelated conceptual matrices," which goes beyond "a simple association." While the artist is reviving traditional methods, they are not combining them with modern or other approaches in a way that "forges a new aesthetic experience."

(D) According to paragraph 1, "Arthur Koestler posits that this phenomenon [creativity] is not divine inspiration" because it "does not create something out of nothing."

Detailed Explanation for Question 1

Skill: The Anticipate Response skill is tested here by asking how someone whose viewpoint is described in the passage would judge the question stem's new, hypothetical scenario.

Question: A new scenario involving an artist who replicates classic techniques is introduced. Koestler is the responder; you need to determine Koestler's likely reaction (his response) by comparing the definition of his bisociation theory of creativity in the passage with the description of the artist's approach in the question stem (which is the new situation).

Passage: Paragraph 1 establishes that for Koestler, true creativity requires "a confluence he termed 'bisociation.'" It is a "revolutionary spark" that results from the "synthesi[s]" of "two … previously unrelated conceptual matrices." When it comes to "artistic expression," this "juxtaposition forges a new aesthetic experience." The artist described in the question stem, however, merely replicates classic techniques, meaning that their work is derivative of a single, pre-existing conceptual matrix. So Koestler would probably conclude that the essential "bi" of "bisociation," the fusion of two disparate modes of thinking in the creative act, is missing from the artist's craft. The correct answer should, therefore, reflect this judgment: The artist may be skillful but not truly creative by Koestler's specific definition.

Answer: **(B)** matches the prediction that Koestler would judge the artist's approach as uncreative for lacking the necessary combination of two disparate ideas, methods, or styles. The other options are inconsistent with Koestler's bisociative definition of creativity.

Paragraph 2

While Koestler's bisociative theory focuses on the dramatic moment of an "intuitive leap," it acknowledges "one should not underestimate ripeness." According to Koestler, this ripeness must develop within the broader cultural and intellectual climate as well as the individual's own conscious reasoning within separate matrices. Once ripe, "the various components which will go into the new synthesis are all lying around and only waiting for the trigger-action of chance, or the catalyzing action of an exceptional brain, to be assembled and welded together." Emphasizing these prerequisites, inventor Thomas Edison is credited with the saying "Genius is one percent inspiration and ninety-nine percent perspiration." Later theorists, such as psychologist Dean Keith Simonton, formalized this "perspiration" model as a process of "Blind Variation and Selective Retention" (BVSR). In this iterative framework, a creator generates a multitude of small variations on an existing idea and, through relentless trial and error, selects the most advantageous ones to form the basis for further adjustments.

Active Reading Check for Paragraph 2

The author introduces the concept of "Blind Variation and Selective Retention" in the second paragraph primarily to:

A. provide a formal model of the effortful aspect of creativity, which the author introduces as an extension of Koestler's concept of "ripeness."

B. present a competing theory of creativity that contradicts the "intuitive leap" of Koestler's bisociation.

C. suggest that the process of innovation is largely up to the random "trigger action of chance."

2. Albert Einstein is apocryphally quoted as saying, "The intuitive mind is a sacred gift and the rational mind is a faithful servant. We have created a society that honors the servant and has forgotten the gift." The passage author would probably react to this claim by:

A. suggesting that, unlike society, Edison actually honors what this quote calls the "gift," while Koestler honors what it calls the "servant."

B. disagreeing because the passage implies that the rational mind and the intuitive mind are simply two different names for the same cognitive process.

C. arguing that the quote's concept of a "sacred gift" reinforces Koestler's view that creativity comes from "divine inspiration."

D. agreeing with the quote's wider premise that it is important to remember the contributions of both the intuitive and rational aspects of the creative process.

Active Reading Check for Paragraph 2: (A)

(A) Paragraph 2 introduces the "relentless trial and error" of BVSR as a formalization of Edison's quote about the importance of "perspiration" in creative genius. The passage author associates this effortful preparation for a breakthrough with the "conscious reasoning" that goes into the individual component of Koestler's "ripeness."

(B) Paragraph 2 says BVSR formalized the "perspiration" proportion of Edison's quote about creative genius while "Koestler's bisociative theory focuses on" the "inspiration" part but "acknowledges" some prerequisites for such an "intuitive leap." So the passage author frames BVSR in continuity with Koestler's framework, with a difference in where attention is focused, rather than an outright contradiction.

(C) Paragraph 2 describes BVSR as a systematic "iterative framework," whereby "a creator generates a multitude of small variations on an existing idea" without intuition as to which will be effective "and, through relentless trial and error, selects the most advantageous ones to form the basis for further adjustments." Within Koestler's theory of creativity, BVSR is consistent with preparatory "conscious reasoning within [a] separate ... matrix" rather than the momentous, intuitive combination of matrices, which can be incited by the "trigger-action of chance."

Question 2: (D)

Answer Choice Explanations for Question 2

(A) The concepts from the quote align with the opposite figures from the passage. Koestler's focus on the "intuitive leap" maps onto the "gift," while Edison's focus on "perspiration" maps onto the rational "servant," although both acknowledge that the other aspect plays a role in creativity.

(B) Paragraph 2 and the question stem quote present two separate aspects of creativity. One is the sudden, revelatory moment: what Koestler calls the "intuitive leap," Edison is said to call "inspiration," and Einstein is said to call the "sacred gift." The other is the preparatory, effortful work: part of what Koestler calls "ripeness," Edison is said to call "perspiration," and Einstein is said to call "faithful servant." Because the passage presents these as distinct concepts with varying significance in the views of Koestler and Edison, they are not simply two names for the same process.

(C) According to paragraph 1, Koestler argues creativity "is not divine inspiration" because it "does not create something out of nothing."

(D) While the passage doesn't explicitly argue that society underappreciates the "intuitive mind," the author is promoting awareness of Koestler's theory, which "focuses on" the "intuitive leap" but also "acknowledges" the importance of effortful preparation, and of Edison's model that "emphasize[s] these prerequisites" as "perspiration" but also recognizes a component of "inspiration." This suggests that by either model the author would agree with the quote's "wider premise."

Detailed Explanation for Question 2

Skill: This question assesses the Anticipate Response skill by requiring you to use the reasoning and attitudes presented by the author in the passage to predict how they would react to a new perspective introduced in the question stem.

Question: The question stem introduces a viewpoint from outside the passage in the form of a quote, often attributed to Einstein, that distinguishes between the intuitive "gift" and the rational "servant." The passage author is the responder; to predict the author's response, start by determining how these two concepts from the quote map onto the different models of creativity discussed in the passage.

Passage: In paragraph 2, Koestler's theory shares the word "intuitive" with the Einstein quote to describe a sudden epiphany and this aligns with the concept of "inspiration" attributed to Edison. The "rational" complement is the gradual preparation that Koestler calls "ripeness" (involving "conscious reasoning") and what Edison is said to call "perspiration" (formalized by the "trial and error" of BVSR). Since the passage explains two models of creativity that both recognize intuition and rationality without favoring Koestler's emphasis on the "gift" or Edison's emphasis on the "servant," the author would likely agree with the quote's wider premise that both aspects of creativity are significant.

Answer: **(D)** is consistent with the prediction; it reflects the balance identified in the author's handling of both components of creativity. The other choices present views that conflict with how the author characterizes the Koestler and Edison models.

Paragraph 3

Edison's own "lightbulb moment" wasn't a simple flip of a switch, but the culmination of countless tests and failures. His team experimented with thousands of materials before settling on a carbonized bamboo filament. The fact that several other inventors globally were on the cusp of a similar invention is powerful evidence for the era's "ripeness"; the essential components were "in the air," waiting for a final synthesis. Edison's bisociative leap connected the circuit with a high-resistance, long-lasting filament, an efficient vacuum sealed within the glass bulb, and a safe system of household electrical power. While Koestler and Edison focus on different aspects of the creative process, they agree the collective, incremental work of a historical moment creates the necessary ripeness, but it is the singular revelation of a prepared mind that ultimately converts potential into illumination.

Active Reading Check for Paragraph 3

The metaphor of "illumination" in the conclusion of paragraph 3 is primarily intended to represent:

A. the light produced when electricity flows through the filament of an Edison bulb.

B. the methodical process of trial and error that precedes a major discovery.

C. the emergence of sudden creative insight that alters understanding of reality.

3. How would the passage author most likely react to the fact that British physicist Joseph Swan developed a working incandescent lightbulb using a carbonized cotton thread filament in a vacuum bulb and publicly demonstrated his invention before Edison?

A. Because the existence of a competitor contradicts the idea of a peerless genius, the author would be confused.

B. Because the contemporary's achievement supports the "ripeness" of the culture for this discovery, the author would be affirmed.

C. Because Swan's incandescent bulb was inferior to Edison's later design, the author would be relieved.

D. Because Swan and Edison both relied on prior scientific discoveries, the author would be uninterested.

Active Reading Check for Paragraph 3: (C)

(A) This is the literal meaning of "illumination" within the lightbulb example, but the question asks for how it is used primarily as a "metaphor." The language in the final sentence of paragraph 3, which notes that a "singular revelation of a prepared mind … converts potential into illumination," indicates that it means a conceptual breakthrough.

(B) Paragraph 3 presents the methodical "countless tests and failures" as the buildup of "potential" that is converted into "illumination," not as the illumination itself.

(C) Paragraph 3 explicitly states that "illumination" is the result of a "singular revelation of a prepared mind," directly linking the metaphor to the moment of sudden creative insight.

Question 3: (B)

Answer Choice Explanations for Question 3

(A) The author does not portray Edison as a peerless genius. In fact, the passage explicitly cites "the fact that several other inventors globally were on the cusp of a similar invention," so the existence of a competitor would not be confusing to the author.

(B) Swan's success is an example that supports the author's argument. Paragraph 3 says "The fact that several other inventors globally were on the cusp of a similar invention is powerful evidence for the era's 'ripeness.'"

(C) The author's argument does not rely on Edison's creativity being superior to his competitors'; in fact, their similar designs support paragraph 3's claim that "the essential components were 'in the air,' waiting for a final synthesis."

(D) The author would be interested because they cite Koestler's theory of "ripeness" in paragraph 2 to explain how "the cultural and intellectual climate" makes ready for a final creative synthesis of prior knowledge from "separate matrices."

Detailed Explanation for Question 3

Skill: By asking how the author would feel about newly presented information based on the context of the passage, this question tests the Anticipate Response skill.

Question: The question stem introduces a new historical fact from outside the passage about an inventor who competed with Edison (the situation). The author is the responder; to determine the author's likely response, review what the passage says about the cultural and intellectual climate surrounding Edison's invention and then assess what impact this new information has on the author's account.

Passage: In paragraph 3, the passage author adopts Koestler's concept of "ripeness" and applies it to Edison's creation of an incandescent lightbulb design by pointing to "the fact that several other inventors globally were on the cusp of a similar invention" as evidence that "the essential components were 'in the air,' waiting for a final synthesis." The new information about Joseph Swan provides a specific example of exactly such an inventor working at the same time as Edison. Therefore, this fact does not challenge the author's argument but instead serves to illustrate the passage's main idea. The correct answer choice must reflect this corroboration.

Answer: Only **(B)** is consistent with how someone would feel about having their argument supported by new evidence. This fits the prediction about the author whose claim about the "ripeness" of Edison's historical environment is "affirmed" by the question stem's example.

Skill and Strategy Summary

Skill Description

- The **Anticipate Response** skill requires you to predict how a responder (the author or another figure from the passage) would likely react to a new, hypothetical situation.
  - Anticipate Response questions make up about 15% of all Reasoning Beyond the Text questions.
- All questions testing this skill involve three components: the responder, the situation, and the response.
- The key to solving these questions is to find a connection in the passage between the responder and the situation.

Question Variations and Examples

- Anticipate Response questions can vary in the following ways:
  - **Identity of the Responder**: The responder is either the author or another perspective discussed in the passage.
  - **Element Requested**: Usually a situation is described in the question stem and the response to it is in the answer choices, but sometimes the response is in the question stem and the situation that prompted it is in the answer choices.
  - **Justification in the Answer**: The response is usually not supported or explained, but in some cases it is accompanied by justification.

Applying the Kaplan Method

- Step 1: Type the Question
  - Identify these questions by looking for a responder from the passage and a new, hypothetical situation, or a hypothetical response, in the stem.
  - Anticipate Response questions are Reasoning Beyond the Text (RBT), making them good candidates to triage (save for *later*) if you are unsure where to find the relevant information in the passage.
  - Be sure to distinguish them from Predict Outcome/Explanation questions, which focus on an objective connection rather than a subjective, personal reaction.
- Step 2: Rephrase the Stem
  - Translate the question into an action plan by identifying the responder, and whether you are looking for the response or a new situation in the answer choices.
  - A quick scan of the answer choices can provide clues about the type of response you should look for (e.g., emotional reaction, value judgment, recommended action, etc.).
- Step 3: Investigate Potential Solutions
  - If the responder is the author, your investigation should focus on finding a connection between the new situation in the stem and a similar topic or broader category already discussed in the passage.
  - If the responder is someone else, the relevant information is usually localized. Go to the part of the passage where that person or group is discussed to find their beliefs and values.
  - Use the information you find to form a prediction about the correct answer.
- Step 4: Match Your Prediction to an Answer Choice
  - Always try to form a prediction before you evaluate the answer choices in detail.

- If the answer choices are responses, your prediction should be targeted. Match the choices against it.
- If the answer choices are situations, your prediction will probably be a broader category. Look for the situation in the choices that fits into that category.
- If you must use the process of elimination, be wary of common traps like **Faulty Use of Detail**, **Opposite**, and **Out of Scope**. Make sure the answer choice refers to the correct responder and is based on the passage text.

CHAPTER 18

PREDICT OUTCOME/ EXPLANATION

In This Chapter

18.1 Skill Description 284
Identifying One-Way Connections........ 285
Following One-Way Connections......... 285
18.2 Question Variations and Examples. . . 286
Direction of Reasoning.................. 286
Where New Information Appears......... 287
18.3 Applying the Kaplan Method....... 289
Step 1: Type the Question................ 289
Step 2: Rephrase the Stem 290
Step 3: Investigate Potential Solutions 291
Step 4: Match Your Prediction to an Answer Choice 291
18.4 Skillbuilder..................... 291
Skill and Strategy Summary 299

LEARNING OBJECTIVES

After Chapter 18, you will be able to:

- Define the Predict Outcome/Explanation skill
- Identify one-way connections in passages and recognize their significance to questions
- Follow one-way connections to reason forward to a likely outcome or backward to a likely explanation
- Recognize common wordings for questions that test Predict Outcome/Explanation
- Apply the Kaplan Method for CARS Questions to Predict Outcome/Explanation questions
- Evaluate your current proficiency with the Predict Outcome/Explanation skill

REASONING BEYOND THE TEXT SKILL

Predict Outcome/Explanation: Apply causal reasoning or another connection from the passage to a new situation.

Approximate Frequency: 15% of Reasoning Beyond the Text questions

The latter half of the 20th century witnessed a profound economic shift in many Western nations, characterized by a process of de-industrialization. As manufacturing jobs, once the bedrock of middle-class stability, were increasingly automated or relocated to regions with lower labor costs, a void was left in the urban employment landscape. This decline in stable, long-term industrial employment did not merely reduce the number of available jobs; it altered the nature of work itself. The erosion of union-based factory work, with its associated benefits and predictable career paths, directly contributed to the rise of what is now termed the "gig economy."

This new economic model is defined by short-term contracts, freelance assignments, and contingent labor, rather than permanent, salaried positions. For the workforce displaced by de-industrialization, the gig economy emerged not as a choice but as a necessity. It offered a patchwork of income streams in place of a single, reliable paycheck. Consequently, the precarity that was once associated with the margins of the economy began to define the mainstream, as workers were forced to trade the security and collective bargaining power of industrial labor for the flexibility—and instability—of independent contracting.

If the widespread adoption of generative artificial intelligence began to automate many tasks traditionally performed by salaried graphic designers, which of the following would be the most likely result, according to the passage?

A. A growing number of former salaried designers would begin competing for temporary design consultant roles.

B. Most displaced designers would find more secure, long-term positions at firms specializing in AI-driven creative work.

C. An increase in independent designers working on a contract basis would lead to a revival of collective bargaining.

D. Design firms would expand their salaried workforce to capitalize on the increased efficiency of the new AI tools.

18.1 Skill Description

Clinical reasoning often involves navigating a chain of cause and effect. Sometimes, you reason forward from a known cause to a likely **outcome**. For example, when a patient with a history of hypertension presents with a severe headache, you immediately consider the potential for a stroke. You are applying an established medical relationship (uncontrolled high blood pressure can cause cerebrovascular accidents) to predict a possible complication.

At other times, you reason backward from a known effect to a plausible **explanation**. A patient with Type 1 diabetes on a new beta-blocker reports dizzy spells. Knowing that beta-blockers can mask the usual symptoms of low blood sugar, you hypothesize that the new medication is the most likely explanation for the patient's symptoms.

Predicting outcomes and finding explanations are two sides of the same cognitive coin. They both require you to master a set of established relationships—the one-way connections between diseases and symptoms, or between drugs and their effects—and apply them to specific clinical scenarios. On the MCAT, the **Predict Outcome/Explanation** skill tests this same ability, asking you to apply a one-way connection from a passage to a new situation.

Identifying One-Way Connections

Predict Outcome/Explanation questions always hinge on a relationship where one idea flows to another. We call these **one-way connections**. Your first and most important job is to find the specific one-way connection in the passage that the question is testing. The best clues for spotting these are the **Connection keywords** discussed in Chapter 3.

While any Connection keyword can be useful, the most high-yield ones for this skill are those that signal **cause and effect**. The author will tell you that one thing happened *because* of another, or that a certain event *led* to a specific result. These words create a directional path that you can follow to the correct answer.

While it might be nice if a passage uses both Cause keywords and Effect keywords to clearly define the terms in the one-way connection, that often isn't necessary. A single keyword of either type can reveal both cause and effect. For example, any statement in the form of "X causes Y" simultaneously identifies the cause (X) and the effect (Y). In short, look both before and after a Cause keyword or an Effect keyword to see if you can identify both sides of the connection. Return to Chapter 3 for additional elaboration on this point.

To see how keywords reveal one-way connections, consider the sample passage from the beginning of the chapter on de-industrialization. The author creates the central one-way connection of the passage in the first paragraph, using an Effect keyword:

> The erosion of union-based factory work, with its associated benefits and predictable career paths, *directly contributed to* the rise of what is now termed the "gig economy."

This keyword "directly contributed to" establishes a clear cause-and-effect relationship that serves as the engine for the rest of the passage. Once you spot this, you can distill the core logic:

- **Cause**: The large-scale loss of stable, union-based jobs
- **Effect**: The rise of a precarious, contract-based economy

By distilling this one-way connection, you have the tool you need to answer any question about it. To recognize that a question is actually asking about a specific one-way connection from the passage, look for similar language in the question stem. For example, a Predict Outcome/Explanation question about a causal connection is almost guaranteed to contain either a Cause keyword or an Effect keyword, such as in the sample question's use of the Effect keyword "result." If a passage contains multiple one-way connections, pay attention to other clues in the stem to make sure you create your prediction based on the right one.

KEY CONCEPT

- **Cause keywords** precede the reason *why* something happened. Be on the lookout for words like *because*, *since*, and *if*; phrases like *due to*; and passive-voice forms of verbs like *caused by*, *produced by*, *explained by*.
- **Effect keywords** precede the *result* of something. Watch for words like *so* and *consequently*; active-voice verbs like *causes*, *produces*, and *explains*; and verb phrases like *leads to*, *results in*, and *contributes to*.

Following One-Way Connections

Once you've identified the right one-way connection, you need to follow it in the direction indicated by the question. This typically involves either reasoning forward from a cause to its effect (predicting an outcome) or reasoning backward from an effect to its cause (predicting an explanation). In either case, you will apply the logic from the passage to a new, analogous situation.

The sample question asks for the "most likely result" if AI automates the jobs of salaried graphic designers. This is specifically an outcome (rather than an explanation), so we need to reason *forward.*

1. Start with the new cause: The question describes the widespread automation of stable, salaried design jobs.
2. Find the analogous cause in the passage and its effect: This new cause is directly analogous to the erosion of stable, union-based factory jobs, which caused the precarity of the gig economy.
3. Predict the analogous effect: Since the causes are analogous, the effects should be too. The effect in the passage was the gig economy, so the most likely result for the designers would be a shift toward a similar system of precarious, independent work.

This is exactly what **(A)** describes: "A growing number of former salaried designers would begin competing for temporary design consultant roles." The stable "salaried" positions are replaced by insecure "temporary" roles, which is a perfect parallel to the passage's one-way connection.

Because answer choices in Predict Outcome/Explanation questions describe situations, they are often wordy, so watch out for the inclusion of ideas that would make an otherwise correct answer go wrong. For example, **(C)** states: "An increase in independent designers working on a contract basis would lead to a revival of collective bargaining." This choice is correct to identify an increase in contract work, which is what makes it tempting. However, suggesting that this would enhance collective bargaining is contradicted by the last sentence of the passage: "workers were forced to trade the security and collective bargaining power of industrial labor for the flexibility—and instability—of independent contracting." Collective bargaining power was traded away forcibly, not increased.

KEY CONCEPT

Cause and effect is a common type of one-way connection, but the MCAT also tests other unidirectional relationships. For example, a passage might state a universal *principle* and describe a specific *application* of that rule, or it might give a general *explanation* for a particular *phenomenon*. The underlying skill is the same: identify the two connected ideas and the direction of the relationship between them, and then apply it. Technically, *evidence* and *conclusion* make up another type of one-way connection, but they are so common in CARS that they are the focus of completely separate skills like Strengthen/Weaken Argument (Chapter 19).

18.2 Question Variations and Examples

Questions that test the Predict Outcome/Explanation skill tend to vary in two primary ways: the direction of reasoning may be forward to an outcome or backward to an explanation, and the new information may appear in the question stem, answer choices, or both.

Direction of Reasoning

With every one-way connection, you can attempt to reason forward (in the direction of connection) or backward (in the opposite direction). For example, a cause always precedes its effect, so reasoning forward for causal relationships begins with a cause and ends with its effect, while reasoning backward moves from effect to cause.

Outcome

Reasoning forward means predicting a cause's effect or another kind of outcome. The question stem will always include a situation, typically a new one described in the stem. The question will ask you to find an expected outcome of the mentioned situation, with answer choices offering descriptions of those potential results.

EXAMPLE QUESTION STEMS

If a government were to implement the economic policies criticized in the second paragraph, the most likely outcome would be:

Suppose that a new trend in fashion rejected the ideal of self-expression through consumption choices. Which of the following positive consequences mentioned in the passage would most likely occur?

According to the logic of the passage, someone who called themselves a pilot despite never flying a plane would be expected to:

The desired outcome is usually a new idea, but sometimes it's something that was already described in the passage, as addressed in the Location of New Information section below.

Explanation

Reasoning backward is the opposite of forward: you move from a situation to the cause of that situation or some other explanation for it. While both variations on the direction of reasoning start with a situation, each treats that situation differently. With predicting an outcome, you treat the situation in the stem like a potential cause that could produce a yet-to-be-seen outcome; with explanations, you treat the situation like a mysterious effect that requires a yet-to-be-discovered explanation.

Explanation questions thus ask you to uncover the explanation that best accounts for the situation while staying in agreement with the passage. Some examples follow.

EXAMPLE QUESTION STEMS

Which of the following, if true, would best explain the sudden decline of the ancient civilization described in the passage?

Suppose a society experiences a rapid increase in social mobility. According to the passage, this phenomenon would most likely be a consequence of:

Imagine the novel discussed in the passage had a different ending in which the protagonist survived. The passage author would most likely justify this alternative narrative decision by:

Where New Information Appears

New information always features in any Reasoning Beyond the Text question, including all those that test the Predict Outcome/Explanation skill. New info can appear in the question stem, the answer choices, or both. These same patterns hold for both outcome and explanation variations.

MCAT EXPERTISE

For both outcome and explanation variations, answer choices strongly tend to be on the long side. Versions that end in a question mark will often have complete sentences or detailed descriptions as correct answers. While not quite as extreme, questions that end with a colon, in which you have to complete the sentence, still tend to have lengthy answers with nuanced details about different situations. Shorter choices occasionally appear with this skill but are very rare.

MCAT EXPERTISE

Scattered variations (see Chapter 6) of Predict Outcome/Explanation are rare and almost always the Roman numeral variety, in which you need to assess three descriptions as possible outcomes or explanations of passage ideas. The new information in these questions consists of the descriptions appearing after each numeral, sometimes with additional new information given before the numerals are listed, providing a shared context for all.

Question Only

Sometimes the question stem will describe a new situation and ask for a specific connection to the passage, such as a passage effect that it could cause or a passage explanation that would best account for it.

EXAMPLE QUESTION STEMS

The emergence of a new, highly contagious virus that primarily affects the elderly would most likely lead to which of the phenomena described in the passage?

Suppose a historian discovers new evidence of widespread peasant revolts in the 14th century. This discovery would be best explained by the author's claim that:

The development of a new form of mass media that allows for instant global communication would, according to the passage, likely result in which of the following?

I. A decrease in the influence of traditional nation-states

II. An increase in the speed of cultural homogenization

III. A decline in the importance of local traditions

MCAT EXPERTISE

When new information only appears in the answer choices, the question stem will generally refer to a situation or other relevant information from the passage with a paraphrase. Paragraph numbers or direct quotations can occur, but both are rare for Predict Outcome/Explanation. Refer back to Chapter 10 on Paraphrase Detail for guidance on locating information in the passage when clues are limited.

Answers Only

In other cases, the question stem will mention a specific situation from the passage, with answer choices containing new outcomes of that situation or new explanations for it. With sentence completion questions (those ending with a colon), some element of the new information could appear in the question stem, but most of the detail will appear in answer choices.

EXAMPLE QUESTION STEMS

The author's critique of Enlightenment rationalism implies that a society based purely on such principles would likely result in:

Based on the passage, the Impressionist painters' break from the Academy would be best explained by which of the following historical developments?

Both Question and Answers

New information may appear in both the question stem and the answer choices. Such questions will give you a new situation and then ask for an explanation or outcome of that situation that will be new as well. While new information appears in both places, these questions are still tied to the passage because they follow the model of a one-way connection from the text. The new cause will be like a cause from the passage, while the new effect will be like the corresponding effect from the passage, so you just need to fill in the missing piece.

EXAMPLE QUESTION STEMS

Suppose a well-known contemporary artist begins producing works that are emotionally detached and highly commercialized. The author would most likely explain this artist's new style as a response to:

Imagine a government sought to suppress free expression through more forceful means than those considered in the passage. Based on the author's argument, one probable consequence would be:

18.3 Applying the Kaplan Method

Step 1: Type the Question

Chapter 6 explains how your first step in attacking a question is to identify its type. This can happen at two levels, one recommended for everyone and a second that's optional after you've completed enough CARS practice. All test takers should aim to identify the broad AAMC skill category (or its Kaplan shorthand): Foundations of Comprehension (surface questions), Reasoning Within the Text (deep questions), or Reasoning Beyond the Text (new info questions).

Identifying the Skill

The second level of typing happens at the skill level. Once you've practiced enough to feel comfortable recognizing every skill in all three categories, you can incorporate a question's skill into your triaging decision.

Like other Reasoning Beyond the Text questions, those that test the Predict Outcome/Explanation skill involve a new situation, often given in the question stem. In a number of cases, the new situation might not seem that "new" because it might rely heavily on ideas from the passage. Consider a question like the following.

> If the author's ideas were applied to a school district, it would be reasonable to expect:

Attached to a passage that never brings up the topic of education, "school district" clearly signals new information. However, in a passage that discussed policies at the level of a classroom or a single school, the expansion to the "district" level would still make this new information. This is important to recognize because the introduction of new information in the question means that the correct answer can extend beyond what is strictly stated or implied in the passage.

If you don't see new information in the question stem, you may instead find topics the passage never mentions in the answer choices when you glance at them. As long as this is true of every choice and not just one or two that are Out of Scope traps (see Chapter 6), you're dealing with Reasoning Beyond the Text. One clue that the answer choices indeed contain new information is the use of hypothetical language like "if," "would," or "could" in the question.

Assuming there is some new information involved, the number one sign of a Predict Outcome/Explanation question in particular is the presence of one or more Connection keywords, especially Cause and Effect keywords. Limiting keywords like "likely," "probable," and "expected" are also common in these questions. See Chapter 3 for more on keywords.

Deciding When to Attack

The default for new info questions is to triage them for *later*. This is especially true for Predict Outcome/Explanation, which tends towards longer question stems and answer choices. The only time they are likely worth attempting *now* is when they're on the shorter side, usually a sentence completion (question ending with a colon) for a relatively short sentence. Be careful though: sometimes short questions can be deceptively difficult, especially in this category, so be willing to pivot if you've spent more than a minute on a question with no clear end in sight.

Step 2: Rephrase the Stem

Once you've identified a question as testing the Predict Outcome/Explanation skill, your next step is to rephrase it into a series of tasks. Generally speaking, the first task will always be finding the relevant cause-effect or other one-way connection from the passage. If the passage contains just one or a few Cause keywords or Effect keywords, this will be quick. The sentences that contain these keywords are likely the ones describing the connection.

If the author instead discusses many causal relationships in the passage, you'll need to pinpoint the one intended by the question. The cause or effect given in the question might exactly match one discussed in the passage, or it might be an example or analogy of one. (See Chapter 20 for explanation of examples and analogies.) Either way, look for similarities between the new information and passage ideas. The relevant connection is the one that's most similar to the new situation, not necessarily at a surface level (the topic could differ) but at the level of its logic or structure.

Some questions become more involved after this first task, but most will just require you to reason in the direction the question provided, toward an outcome or toward an explanation. The process is largely similar with both, though there are questions that will occasionally require more reasoning steps to reach the correct answer.

Let's consider two examples to see some variations in how these questions can be rephrased.

> Suppose a well-known contemporary artist begins producing works that are emotionally detached and highly commercialized. The author would most likely explain this artist's new style as a response to:

The answer choices could be long or short depending on what the passage says, which should affect the length of your prediction but not the way you rephrase the question. This is one way to approach the tasks:

- Find a situation similar to the artists in your distillation or the passage, then look for Cause or Effect keywords that indicate what caused the situation (an explanation), watching especially for any type of reaction against ("response to") something.
- Predict that this something reacted against will be identical to or structurally similar to the explanation in the correct answer.

This general format works regardless of how close the new situation is to the passage, but the difficulty tends to increase when there is greater distance.

With other questions that test this skill, the process will be similar but distinct.

> The author's critique of Enlightenment rationalism implies that a society based purely on such principles would likely result in:

This is relatively short for Predict Outcome/Explanation, but stems like these are often accompanied by more elaborate answer choices. Again, this affects the prediction more than rephrasing.

- Use your distillation to find the author's critique as described, then look for language that suggests consequences or other outcomes (probably negative ones).
- Apply the consequences to a society-wide level, most likely by extending them from an individual case to a collective one, and use that as a predicted outcome.

In both cases, you start by looking for the one-way connection and specify whether it's an explanation or an outcome. Then you find a way to apply that connection to the situation in the question.

Step 3: Investigate Potential Solutions

With a plan in place, you can approach these questions strategically. You'll try to isolate a specific one-way connection in the passage and just reread the text that describes the connection in detail. Once you've found the connection, think about whether the information provided in the stem is the cause (in which case you need an outcome) or the effect (in which case you need an explanation).

Once you know what you need and how the one-way connection is described in the passage, you can formulate a prediction. If you're looking for an outcome, predict that you'll see something identical or similar to the relevant effect from the passage. For an explanation, predict an identical or similar cause. Expect that the correct answer will be adapted to the subject matter and other characteristics of any new situation described in the question.

Step 4: Match Your Prediction to an Answer Choice

With this skill, the correct answer could be something identical to what's described in the passage or just similar in some way. Chapter 20 explains how answer choices can be examples or analogies of ideas in the passage, and you'll find the subskills discussed in that chapter relevant here as well. Be a bit flexible about finding a match, but watch out for anything that contradicts the passage.

Because of their often-lengthy answer choices, Predict Outcome/Explanation questions are susceptible to wrong answer traps that can be introduced by single words or short phrases, such as **Opposite** and **Distortion**. Though the choices are often long, be sure to pay attention to every word if a choice seems like a match to you, in order to avoid these traps.

If you weren't able to make a good prediction, try to connect each answer choice to the situation discussed in the passage and see which best fits. If you're looking for an outcome, ask yourself if you could imagine the passage author describing the cause in the stem leading to the effect in the answer choices. For explanations, would the explanation in the answer for the situation in the stem be consistent with how things are explained in the passage?

18.4 Skillbuilder

Use the following shortened passage to practice the Predict Outcome/Explanation skill. The reading is scaffolded to reinforce good active reading habits and to let you devote more of your attention to practicing your critical thinking skills. It includes Active Reading Checks with each paragraph to evaluate how well you're uncovering important passage information at every level. Answer both the Active Reading Check and the CARS question that accompanies each paragraph before continuing. You can check your answers on the next page before you move on to paragraph 2, and the same for paragraph 3.

This page is intentionally blank. Chapter continues on the next page. ▶ ▶ ▶

Paragraph 1

The Trolley Problem, introduced by philosopher Philippa Foot in 1967, contrasted two dilemmas: a train conductor choosing whether to switch from a track with five endangered people on it to a track with only one, and a surgeon considering whether to kill one healthy patient and harvest organs to save five others. Years later, Judith Jarvis Thomson sharpened the first thought experiment into its most famous form: the choice is made by a bystander who can pull a lever to divert the trolley. Thomson also added the iconic "footbridge" variation in which the bystander must choose whether to push a large stranger off a bridge and onto the tracks in order to stop the trolley and save five people. The starkly different responses—most approve of pulling the lever, while almost all abhor pushing the man—have demanded explanation ever since.

Active Reading Check for Paragraph 1

Why does the author bother to mention both Philippa Foot and Judith Jarvis Thomson?

A. To emphasize that two philosophers were needed to complete the Trolley Problem

B. To show that women have made important contributions to philosophy

C. To illustrate how a famous thought experiment has evolved over time

1. To clear three students falsely accused of misconduct, a dean deliberately frames another innocent student for the offense. According to paragraph 1, how would the community most likely react if this action were exposed?

A. General approval for saving the three innocent students

B. Split opinion about whether the ends justified the means

C. Widespread skepticism about the dean's underlying motivations

D. Virtually universal condemnation of the dean's actions

Active Reading Check for Paragraph 1: (C)

(A) This interpretation implies that the author is trying to highlight the complexity or difficulty of the Trolley Problem, but there is no evidence in the text for that. Furthermore, there is no suggestion that the Trolley Problem is in some way now "complete."

(B) While it is true that Foot and Thomson are both women, the focus of the paragraph is on the development of the thought experiment itself, not on the philosophers' personal characteristics.

(C) The author first introduces Philippa Foot's original 1967 version of the Trolley Problem and then notes that "years later, Judith Jarvis Thomson sharpened the first thought experiment" and "added the iconic 'footbridge' variation." This chronological presentation is intended to show the evolution of the thought experiment.

Question 1: (D)

Answer Choice Explanations for Question 1

(A) The passage states that approval is the typical reaction to the pulling-the-lever scenario, not the "footbridge" scenario, which, like the dean's action, involves personally hurting an innocent person.

(B) Because the dean's action involves directly harming an innocent person, it is clearly analogous to the "footbridge" variation of the Trolley Problem, in reference to which the passage says "almost all abhor" the idea of pushing someone onto the track.

(C) The passage discusses moral judgments about actions themselves, not motivations. Moreover, there is nothing in the question stem that suggests the dean's motives were not altruistic.

(D) Because they involve purposefully and personally hurting someone else in a situation where his options aren't strictly limited, the dean's actions are directly parallel to pushing the man onto the track in the "footbridge" version of the Trolley Problem, which the passage states is met with near-universal disapproval.

Detailed Explanation for Question 1

Skill: Because this question asks you to take the principles and patterns described in the passage and use them to predict the most likely outcome of a new situation, it is testing the Predict Outcome/Explanation skill.

Question: The question asks you to predict the community's reaction to the dean's behavior. First, analyze that behavior: the dean "deliberately frames another innocent student" to save three others. Your task is to determine what in paragraph 1 most closely resembles that action, and then predict the corresponding public reaction.

Passage: Paragraph 1 describes two core scenarios that elicit opposite reactions. The first is "pull[ing] a lever to divert the trolley," which "most approve of." The second is "push[ing] a large stranger off a bridge," an action that "almost all abhor." Why? There are two immediately apparent differences between the actions. In the first scenario, the bystander is presented with only two rigidly defined choices, neither of which involves *personally* harming an innocent person. The second scenario seemingly involves many possible choices, and proactively and deliberately harming an innocent person who was not otherwise in danger. Framing an innocent student for cheating is much more analogous to the latter action, so it makes sense to expect that the vast majority of people would disapprove of it. Scan the answer choices looking for one that articulates this idea.

Answer: Only **(C)** and **(D)** involve largely negative public reaction, but **(C)** focuses on motives, and involves a mild rejection ("skepticism"), whereas the passage uses the much stronger Negative keyword "abhor," and focuses on the dean's act itself, as does **(D)**: "virtually universal condemnation" is correct.

Paragraph 2

One influential interpretation of this result centers on non-maleficence—the philosophical proscription against directly, actively hurting people as a means to an end. An alternative view, however, suggests our judgment is guided by more pragmatic considerations. Pulling a lever is a simple act, and we trust its consequences are predictable. Pushing a person onto the track, however, is physically complex and chaotic, filled with variables that make our internal sense of risk skyrocket: Maybe hitting the man won't stop the trolley, or maybe the five endangered people can evade the trolley without help. This suggests our decision is deeply connected to an intuitive calculation of a given plan's likelihood of going awry.

Active Reading Check for Paragraph 2

What is a major difference between the two explanations the author presents in this paragraph?

A. One explanation involves a philosophical rule, while the other involves a practical judgment.
B. One explanation primarily applies to the Trolley Problem, while the other can be applied to any ethical dilemma.
C. One explanation is older and opposed by the author, while the other is newer and supported by the author.

2. Research shows that most people find actions that harm others much more acceptable when performed indirectly, from a distance. This finding is:

A. consistent with the non-maleficence explanation but inconsistent with the risk-assessment explanation.
B. inconsistent with the non-maleficence explanation but consistent with the risk-assessment explanation.
C. consistent with both the non-maleficence explanation and the risk-assessment explanation.
D. inconsistent with both the non-maleficence explanation and the risk-assessment explanation.

Active Reading Check for Paragraph 2: (A)

(A) The passage introduces the first explanation (non-maleficence) as a "philosophical proscription"; in other words, a rule. It introduces the second explanation as being based on "pragmatic considerations" of a "plan's ... likelihood of going awry," which is a practical judgment.

(B) The passage presents *both* explanations as *general* rationalizations for ethical judgments. In any event, an explanation relevant only to unrealistic hypothetical scenarios such as the Trolley Problem would be largely useless and uninteresting.

(C) The author presents both explanations neutrally, using phrases like "influential interpretation" and "alternative view," without indicating a clear preference for either one. Furthermore, although the passage discusses the non-maleficence explanation first, there are no implications about when either explanation actually originated.

Question 2: (C)

Answer Choice Explanations for Question 2

(A) The research described in the question stem is not inconsistent with the risk-assessment explanation. The more distance that intervenes between an action and its consequences—in terms of both time and space—the less accurately those consequences can be predicted. Thus, actions that may hurt another person will seem more acceptable when they are indirect and distanced, because it is less certain that the person will actually be hurt.

(B) The finding described in the question stem is *not* inconsistent with the non-maleficence explanation: the passage explicitly states that this explanation hinges on how "actively" and "directly" one hurts other people.

(C) The finding aligns both with the principle against direct harm and with the idea that our moral calculus includes estimations of how predictable a given consequence is—the more indirect and distant the prospect of a given action hurting another person, the less likely we are to think that person will really be hurt, and the more acceptable the action will seem.

(D) The finding is consistent with *both* theories—it aligns with the idea that one should avoid "directly, actively hurting people," as well as the idea that the more unpredictable the consequences of a given action are, the less likely we are to take account of those consequences in making moral decisions.

Detailed Explanation for Question 2

Skill: This question tests the Predict Outcome/Explanation skill because it asks you whether theories presented in the passage can explain a new finding in the question stem.

Question: The question points to a general research finding: indirect/distant harm is more acceptable to people than up-close/personal harm. Like the various versions of the Trolley Problem, this research involves thinking about hurting other people; unlike the Trolley Problem, however, it does not posit any counterbalancing positive consequences, and this makes comparing it to the Trolley Problem a bit tricky. Moreover, the stem doesn't provide specific guidance about what needs to be determined regarding the research results. A brief glance at the answer choices resolves the latter issue, though; your task is to determine whether or not the research is consistent with each of the two explanations from paragraph 2 (non-maleficence and risk assessment).

Passage: First, consider non-maleficence, as articulated in the passage, which defines maleficence as "directly, actively hurting people as a means to an end." The finding that people prefer actions that harm others "indirectly, from a distance" is almost a direct paraphrase of the non-maleficence principle, and thus is clearly consistent with it. Next, consider risk assessment: According to that principle, people should find actions with *less* predictable negative consequences preferable to actions with *more* predictable negative consequences. All other things being equal, actions performed "indirectly, at a distance" introduce more intervening variables between cause and effect than do actions performed up close and personal. As such, actions likely to harm others should seem more acceptable when performed indirectly, just as the researchers found. The finding is consistent with both models, so look for the corresponding answer choice.

Answer: **(C)** correctly states that the finding is consistent with both explanations.

Paragraph 3

The risk-assessment model is even more powerful when applied to the surgeon's dilemma. The rejection of the organ-harvesting scenario is nearly unanimous, and while that plan can be seen as the ultimate violation of using someone as a means, common sense also indicates that it's very risky. Will the transplants succeed? Even so, will the five people die soon anyway? Are there other potential donors? There are countless ways for this scheme to backfire and produce devastating unintended consequences. Even if the experimenter asks subjects to assume a guaranteed outcome, our intuition, honed by a lifetime of experience, flags the scenario as inherently unstable, and regardless of whether we consciously accept the experimenter's guarantee, our subconscious distrust is so profound that it inevitably influences our decision making. It's interesting to speculate about how many of our moral judgments may be, at least in part, predicated upon similar analyses.

Active Reading Check for Paragraph 3

What is the author's principal speculation in this paragraph?

- **A.** Many of our ethical beliefs are probably flawed because they are based on faulty risk assessments.
- **B.** Our gut feelings about right and wrong may often be based on subconscious calculations of risk.
- **C.** Experimenters should find ways to improve their outcome guarantees so that they can better study moral decision making.

3. Based purely on ideas expressed in the passage, which of the following is most likely to deter a person from taking a given action in order to achieve a legitimate goal?

- **A.** Months will pass before the anticipated results of the action can occur.
- **B.** The action is technically illegal, although the law is never enforced.
- **C.** The action will harm fewer people than the number of people it helps.
- **D.** Many other people are available who could take the same action instead.

Active Reading Check for Paragraph 3: (B)

(A) This contradicts the passage. The author calls our intuitive risk assessments a form of "common sense" honed by a "lifetime of experience." The passage never suggests that this faculty is "faulty" or that the beliefs derived from it are "flawed."

(B) The final sentence of the passage speculates (the author even uses the word "speculate") that "many of our moral judgments" may be "predicated upon similar analyses" to the "intuitive" and sometimes "subconscious" risk assessment of the surgeon's dilemma discussed in the rest of paragraph 3.

(C) The author's speculation, contained in the passage's final sentence, concerns the nature of human judgment; there is no recommendation for improving experimental methods.

Question 3: (A)

Answer Choice Explanations for Question 3

(A) A long time delay between an action and its hoped-for consequences would most probably increase the perceived complexity and uncertainty of a plan, which paragraph 3 argues should trigger our intuitive distrust and deter action.

(B) Note first that the question stem asks you to consider the scenarios "based purely on ideas expressed in the passage." The passage never discusses or suggests a connection between our intuitive moral judgments and the legality or illegality of our actions.

(C) According to the passage, this fact would serve as an *incentive* to act, not a deterrent.

(D) Note first that the question stem asks you to consider the scenarios "based purely on ideas expressed in the passage." This answer choice is a reference to the *bystander effect*, and although the word "bystander" is used in the passage, that psychological phenomenon is not discussed.

Detailed Explanation for Question 3

Skill: Because it asks you to use the principles in the passage to predict which situation is most likely to lead to a specific outcome (in this case, deterring a person from acting), this question tests the Predict Outcome/Explanation skill.

Question: The question asks you to judge, "based purely on ideas expressed in the passage," which scenario would most likely deter someone from taking an action. To do this, you will have to examine the relationship between the four scenarios described in the answer choices and the passage's discussion of the psychological mechanisms that influence moral decisions. The first step in answering, therefore, should be to make sure you have a firm grasp of that passage discussion.

Passage: Paragraphs 2 and 3 focus heavily on the risk-assessment model. It argues that people possess a powerful "distrust" of complex schemes with many variables, because our intuition recognizes some situations as "inherently unstable." Earlier in the passage, there is a shorter discussion of the "non-maleficence" model, which basically says that we feel it's wrong to hurt other people as a "means to an end," even if that end is something good. With that brief review in mind, it is time to turn to the answer choices, remembering that evaluating them may require revisiting the passage again and checking on various details.

Answer: **(A)** describes a plan with a long time delay between the action and its consequences. This long delay between action and result should increase the plan's complexity and uncertainty, triggering the distrust that is integral to the risk assessment model, and thus deterring action. Right away this seems like the correct choice, but you should still briefly survey the other options to make sure you aren't missing anything. Both **(B)** (legality) and **(D)** (bystander effect) are completely outside the scope of the models described in the passage, and **(C)**, if anything, would be seen as a reason to act rather than a deterrent to action since it involves helping more than harming. **(A)** is definitely correct.

Skill and Strategy Summary

Skill Description

- The **Predict Outcome/Explanation** skill involves the application of one-way connections described in the passage to new situations provided in the question.
  - Predict Outcome Explanation accounts for about 15% of Reasoning Beyond the Text questions.
- **One-way connections**, such as **cause-effect**, can be recognized in both the passage and questions through the use of **Connection keywords** like **Cause keywords** and **Effect keywords** (see Chapter 3).
- To apply a one-way connection in a new situation, identify your starting point (for example, the cause or the effect) and then reason forward (to the effect or other outcome) or backward (to the cause or other explanation) as appropriate.

Question Variations and Examples

- Predict Outcome/Explanation questions can vary in the following ways:
  - **Direction of Reasoning**: Outcome questions move forward (for example, from cause to effect), while Explanation questions move backward (for example, from effect to cause).
  - **Where New Information Appears**: New information might appear only in the question stem and ask for a passage outcome/explanation, or it might appear only in the answer choices as outcome/explanation for something from the passage, or it might appear in both question and answer choices, such as when the cause and effect are both new but analogous to ones in the passage.

Applying the Kaplan Method

- Step 1: Type the Question
  - Recognize the Reasoning Beyond the Text skill category by the presence of new information in the question or choices.
  - Identify the Predict/Outcome Explanation skill by the use of wording that suggests one-way connections, such as Cause keywords and Effect keywords.
  - As new info questions, the default triage decision should be to save these questions for *later.*
- Step 2: Rephrase the Stem
  - Identify the specific one-way connection that the question is based on, along with your starting point, which will also tell you whether you're moving forward or backward.
- Step 3: Investigate Potential Solutions
  - First, find the text from the passage that describes the relevant one-way connection, using your distillation (outline or highlights) if needed.
  - Predict by isolating the most important features of the analogous outcome or explanation from the passage, or otherwise try to apply the one-way connection in the direction needed.
- Step 4: Match Your Prediction to an Answer Choice
  - Choose the choice that is most similar to the cause, effect, or other corresponding term from the passage.
  - If there's no close correspondence between the choices and ideas from the passage, try to relate each choice to the new information and select the option that best connects in the correct direction (forward or backward) without contradicting the passage.
  - Watch out for words or phrases that can make an answer wrong, as can occur with the **Opposite** and **Distortion** wrong answer pathologies.

CHAPTER 19

STRENGTHEN/WEAKEN ARGUMENT

In This Chapter

19.1 Skill Description 302
Identifying the Source of Claims 305
Recognizing the Logical Relationship 306
Predicting the Missing Pieces 307
19.2 Question Variations and Examples . . . 308
Element Requested 308
Where New Information Appears 309
Affirmative or Negative Relationship 311
Location Clues 311
19.3 Applying the Kaplan Method 312
Step 1: Type the Question 312
Step 2: Rephrase the Stem 313
Step 3: Investigate Potential Solutions 313
Step 4: Match Your Prediction to an Answer Choice 314
19.4 Skillbuilder 314
Skill and Strategy Summary 321

LEARNING OBJECTIVES

After Chapter 19, you will be able to:

- Define the Strengthen/Weaken Argument skill
- Assess the logical connection between new claims and passage arguments
- Recognize common wordings for questions that test Strengthen/Weaken Argument
- Apply the Kaplan Method for CARS Questions to Strengthen/Weaken Argument questions
- Evaluate your current proficiency with the Strengthen/Weaken Argument skill

REASONING BEYOND THE TEXT SKILL

Strengthen/Weaken Argument: Characterize the logical relationship between a new claim and arguments from the passage.

Approximate Frequency: 50% of Reasoning Beyond the Text questions

For centuries, the epic poems of the *Iliad* and the Odyssey were attributed to a single ancient Greek poet named Homer. Revered as the foundational genius of Western literature, he was called the one who "has taught Greece" by Plato, "poet sovereign," king of all poets, by Virgil in Dante's *Divine Comedy*, and the "greatest of poets" by Alexander Pope in the preface to his translation of the *Iliad*. This "Unitarian" view posits that both epics are a unified, coherent work of art, the product of a singular creative genius. Proponents of this theory point to the consistent characterizations of heroes like Achilles and Odysseus, the intricate, overarching plot structures, and the masterful use of epic similes as evidence of a single author's deliberate craftsmanship.

However, starting in the 19th century, the "Analyst" school of thought began to challenge this traditional attribution. Analysts argue that the Homeric epics are instead the culmination of a long and fluid oral tradition, compiled over generations. Their primary evidence lies within the texts themselves: they point to narrative contradictions, stylistic variations between different books of the epics, and anachronisms, such as separate passages describing both large battle shields typical of the late Bronze Age when the poems are set and smaller shields of the type found during the early Iron Age when the poems were written. These features, they contend, are not minor flaws expected in a work of this magnitude, but rather reflect the layering of different elements that accumulated from storytellers across the time span of oral tradition.

Which of the following discoveries, if true, would most weaken the "Unitarian" view of Homeric authorship?

A. The *Iliad* and *Odyssey* include words already considered archaic during the early Iron Age and words that only entered the Greek language during that period.

B. Archeological excavations at the site of ancient Troy reveal fortifications discrepant from the descriptions of the city walls in the *Iliad*.

C. Other works sometimes attributed to Homer in antiquity show quantitative differences in metrics of literary style compared to the *Iliad* and *Odyssey*.

D. The goddess Athena aids Achilles during the Trojan War in the Iliad and assists Odysseus on his journey home in the *Odyssey*.

19.1 Skill Description

In your career as a physician, you will order additional laboratory tests, radiologic imaging, or specialist consultations to rule out or confirm likely diagnoses based on preliminary history taking, physical examination, and routine test results. Your job is to determine if new information confirms (strengthens) or contradicts (weakens) the suspected cause of your patient's problem. Does their high white blood cell count support the diagnosis of pneumonia, or does their clean chest X-ray challenge it? Is an ECG finding of ST segment elevation indicative of myocardial infarction, or does the patient's normal blood troponin level point to an alternative etiology for chest pain? The ability to integrate new facts into an existing line of reasoning is crucial to the practice of medicine.

It's no wonder that the **Strengthen/Weaken Argument** skill is tested so frequently on the CARS section of the MCAT. Medical schools are interested in recruiting students who can process information they have elicited from patients and go a step further to identify subsequent diagnostic steps. A good medical school candidate is someone who can tolerate uncertainty and be open to new data during the management of complex clinical situations, rather than fixate on their first impressions and fall prey to confirmation bias.

The elaborative interrogation approach, introduced in Chapter 4, encourages you to treat each passage much like you would take medical histories of the patients in your care on the wards (maybe saving a few of the difficult cases for the end to give them extra attention in your limited time). As you gain practice in reading passages more deeply, you'll pay more attention to elements of the passage's architecture, such as how authors build their arguments. With enough experience, you may even begin to imagine what additional information could reinforce or refute the conclusions presented in the passage as you read.

The sample question at the beginning of this chapter is a prime example of the Strengthen/Weaken Argument skill in action. It asks you to find a new piece of information that, "if true, would most weaken the 'Unitarian' view of Homeric authorship." Clues like "if true" and the subjunctive "would" suggest the answer choices are hypothetical new developments that could change (in this case, cast doubt on) how you originally interpreted the arguments presented in the passage.

If you actively read and distilled the passage, you're more likely to recall what the "Unitarian" viewpoint is in the debate over who authored the Iliad and Odyssey, or at least where to find that theory in the passage. The first paragraph presents it as a longstanding consensus, which "posits that the epics are a unified, coherent work of art, the product of a singular creative genius." This conclusion is signaled by what Chapter 3 would call a Conclusion keyword: "posits."

Your task, therefore, is to find the new revelation among the answer choices that makes this "single author" belief less likely to be true. A good prediction would include any new information that challenges this conclusion head-on or (more likely) does one of the following:

- It discredits evidence the author cited as support for the theory
- It reinforces counterpoints the author cited as problems with the theory
- It has one of the opposite effects on the opposing theory (bolstering its evidence or challenging its flaws)

The correct answer, **(A)**, states that the poems contain a mix of very old ("archaic") words and newer words from a later period. How does this affect the single-author theory? A single person writing at a single point in time would use the language of that specific time. A mix of vocabulary from different eras strongly suggests that the poems were compiled over an extended period by different people, which directly supports the "Analyst" view from paragraph 2 and undermines the "Unitarian" view. It's a powerful weakener of the argument in question.

Notably, **(A)** is analogous (or similar) to evidence that the author cites as support for the opposing "Analyst" theory within the text. In the same way that different passages of the *Iliad* and *Odyssey* describing the designs of battle shields from both the late Bronze Age and the early Iron Age "reflect the layering of different elements that accumulated from storytellers across the time span of oral tradition," so

REAL WORLD

Evidence-based medicine relies on constantly evaluating how new research findings strengthen or weaken established treatment protocols. A new clinical trial might provide strong evidence to adopt a new medication (strengthening the argument for its use) or reveal a side effect that challenges its place as a first-line treatment (weakening the argument). Doctors must constantly assess these logical relationships to provide the best standard of care.

MCAT EXPERTISE

Since the Reasoning Beyond the Text (RBT) category accounts for roughly 40% of questions in the CARS section, and the Strengthen/Weaken Argument skill is tested by roughly 50% of all RBT questions, this skill is central to about 20% of CARS questions overall. It's not uncommon to encounter 10 or 11 such questions on Test Day, so mastering this skill is critical for a strong CARS score!

too do "stylistic variations," including the use of words that did not belong in either the time when the poems are set or when they were written.

Now consider a deceptively tempting wrong answer. **(D)** points out that the goddess Athena plays a consistent role supporting the heroes of both epics. Does this weaken the single author theory? Paragraph 1 states that proponents of the Unitarian viewpoint cite "consistent characterizations of heroes" as evidence for (not against) their theory. A specific textual example of this evidence would therefore strengthen the Unitarian view. This is a classic Opposite trap: it has a strong logical impact and sounds reminiscent of the passage reasoning, but it's the opposite of what the question asks for.

The other two choices seem plausible. **(B)** misses the target. The "discrepancy" in Troy's fortifications could weaken some other argument, perhaps discrediting the historical authenticity of the epics, but it is not relevant to the debate over whether they had one author or several across generations.

Similarly, **(C)** distorts the passage's arguments by alluding to an example that could be confused for the kind of evidence cited as support for the "Analyst" view in paragraph 2: "stylistic variations between different books of the epics." However, these "books" refer to the subdivisions (like chapters) of the *Iliad* and *Odyssey*, rather than other works attributed to Homer in addition to these two epics. Finding "quantitative differences in metrics of literary style" in comparison to other outside works actually suggests an internal stylistic consistency within the *Iliad* and *Odyssey* themselves.

As this sample question reveals, the Strengthen/Weaken Argument skill involves the ability to integrate new information back into the logic of an argument from the passage. An **argument**, as defined in Chapter 3, is fundamentally a logical structure made up of a **conclusion** and the **evidence** that justifies that conclusion. To keep the terminology simple, this book generally uses the terms evidence and conclusion in the affirmative sense that information supports or confirms a specific claim. When the reasoning is flipped, we instead describe a **counterargument** in which a **target** is challenged by **counterpoints**, contrary evidence that makes the target claim less likely to be true.

Thus, evidence can be thought of as strengtheners of conclusions in arguments and counterpoints can be thought of as weakeners of targets in counterarguments. This is not necessarily what those components will be called on the test. Occasionally the test maker uses wording like "evidence that" or "evidence for" to indicate a strengthening relationship, and they may use wording like "evidence against," "counterevidence," or "counterexample" to indicate a weakening relationship. More often, you will find synonyms of the words "strengthen" or "weaken" to indicate the relationship.

All of these terms are relative to one another. The logical support structure for the passage's overall thesis could be called an argument, but so could paragraph- or sentence-level conclusions with increasingly granular evidentiary support. In this way, a claim could be the conclusion of a lower-level argument, which then becomes evidence for a wider conclusion. The evidence for a conclusion could also be a counterpoint against a competing target. This is explained with some examples in the discussion of Logic keywords in Chapter 3.

Your primary task is to identify the two parts of the argument or counterargument: the conclusion or target and the evidence or counterpoint. Of course, you can only assign the specific labels after you know whether the relationship is weakening or strengthening. Sometimes you won't know the nature of the relationship and will instead have to determine how one new idea relates to an

REAL WORLD

The discipline of logic uses the term "premises" to refer to the declarative sentences or "propositions" that lead to a "conclusion" in a valid argument. While you may have been taught other labels for the parts of an argument, recognizing the relationship between these elements is more important than what you call them for answering CARS questions.

idea from the passage. While the answer will usually be some variation of strengthen or weaken, in rare cases there will be other relationships, addressed later in this chapter.

Identifying the Source of Claims

Because the Strengthen/Weaken Argument skill is part of the Reasoning Beyond the Text category, every question will involve a claim that did not appear in the passage. The new claim could be operating as any of the argument elements discussed above.

Before worrying about the logical relationship, your first job is to determine the source of the claims you are being asked to evaluate. For these questions, one part will be new to the question, and the other will come from the passage. The new element could appear in either the question stem or the answer choices, and the passage element will be referenced in the opposite location.

The new element, the touchstone for Reasoning Beyond the Text, is often signaled by hypothetical language, acknowledging that the question stem is adding to the line of reasoning laid out in the passage, and this addition should be accepted as granted for the sake of argument. When the new claim is not hypothetical, the question might directly call it "additional information" or a "new example."

However, this isn't always made explicit. Occasionally, the question stem will present a new claim outright as a truth without any warning. This could be a factual claim that didn't come up in the passage but is somehow relevant, like a real quote that could support or challenge a passage viewpoint or a verifiable example that matches or conflicts with a passage principle. Sometimes these new elements are specific, like "Dr. Martin Luther King Jr. wrote 'Injustice anywhere is a threat to justice everywhere'" or "In *The Canterbury Tales*, Chaucer's Wife of Bath uses her knowledge of the Bible to justify her actions and her views on marriage, reinterpreting passages on celibacy and marriage to suit her perspective." In other cases, these new elements will introduce a school of thought by saying something like "it has been argued..." or "some critics contend..."

Because the new component did not appear in the passage, the question needs to be specific enough for you to be able to assess its relevance. A less common way the new component could appear is as a description of the type of new information rather than stating the new information itself. This could be a summary of the nature of the new information or an appeal to someone with specialized insight on the subject (rather than specifying the content of their input). Such a question could broadly refer to "examples of bourgeois leisure in impressionist paintings" rather than specifying "Renoir's *Luncheon of the Boating Party* depicts a middle-class group socializing in an informal setting."

In contrast to the required specificity of the new element, it is much more common for questions to refer to the preexisting passage element very gener-

BRIDGE

In the same way that the passage author constructs arguments within the text by supporting conclusions with evidence and considering potential counterarguments, any of these elements can also be newly introduced in the question, and the test could ask for a determination of how they are relevant to the passage's established logic. Questions about the logical connections between original parts of the passage test the Evaluate Reasoning skill (Chapter 14) of the Reasoning Within the Text AAMC skill category, and the strategic approach is largely similar. To build your proficiency, pay close attention to how authors construct arguments as you read, and treat every Evaluate Reasoning question you encounter as valuable practice for the Strengthen/Weaken Argument skill.

KEY CONCEPT

Certain words and phrases are reliable clues that the question stem or answer choices are introducing new, hypothetical information from outside the passage. Be on the lookout for conditional language such as:

- if true
- if verified
- suppose that
- assume that
- would
- could

ally. Language like "the author's claims," "the passage thesis," "the passage author's conclusions," "the argument made in the passage," or simply "the passage" mean that the question isn't specifying a particular claim or position from the passage. However, even when the question asks about the passage broadly like this, the relevance of the new information could be at a paragraph- or sentence-level argument rather than directly engaging the passage's overall thesis or main idea.

Sometimes the question will narrow the scope of the passage element to a specific topic and/or viewpoint, and might even provide a paragraph reference, for example "the 'Unitarian' view of Homeric authorship," "Nkrumah's position (paragraph 3)," "the passage author's point about campaign finance regulations," etc. The topic could be named without citing the passage like "da Vinci's influence." You can recognize that this is the preexisting element, the piece that comes from the passage, through your recollection that it was discussed in the passage or by the lack of any suggestion that it is a hypothetical new finding.

Occasionally, the question will paraphrase a specific claim or summarize a position from the passage. This could be worded as "the author's assertion that true folk music is an act of communal creation" or "Muir's view that wild nature has a right to exist, independent of its usefulness to humans" or "the author's advocacy for judging historical figures by the moral standards of their own time."

When these appear in the answer choices rather than the question stem, the right answer is the component of the passage with the specified relevance to the new element introduced in the question. Wrong answers could be actual author claims from the passage that are not relevant or do not have the specified relationship to the new element, or they could be inaccurate distortions of a viewpoint from the passage or one that did not appear in the passage at all.

Recognizing the Logical Relationship

Once you have identified that the question is evaluating the logical relationship between an element from the passage and a new one introduced in the question, the next step is to find where that relationship is characterized. Is it specified in the question stem or to be determined in the answer choices? You may be asked to seek a claim that has the desired relationship or you may be asked to determine the relationship between the new and passage components yourself. When the relationship appears in the answer choices, the question stems will generally ask for the "impact," "effect," or "relevance."

Another way of thinking about this is to label the parts as evidence/conclusion or target/counterpoint. These labels imply their relative relationship. The evidence strengthens a conclusion; a counterpoint weakens the target. Often questions use the actual words "strengthen" and "weaken," but synonyms are also common.

The relationship is not always indicated by a verb. Sometimes a noun is applied to one part of the argument to specify its role. For example, the verb "support" is synonymous with "strengthen" ("this finding most strongly supports..."). However, the noun "support" could also appear ("provides the strongest support for...").

As mentioned previously, the noun "evidence" is generally used in a positive sense as a strengthener, typically paired with "for" or "that" to clarify the relationship ("is evidence that..." or "provides evidence for..."). It is possible

MCAT EXPERTISE

Synonyms of "strengthen" include terms such as *support, affirm, justify, validate, reinforce, substantiate, corroborate, bolster, bear out, give credence to, uphold*, etc.

Synonyms of "weaken" include terms such as *challenge, undermine, damage, disprove, oppose, lose relevance, violate, invalidate, contradict, refute, rebut, counter, dispute, be at odds with, cast doubt on, discredit*, etc.

a question could ask for "evidence against" to indicate a weakening relationship, but terms like "counterevidence" or "counterexample" are plainly negative.

Rather than identifying one element as having the impact (evidence/counterpoint) and the other as being impacted (conclusion/target), occasionally the direction of the impact is unspecified. In these cases, the question may ask for elements that are "consistent" or "inconsistent," that are "in agreement" or that "disagree." Another possibility is "no impact" or irrelevance. These are often one of the answer choices for questions that ask if/how new information is relevant without specifying the desired relationship. Be certain before selecting that the new element has no relevance to the passage by ruling out the possible relationships suggested in the other answer choices.

Miscellaneous logical impacts beyond strengthening or weakening are less frequently listed in answer choices but deserve serious consideration. When they do appear, first confirm they aren't a synonym for strengthen or weaken in disguise. For example, to "complicate" an argument might be a specific way of weakening the connection between evidence and conclusion. Suggesting an assessment was "overestimated" or "underestimated" also calls its veracity into question.

Some logical impacts don't necessarily strengthen or weaken. For instance, a new claim might extend, broaden, or generalize the passage's point to a wider set than the author intended. The opposite could also occur: narrowing the author's claim to exclude a subset by finding an "exception to the rule."

Predicting the Missing Pieces

By identifying what is given in the question stem and what is uncertain in the answer choices, you can find an option that aligns the new and passage elements and the relationship between them. In Reasoning Beyond the Text questions, especially when the new element appears in the answer choices rather than the question stem, formulating a focused prediction of what to look for can be challenging, but a general prediction can still help you save time and avoid traps.

One powerful strategy is to predict the type of missing element rather than the exact content. The previous section on "identifying the source of claims" mentioned an infrequent variation where a category or type of new information is described rather than a specific claim. With many Strengthen/Weaken Argument questions, you'll want to aim for that kind of generality for your answer choice prediction. With a broad prediction, you just select the specific answer that falls into the general category that you predicted.

A second, related strategy is to imagine a specific, concrete example of what is missing from the argument and then evaluate the answer choices based on how analogous they are to what you imagined. Could they bear the same load in the new logical structure? Remember that the relationship between the new element and the passage element is more important than anticipating the details.

The sample question at the beginning of this chapter demonstrated how this is done. The task was to weaken the "Unitarian" view. A strong general prediction, therefore, was to look for something that would undermine support for the single-author theory or bolster support for the multi-author "Analyst" theory. The correct answer matched this prediction as analogous to evidence advanced

BRIDGE

As you will learn in Chapter 20 on the Imagine Example/Analogy skill, recognizing when a new situation is analogous to an idea from the passage is a critical reasoning ability. If you can identify that a new piece of information is an example of or analogous to evidence the author used to support their conclusion, you can predict that this new information will also serve as a strengthener. Conversely, if it is analogous to (or exemplifies) a counterpoint, it will likely function as a weakener.

by the opposition in the passage. Put yourself in the shoes of the passage author and imagine how they would incorporate the new element into their existing reasoning.

19.2 Question Variations and Examples

While the core task of a Strengthen/Weaken question is always to assess the relevance of new claims, the MCAT can present the components of the argument (the passage element, the new element, and their logical relationship) differently. Besides the basic variation between strengthening and weakening, questions can vary with respect to: the element requested as an answer, the location of new information, whether a connection or its absence is sought, and the presence or absence of location clues.

Element Requested

In Strengthen/Weaken Argument questions, the element of the logical relationship that appears in the answer choices can vary: the answer may be the element that strengthens/weakens, the element that is strengthened/weakened, or a characterization of the logical relationship between new information and the passage (strengthening, weakening, or some other description).

Answer Strengthens or Weakens

In this common format, the question stem mentions a claim, and the correct answer choice strengthens or weakens that claim. Each question will ask either for a strengthener or a weakener.

BRIDGE

As described in Chapter 15 on the Make Deduction skill, arguments often rely on assumptions. These hidden connections between evidence and conclusions create a key strategic opportunity for answering questions that test the Strengthen/Weaken Argument skill. An effective way to strengthen an argument is to introduce a new claim that reinforces this unstated connection. Conversely, one of the most effective ways to weaken an argument is to introduce a new fact that contradicts or invalidates an assumption.

EXAMPLE QUESTION STEMS

Which of the following statements, if true, would most strengthen the author's view regarding the theme of alienation in 1970s cinema?

Which of the following findings would most seriously challenge the author's central claim?

Some archeologists contend that English coastal defenses during the Viking era were more sophisticated than previously believed. Which evidence in the passage provides the strongest support for this claim?

In most of these examples, the question stem specifies the desired effect (such as strengthen/support or weaken/challenge) and refers to a conclusion or target from the passage. Sometimes this passage reference is specific, offering a brief paraphrase of the position like "the author's assertion that true folk music is an act of communal creation." More often, however, the reference is general, using broad phrases like "the author's thesis," "the passage argument," or "the author's point about" some topic.

Your task is to find the correct new piece of evidence (a strengthener) or counterpoint (a weakener) in the answer choices that produces the desired effect. In rarer cases, the conclusion or target is a new piece of information (like in the third stem above) with answer choices that come from the passage, but they operate according to a similar logic.

Answer Is Strengthened or Is Weakened

This is the reverse of the previous format and is much less common. The question stem mentions a claim that either strengthens or weakens the correct answer choice, depending on what the question requests.

EXAMPLE QUESTION STEMS

If the population of settlements north of the Arctic Circle were the same in the summer and winter months, this information would most strongly support the author's assertion that:

Assume that a high level of social trust in a society is correlated with economic prosperity. This would most weaken the author's claim that:

In this variant, the question stem almost always introduces new information, and the correct answer is a passage claim that's strengthened (or weakened) by that new information.

Answer Characterizes Impact

This format is quite common as well. The correct answer identifies new information's impact, typically that it strengthens, weakens, or is irrelevant to arguments made in the passage.

EXAMPLE QUESTION STEMS

A newly discovered diary of Åberg reveals that she secretly despised the rural lifestyle she praised in her books. What is the relevance of this information to the passage?

Suppose that adhering to the principle of deontology could lead to a preventable global catastrophe. How would this possibility affect passage claims?

Where New Information Appears

Questions testing the Strengthen/Weaken Argument skill can also vary based on where the new information appears.

Question Only

This format is very common and can include all of the various relationships between the question stem and correct answer described above.

KEY CONCEPT

Words like "suppose," "would," and "if" are reliable clues that a question stem is referring to new information. When one of those words appears at the beginning of the stem, it typically signifies that the question stem is introducing a new claim. When they appear toward the end of the stem, they usually indicate that the answer choices involve new claims.

EXAMPLE QUESTION STEMS

The discovery that ancient scrolls were often edited for political purposes would have what effect on the author's argument?

If it were discovered that a majority of artists in the Renaissance were primarily motivated by financial gain, this finding would most directly weaken which of the following claims made in the passage?

It has been argued that economic inequality is a necessary component of technological innovation. Which of the following examples from the passage would most support this belief?

Answers Only

This variation is also common, and it almost always involves questions where the correct answer has a desired effect on the question stem, as described above.

MCAT EXPERTISE

In Strengthen/Weaken questions that have new information in multiple places, the stem typically provides a starting piece of new information that creates a shared context for all of the new details in the answer choices. You must then find the answer choice that, when combined with the information in the stem, has the desired effect on the passage claim. This can create a multi-step logical chain. For instance, if the new context in the stem weakens the author's argument, the answer choices might essentially ask you to find a "weakener of the weakener"—an additional fact that counters the stem's new information to help the author's original position remain valid.

EXAMPLE QUESTION STEMS

The author's argument that the invention of the printing press was the primary cause of the Protestant Reformation would be most strengthened by the discovery that:

The author's causal explanation for the decline of civic engagement in Western democracies would be most challenged if a new study found that:

Both Question and Answers

This format is rare, and the logic of the question typically involves combining a new claim in the question stem with a new claim in the correct answer to create a desired effect on a passage argument.

EXAMPLE QUESTION STEMS

A new economic analysis reveals that the income gap between university graduates and non-graduates remained static during the mid-20th century. This additional information would most reasonably help to explain the author's claim about the role of public universities in social mobility if:

Suppose present-day meatpackers were surveyed about their support for labor unions. Which of the following findings would most challenge Sinclair's depiction of occupational safety?

Affirmative or Negative Relationship

While most Strengthen/Weaken Argument questions ask for relationships that do exist between the passage and new information, some ask for a relationship that does *not* exist.

Affirmative Relationship

This is much more common. These questions ask for the answer choice that establishes a particular relationship with the passage and/or information introduced in the question stem.

EXAMPLE QUESTION STEMS

Based on the criteria for "great art" discussed in the passage, the author would most likely reject the argument that a new, popular art form is artistically significant if it were shown that:

Which of the following observations would most strengthen the theory of linguistic relativity presented in the passage?

Negative Relationship

In this rare variant, questions ask for the choice that does not establish a particular relationship.

EXAMPLE QUESTION STEMS

Which of the following findings, if true, would LEAST support the author's thesis?

If it were proven that a large, isolated society flourished for centuries without any concept of private property, this discovery would weaken all of the following theories EXCEPT:

Some historians argue that major technological innovations are driven primarily by state funding rather than private enterprise. Which of the following examples from the passage would NOT challenge that thesis?

MCAT EXPERTISE

Questions that ask about the absence of a relationship by using language like "EXCEPT," "NOT," and "LEAST" are inherently more challenging, and they require you to evaluate all four answer choices against the same criterion. Instead of searching for one correct answer, you must find the three that fit to eliminate them. This tendency to need to search in a greater number of places in the passage is why we sometimes refer to these as "scattered" variants. It is almost always a good strategy to save scattered questions for the end of the set.

Location Clues

Strengthen/Weaken Argument questions that ask about specific concepts from the passage can also be categorized based on whether they indicate where the concept is discussed.

No Paragraph Reference

The great majority of questions do not indicate which paragraph ideas mentioned in the question stem appear in, so you must locate the topic or claim yourself.

EXAMPLE QUESTION STEM

Which of the following hypothetical findings, if true, would most seriously challenge the author's central claim regarding the function of myth in pre-literate societies?

Paragraph Reference

For these variants, the question stem directly states the paragraph that mentions a claim or concept that the stem references.

EXAMPLE QUESTION STEM

Which of the following discoveries would offer the strongest support for the author's hypothesis about the fall of the Roman Empire (paragraph 4)?

Questions that provide a paragraph reference usually fall under the previously described variants where the correct answer strengthens (or weakens) the question stem, and where new info only appears in the answer choices.

19.3 Applying the Kaplan Method

Step 1: Type the Question

If reading the question stem thoroughly and glancing at the answer choices reveals new information from outside the passage, you are dealing with a question in the Reasoning Beyond the Text skill category, or a new info question. Conditional wording and other markers of new information are detailed in the "Identifying the Source of Claims" section earlier in this chapter. This feature distinguishes it from both Foundations of Comprehension (surface questions) and Reasoning Within the Text (deep questions). Even when the specific skill is not immediately apparent, recognizing the category informs your expectation of difficulty and triage decision.

Identifying the Skill

When you are asked to incorporate that new information into the logical structure of the passage, you need to use the Strengthen/Weaken Argument skill. In addition to presenting one new part of an argument and one from the passage, the question will involve how they connect. Keywords that ask about this relationship include synonyms of "strengthen" and "weaken," "consistent" and "inconsistent," or neutral effects such as "relevance" or "impact." A more comprehensive listing of relationship terms can be found in the "Recognizing the Logical Relationship" section earlier in this chapter.

Deciding When to Attack

Reasoning Beyond the Text skill questions are often among the most complex and time-consuming on the CARS section because they require you to perform a new logical operation, not just locate information or analyze an existing argument. As such, the best strategy is usually to save these questions for *later* in the set. Secure your points on more straightforward Foundations of Comprehension and Reasoning Within the Text questions first, then return to tackle these more complex challenges with a solid understanding of the passage.

You might choose to attack a Strengthen/Weaken question *now* if the passage claim being targeted is very specific (perhaps with a paragraph reference), you have a strong grasp of it from your initial reading, and the answer choices are short and direct.

Step 2: Rephrase the Stem

After typing the question, your next goal is to translate the test maker's language into a simple, concrete mission for yourself. For this skill, your rephrased task must clearly identify three components: the passage element, the new element, and the logical relationship between them.

Rephrase the question to plainly state which of these pieces the question stem provides and which piece(s) you need to identify in the answer choices. This clarifies your task.

For example, if the question stem is:

> Which of the following statements, if true, would most undermine the author's claim that Impressionism was primarily a rejection of academic tradition?

This question provides the passage element (the claim that "Impressionism was a rejection of academic tradition") and the relationship ("undermine"). Your rephrased task is:

- Find a new fact in the answer choices that weakens the author's claim about Impressionism.

On the other hand, if the question stem is:

> A newly discovered letter reveals that Claude Monet sold several paintings to the French Academy in 1865. This finding has what effect on the passage's argument?

In this case, the new element is specified in the stem. Your task is:

- Determine the relationship between this new fact about Monet and the passage's argument, then find the answer choice that correctly describes it.

Step 3: Investigate Potential Solutions

With your mission clear, you should have a sense of how focused your prediction of the answer choice can be. If the answer choices contain the passage element and/or the logical relationship, you might be able to form a focused prediction about those missing pieces. If the answer choices contain the new element, a more general prediction is required, as the possibilities are endless.

Use the outline or highlights of your distillation to consider the passage element of the question. Is the passage referenced generally, or is a particular topic mentioned, or even a direct claim paraphrased? Is there a paragraph number referenced? Knowing the general structure of the author's argument might be enough to evaluate the relevance of the new information, but sometimes paragraph- or sentence-level claims are the point of impact, even when the question refers to the passage argument generally. Your distillation can help you navigate directly to the relevant text for a quick, targeted review.

In addition to the specific or general passage element referenced in the question, be on the lookout for elements of the passage analogous to the question's new claim that might have the same logical impact. For example, is a new piece of evidence somehow similar (or contrary) to an example or a type of evidence cited as a strength (or weakness) in a passage argument?

This is the time to apply the strategy outlined in the "Predicting the Missing Pieces" section of this chapter. Whether you are working from your distillation alone or from a quick review of the text, your goal is to imagine the missing link. While you can't predict the exact content of a new claim, you can almost always predict its logical role. This general prediction is your most powerful tool for navigating the answer choices and avoiding traps when the new element appears in the answer choices.

Step 4: Match Your Prediction to an Answer Choice

Armed with a focused or general prediction, you can now efficiently assess the answer choices. Systematically compare each option to your prediction, eliminating those that do not reflect the correct logical relationship. Be especially wary of common wrong answer traps that are prevalent for this skill.

The **Opposite** wrong answer pathology is especially common with this skill (e.g., a choice strengthens when you were asked to weaken). This was demonstrated by **(D)** in the sample question at the beginning of the chapter.

Another frequent wrong answer pattern in Strengthen/Weaken Argument question is an answer that strengthens or weakens a different argument or claim than the one the question is addressing. This could be a form of the **Faulty Use of Detail** pathology tailored to RBT questions. **(B)** in the sample question is a good example. It introduces the topic of historical authenticity, which is irrelevant to the passage's central debate about authorship.

Distortion, such as an extreme claim, is not uncommon in answer choices with this skill. Like Faulty Use of Detail, this pathology can be tempting because it uses familiar language from the passage. **(C)** in the sample question applied this misdirection to describe what seemed like (but actually wasn't) an example of a type of evidence cited for one theory in the passage.

One other pattern to be wary of is an answer that requires you to make additional speculation in order to justify it. Such a choice is tempting because it seems highly plausible, despite being unsupported by the text. When the mental gymnastics get too strenuous, reconsider other options before talking yourself into a tenuous logical connection.

19.4 Skillbuilder

Use the following shortened passage to practice the Strengthen/Weaken Argument skill. The reading is scaffolded to reinforce good active reading habits and to let you devote more of your attention to practicing your critical thinking skills. It includes Active Reading Checks with each paragraph to evaluate how well you're uncovering important passage information at every level. Answer both the Active Reading Check and the CARS question that accompanies each paragraph before continuing. You can check your answers on the next page before you move on to paragraph 2, and the same for paragraph 3.

Paragraph 1

Proponents of public and philanthropic arts funding frequently cite as justification for this investment the economic activity that ensues when the community supports theaters, museums, concerts, and festivals. To make this argument, they point to the purchases of various materials and supplies involved in making art, often from local businesses, and to the hiring by arts venues for a variety of box office, security, and other positions. Moreover, prestigious arts venues and events attract tourists who boost the economy with their spending on transportation, lodging, and retail. No one would deny, for example, that New York City realizes a significant commercial multiplier effect from attractions such as the Broadway theater district, the Metropolitan Museum of Art, and the Statue of Liberty. Yet estimates of these economic benefits are often overstated, and justifications of arts funding that rely on projections of economic growth may lead to a misdirection of resources.

Active Reading Check for Paragraph 1

What is the author's opinion of arguments for arts funding that rely on the economic benefits that arts bring to a community?

A. Examples such as New York City's world-famous artistic legacy provide convincing support for such arguments.

B. These arguments are unreliable because they exaggerate the purported economic benefits of arts funding.

C. Though valid, such arguments are incomplete because they ignore the non-economic benefits of the arts.

1. The assertion that the economic activity stimulated by arts funding justifies this use of resources would be supported most persuasively if which of the following statements were true?

A. Regions that surround urban hubs of artistic activity tend to become economically depressed due to tourists favoring the city over its surroundings.

B. Arts events provide entertainment opportunities as enjoyable, educational, and healthful as any other recreational activities.

C. Communities that experience a significant multiplier effect from arts investment have an unusual set of demographic characteristics.

D. Those who allocate funding for projects intended to promote economic growth are most likely to approve proposals to support the arts.

Active Reading Check for Paragraph 1: (B)

(A) The author acknowledges the validity of this evidence for the economic benefits that the arts can bring to a community. However, the author does not conclude that this evidence is "convincing," instead ending the paragraph on a skeptical note.

(B) The author introduces these arguments in the first sentence of the passage and then describes some evidence used by others to support them. However, in the last sentence of paragraph 1, starting with the keyword "yet," the author states their own, contrasting opinion, which is that "these economic benefits are often overstated," or exaggerated. The author goes on to assert that they may result in "a misdirection of resources," indicating that they are unreliable.

(C) While the author is skeptical of the arguments based on economic benefits, they do not say these arguments are flawed because they overlook potential non-economic benefits. In this paragraph, the author does not mention non-economic benefits that the arts may bring to a community.

Question 1: (D)

Answer Choice Explanations for Question 1

(A) If an urban area such as New York City enjoyed economic benefits as described in the passage, but the surrounding region experienced less economic activity as a consequence, this would suggest there's a tradeoff to arts funding, a cost that accompanies any benefits. This choice would weaken the argument, not strengthen it.

(B) This statement does not address the argument, which is about economic benefits. Also, saying that the arts are merely as good as other options does not support funding the arts instead of those other activities. This choice would not strengthen the argument.

(C) If a community needs "unusual" demographics in order to benefit economically from spending on the arts, then most communities will not enjoy the positive economic effects from arts activity that, say, New York City experiences. This choice would weaken the argument, not strengthen it.

(D) Funding proposals that are not approved will have no effect on the community. If proposals for arts funding are more likely to be approved than proposals to fund other activities, then arts funding is more likely to generate economic benefits. This information strengthens the argument of the "proponents of public and philanthropic arts funding."

Detailed Explanation for Question 1

Skill: This question asks you to consider an argument made in the passage and evaluate new information, presented in the choices, to select the fact that is most likely to strengthen that argument. Therefore, this is a Strengthen/Weaken Argument question.

Question: The question refers to a claim made in the passage that arts investment is justified by the economic activity that ensues. This is the claim that the author attributes to "proponents of public and philanthropic arts funding." You are looking for a choice that supports, or strengthens, this claim.

Passage: The first sentence states the claim that this question addresses. Then most of paragraph 1 describes the evidence supporting the claim: artistic activity results in purchases of goods and hiring of staff, and it attracts tourists who spend money, both of which can be observed in cities such as New York. Information that supports the cause-and-effect relationship between arts funding and these economic benefits will strengthen the argument. Choices indicating that arts funding does not generate such positive economic outcomes or that alternative uses of this money would generate better economic outcomes, or choices that are simply irrelevant to this argument, will be incorrect. Because the answer choices consist entirely of new information, a precise prediction is impossible, making the process of elimination the best strategy.

Answer: **(A)** weakens the argument by providing information that arts activity actually depresses the economy of surrounding areas. **(B)** does not address the argument about economic benefits or provide any reason to spend money on the arts instead of on something else. **(C)** weakens the argument by indicating that many communities will not experience a "multiplier effect" (economic benefits) from the arts. **(D)** strengthens the relationship between arts funding and economic activity by saying that arts investment is more likely than other proposals to be approved, making it correct.

Paragraph 2

It is true that arts organizations generate economic activity directly, by creating jobs, and indirectly, by stimulating spending at local businesses. However, this often represents a substitution effect rather than a net economic gain, with every dollar invested in the arts exacting an opportunity cost where it is not invested. For instance, money spent on a theater ticket and a preshow dinner might otherwise have been spent on another leisure activity with a comparable multiplier effect. Similarly, funds directed toward the arts could instead be invested in initiatives like parks development, housing support, or small business incubation, each of which would also generate jobs and economic activity. The same is true of the other instrumental effects of a robust arts scene, which may include improved educational outcomes for youth and better mental health for older adults and individuals with chronic health conditions; all could be achieved at least equally well by investment in, for example, education or healthcare.

Active Reading Check for Paragraph 2

In the context of the passage, the term "substitution effect" in sentence 2 most likely refers to:

A. an economic outcome from investment in one area that could be achieved by investing in other areas instead.

B. the investment of resources in the arts in such a way that the costs equal or outweigh the benefits.

C. the replacement of spending on artistic or cultural experiences with spending on other leisure activities.

2. Suppose that funds made available for housing and small business development often go unused during times of economic uncertainty. How would this fact affect the author's claims?

A. It would reinforce the claim about the multiplier effect of spending on housing and small business.

B. It would undermine the claim about the substitution effect inherent in support of the arts.

C. It would support the claim about the equivalence of the benefits of arts and non-arts investments.

D. It would challenge the claim about the non-economic instrumental effects of spending on the arts.

Active Reading Check for Paragraph 2: (A)

(A) The term "substitution effect" appears in the second sentence of paragraph 2, which states that arts spending "often represents a substitution effect rather than a net economic gain." The author provides several examples where spending on something other than the arts results in comparable economic effects.

(B) The author does not compare the cost of arts investments to the value of their benefits. Instead, the comparison is between the results of spending on the arts and the outcomes of investing money in other sectors.

(C) Spending money on other leisure activities instead of "on a theater ticket and a preshow dinner" is one example used to illustrate the substitution effect. However, "substitution effect" refers to the results of spending in one area rather than another—a failure to generate "a net economic gain"—and not the decision about what to spend money on.

Question 2: (B)

Answer Choice Explanations for Question 2

(A) The author says that spending on housing and small business has a similar economic effect as spending on the arts. However, if the funds for these initiatives go unused, they will have no economic impact. Thus, this information weakens the author's claim about the multiplier effect of these funds.

(B) The author claims a "substitution effect" occurs because spending in other sectors, such as housing and small business, has the same economic benefits as spending on the arts. However, if available funds for these investments are not spent in the community, they will not have the beneficial effect described, and the author's argument is weakened.

(C) The author says that spending on housing and small business has a similar economic effect as spending on the arts. However, if the funds for non-arts activities go unused, they will have no economic impact. Thus, this information weakens the author's claim about the equivalency of these investments.

(D) This choice refers to the "non-economic" effects of arts spending, which the author describes as "improved educational outcomes for youth and better mental health for older adults and individuals with chronic health conditions." The information in the question stem only concerns the availability of funds for non-arts activities, so it has no impact on the author's claims about certain kinds of benefits of the arts.

Detailed Explanation for Question 2

Skill: This question introduces a new fact and asks you to evaluate its effect on the author's argument in the passage. You must determine whether it strengthens or weakens the author's claims, so this is a Strengthen/Weaken Argument question.

Question: The question introduces a new piece of information: that funding for things other than the arts sometimes goes unused. It asks you to evaluate the effect this new information has on the author's argument in the passage. A scan of the verbs in the choices shows that two say the new evidence strengthens the argument ("reinforce," "support") and two say the new evidence weakens the argument ("undermine," "challenge").

Passage: Funding for non-arts activities is discussed in the last two sentences of paragraph 2. Here the author claims that investment in a variety of areas would produce the same outcomes as funding the arts and, therefore, that arts funding has no advantage over these expenditures. Specifically, in the next-to-last sentence, the author says that spending on housing and small business development would have the same economic effects as arts spending. The new information in the question stem suggests, however, that these funds are not always spent when available. If such monies do not flow into the community, they will not have the beneficial effects attributed to them. Thus, in at least some circumstances, such funding may not be equivalent to arts funding, and the author's argument is weakened.

Answer: The fact that available monies for housing and small business may not be spent does not strengthen any part of the author's argument, which hinges on the benefits realized when such investment does occur. Therefore, eliminate **(A)** and **(C)**, which describe strengthening an argument. Eliminate **(D)** because it deals with "non-economic" effects when the author's point is about the economic effects of such spending. **(B)** matches the prediction, as it correctly characterizes the effect of the new information on the author's argument.

Paragraph 3

Given this substitution effect, arguments for arts funding should rely less on benefits that can be realized through other means and instead invoke the intrinsic benefits unique to the arts. A mural that transforms a graffiti-defaced wall into colorful scenes from around the city, a chorus of schoolchildren filling a local park with song, or a performance from the classical theater repertoire—to name just a few examples—can expand individuals' capacity for empathy, engage their minds in rapt absorption, and express communal concerns. The arts serve as a mirror reflecting the community's shared humanity and a lantern illuminating the inner lives of community members, an outcome that other spending priorities cannot claim.

Active Reading Check for Paragraph 3

Based on the examples given in the passage, which of the following would be most likely to demonstrate the "intrinsic benefits" of art that the author mentions?

A. A dance company announces that, in addition to paying its guest stars, it will now pay the dance students in the corps a regular salary.

B. Multimedia artists craft giant papier-mâché puppets for a parade in which the puppets act out key events from the city's history.

C. Members of a ceramics cooperative purchase clay, glazes, and tools from a local merchant and eat lunch at the café next door.

3. Attendance at museums and theaters has trended steadily downward for a number of years. What is the relevance of this fact to the argument in the passage?

A. It weakens it by suggesting that arts venues are conveying diminished intrinsic benefits to the community.

B. It weakens it by indicating that investment in non-arts sectors is increasing in importance to the community.

C. It strengthens it by suggesting that some arts venues will cease operations without increased public or philanthropic investment.

D. It strengthens it by indicating that proponents of arts funding have not sufficiently promoted the arts' intrinsic benefits.

Active Reading Check for Paragraph 3: (B)

(A) The passage does not address whether greater arts funding could result in increasing payments to artists. Moreover, the examples of "intrinsic benefits" in the last paragraph concern psychological and social benefits, not economic benefits.

(B) In discussing "intrinsic benefits," the author gives examples of art that promote psychological and social enrichment. One example is of "a mural [of] colorful scenes from around the city," and the author says that art can "express communal concerns." Therefore, a parade of large puppets that brings the city's history to life—a history that likely influences how the city is experienced by its residents today—is similar to the example in the text.

(C) This is an example of the kind of local economic activity that investment in the arts could generate, but it does not reflect the "intrinsic benefits" described in the last paragraph. Here, the author discusses psychological and social benefits.

Question 3: (A)

Answer Choice Explanations for Question 3

(A) With fewer people exposed to art, fewer people will gain the intrinsic benefits described by the author, such as "expand[ed] capacity for empathy and engage[ment] ... in rapt absorption." Since the author's recommendation to arts proponents rests on arts' ability to convey such benefits, declining attendance weakens the author's argument.

(B) Whether investment in "non-arts sectors" is becoming more or less important is not directly indicated by the new evidence provided, which is only about a trend in the arts.

(C) While it is reasonable to assume that some arts venues are experiencing a negative financial impact from lower attendance, the idea that they will "cease operations" and that the only way to save them is with increased investment is more extreme than is warranted by the evidence.

(D) No information is given about why attendance is falling, so it is not indicated that advocates for arts funding have failed to articulate any particular message.

Detailed Explanation for Question 3

Skill: This question introduces a new fact and asks you to evaluate its effect on the argument in the passage. You must determine whether it strengthens or weakens the author's conclusion, and how it does so, so this is a Strengthen/Weaken Argument question.

Question: The question introduces a new piece of information about a downward trend in attendance at certain arts venues. Your task is to evaluate the information's effect on the author's argument. A scan of the verbs in the choices shows that two say the new evidence weakens the argument and two say the new evidence supports the argument.

Passage: The passage does not discuss attendance at arts events. However, it does talk about the effects of the arts on people and their communities. In paragraph 2, the author asserts that the arts' economic benefits for people and their communities are no greater than those of other sectors, but in paragraph 3, the author concludes that the "intrinsic benefits unique to the arts" are a valid basis for advocating for arts funding. As described in the passage, these intrinsic benefits involve changes in the psychological state of people who view art or attend artistic performances. If, as the question stem states, fewer people are visiting museums and theaters, then the art available in these venues will have less impact. If art is less beneficial for the community because the audience for art is shrinking, then the author's recommendation that proponents of arts funding base their appeals on these benefits is weakened.

Answer: **(A)** matches the prediction, correctly characterizing the effect of the new evidence on the argument. Although **(B)** says the new information weakens the argument, it raises a point about the importance of investment in "non-arts sectors," and the new information speaks only to a trend in the arts. **(C)** and **(D)** state the argument is strengthened rather than weakened, contrary to the prediction.

Skill and Strategy Summary

Skill Description

- The **Strengthen/Weaken Argument** skill asks you to find specific kinds of logical connections between new ideas and passage arguments.
  - Strengthen/Weaken Argument accounts for about 50% of Reasoning Beyond the Text questions.
- Every question involves a new element (from the stem or choices) and a passage element. Your first task is to identify the source of each, then assess their logical relationship.
  - Arguments are composed of evidence (which strengthens) and a conclusion.
  - Counterarguments are composed of counterpoints (which weaken) and a target.
- While many questions strengthen or weaken an argument's stated evidence or conclusion, a powerful alternative focuses on its assumptions—the unstated logical connections between them.

Question Variations and Examples

- Strengthen/Weaken Argument questions can vary in the following ways:
  - **Element Requested:** The correct answer can be a strengthener/weakener, something that gets strengthened/weakened, or a description of a logical relationship (strengthening/weakening/etc.).
  - **Where New Information Appears:** New information can appear in the question stem, the answer choices, or both.
  - **Affirmative or Negative Relationship:** Most questions involve an accurate way of describing the relationship between the passage and new information, while a few ask for a relationship that does not exist.
  - **Location Clues:** Sometimes the question stem directly refers to a specific paragraph, though it usually does not.

Applying the Kaplan Method

- Step 1: Type the Question
  - Recognize the skill by the presence of new information and keywords like *support*, *challenge*, *impact*, or *effect*.
  - As complex new info questions, it is usually best to triage them for *later* in the question set.
- Step 2: Rephrase the Stem
  - Translate the question into a clear mission by identifying the three core components: the passage element, the new element, and their logical relationship.
  - Determine which of these three components you are being asked to find in the answer choices.
- Step 3: Investigate Potential Solutions
  - Begin with your distillation (outline or highlights). Use it to form a general prediction about what the correct answer needs to accomplish.
  - If the question involves a specific passage claim, use your distillation to quickly navigate to the relevant text for a targeted review.
- Step 4: Match Your Prediction to an Answer Choice
  - Systematically compare each option to your prediction.
  - Watch out for common wrong answer traps for this skill, including **Opposite**, **Faulty Use of Detail**, and **Distortion**.

CHAPTER 20

IMAGINE EXAMPLE/ANALOGY

In This Chapter

20.1 Skill Description 324
Examples: Applying a Given Category 325
Analogies: Applying a New Category 327
20.2 Question Variations and Examples . . 328
Element Requested 328
Affirmative or Negative Relationship 329
20.3 Applying the Kaplan Method 330
Step 1: Type the Question. 330
Step 2: Rephrase the Stem 331
Step 3: Investigate Potential Solutions 332
Step 4: Match Your Prediction to an Answer Choice. 332
20.4 Skillbuilder. 333
Skill and Strategy Summary 339

LEARNING OBJECTIVES

After Chapter 20, you will be able to:

- Define the Imagine Example/Analogy skill
- Recognize examples of categories from the passage
- Identify analogies by looking for another example of a passage idea's broader category
- Recognize common wordings for questions that test Imagine Example/Analogy
- Apply the Kaplan Method for CARS Questions to Imagine Example/Analogy questions
- Evaluate your current proficiency with the Imagine Example/Analogy skill

REASONING BEYOND THE TEXT SKILL

Imagine Example/Analogy: Identify new examples of categories defined in the passage or analogies of passage concepts.

Approximate Frequency: 20% of Reasoning Beyond the Text questions

Social dynamics can lead to a particularly thorny difficulty when multiple individuals rely on a shared, limited resource for their economic well-being. The principle known as the "tragedy of the commons" describes a paradox in which individuals, acting in their own self-interest, ultimately deplete the resource, even when doing so is detrimental to the collective group, including themselves. The classic illustration of this concept is a pasture, or "commons," open to all local herders. For any single herder, the incentive to add another animal to their personal flock is compelling; they alone reap the full financial benefit from that animal. The cost, however—a slight increase in overgrazing—is distributed among all herders and is thus a fractional, almost negligible, burden on the individual. Unfortunately, when every herder follows this logic, the result is a collective disaster born from a series of individually rational decisions.

The destructive outcome is not merely the result of inherent human greed but, rather, the product of a system that lacks clear regulation or ownership over a communal asset. The core of the problem lies in the misalignment between individual incentives and the long-term welfare of the group. In such a system, the benefits of exploitation are privatized, while the costs of that exploitation are socialized. This dynamic creates a powerful temptation to consume the resource before someone else does, making conservation seem foolish from a purely individualistic standpoint. The tragedy is therefore the seemingly inescapable ruin of the resource when individuals are trapped in a system that makes cooperation difficult and overconsumption the most logical short-term strategy.

Based on the passage, which of the following scenarios best exemplifies the "tragedy of the commons"?

- **A.** A major sale on a valuable item entices a shopper to buy far more of the item than their family can consume, compelling them to curb expenditures in other budget areas.
- **B.** Multiple independent fishing fleets intensively harvest fish in unregulated international waters, leading to a collapse of the fish population that ultimately harms all fleets.
- **C.** A timber company clear-cuts a forest on its own land to maximize short-term profits, leading to soil erosion that damages the company's long-term prospects.
- **D.** A caterer preparing a buffet dinner for a large event overestimates the number of attendees and is forced to discard a significant amount of uneaten food after the party.

20.1 Skill Description

Applying the **Imagine Example/Analogy** skill is much like the process of clinical diagnosis. A physician learns to appreciate diseases as abstract **categories** of illness, each defined by a cluster of signs and symptoms. When a patient presents with a specific set of findings, the physician's task is to recognize that this concrete case is a real-world **example** of that classic disease category. You use the same skill when a CARS question has you identify a new example of some category introduced in the passage.

This skill of coordinating examples and categories is also the basis of finding **analogies**. Say an author is describing the way DNA encodes for proteins, and a question asks you to find an analogy for this process. Your first step should be to think, what broader abstract category does DNA encoding proteins fall into? One answer would be: instructions for creating a final product. What's another real-world example of instructions for a final product? Blueprints (in architecture) and recipes (in cooking) are two common examples in this category, and both are commonly used as analogies for DNA.

When you use the Imagine Example/Analogy skill, you'll ultimately be relating examples to categories in one of two ways:

- When imagining examples, you apply a *given* category. The passage defines the category explicitly (through stated criteria) or implicitly (through given examples, contrasts, or other clues). An example is a new idea that fits into the category as defined.
- When imagining analogies, you apply a *new* category, one that you have to provide. The passage gives you a description of something, and you determine what broader abstract category it provides an example of. You do this by ignoring more superficial characteristics and isolating the formal or structural features of the example (like the way we ignore the biochemical details of DNA when characterizing it as "instructions"). Once you've identified those structural criteria, an analogy will just be another example that fits into that same new category.

Examples: Applying a Given Category

The most straightforward application of this skill is finding an example of a category that's provided in the passage. These categories might be defined explicitly through a list of criteria, a formal definition, or an informal description. Alternatively, a category might only be defined implicitly, perhaps by contrasting it with opposing categories or by providing a list of examples without additional explanation. Regardless of how the category is defined, you should try to distill its essence into a brief checklist of criteria that you can use to evaluate potential examples.

The way an author defines a category can vary, affecting how you build your checklist.

Categories with Explicit Definitions

The "tragedy of the commons" passage provides a clear definition of a category with several key features. Your first task is to distill this into a mental checklist. The tragedy involves:

1. A shared, limited resource that lacks clear regulation or ownership.
2. Multiple individuals acting independently in their own rational self-interest.
3. A system where the benefits of exploitation are privatized but the costs are socialized.
4. A negative collective outcome where the resource is depleted, harming the entire group.

To find the correct example, you must evaluate each answer choice against this checklist. In **(C)**, a timber company clear-cuts a forest, but it is on the company's own land, so the resource is not shared. In **(D)**, a caterer discards food, but the resource (the buffet) is not depleted by the collective actions of self-interested individuals. The correct answer, **(B)**, is a perfect match: the unregulated international waters are a shared resource, each fleet acts in its own self-interest, and the collective result is the collapse of the fish population, which harms all fleets.

While the sample question presents a more complex definition, often the definition is simpler, requiring a shorter checklist. Such a definition is provided in this excerpt from a passage:

> Richard Wagner is particularly known for his usage of leitmotif—a recurring musical phrase that becomes associated with a specific character, object, or idea—to foreshadow events.

Here, the checklist for an example of the "leitmotif" category is straightforward: (1) a recurring musical phrase and (2) an association with a character or idea.

Categories with Implicit Definitions

While a stated set of criteria makes it easy to define a category, sometimes CARS authors only provide more indirect or "implicit" definitions. One way this is done is by providing a list of examples instead of a formal definition:

> To understand the aesthetic of kitsch, one need not consult a dictionary but rather observe the items that populate a certain stratum of popular taste: the ceramic garden gnome smiling blankly from a manicured lawn; the velvet painting of Elvis Presley; the souvenir snow globe encasing a miniature, glittering Eiffel Tower. The experience extends to the mass-produced figurine of a tearful child, the sentimental landscape printed on a tin serving tray, or the inspirational quote rendered in flowing script over a stock photo of a sunset.

Here, the author never explicitly defines the category of "kitsch." Instead, the reader must recognize the common threads linking the examples—sentimentality, mass production, and a lack of irony or critical depth—to understand the category.

Another common way that categories are defined implicitly is by contrast with a different category that is more clearly defined:

> Historians classify sources based on their relationship to the events being studied. A primary source is an account that offers a direct window into a particular moment in the past. To qualify as a primary source, a document must meet two essential criteria: it must have been created at the time of the events it depicts, and it must originate from a direct participant or eyewitness. A secondary source, by contrast, fails to meet these fundamental requirements of immediacy and direct experience.

The passage defines a secondary source only by what it is not. To get a working definition, just find the opposite of the two criteria provided for primary sources, like so:

1. **Primary source**
   - Written during the time period
   - By a direct participant or eyewitness
2. **Secondary source**
   - Written after the time period
   - By someone who wasn't at the event

Be careful how you conceptualize the opposite: in this case, "after" is effectively the opposite of "during" because "before" is not an option for historical accounts of events. If a question asked you for an example of a secondary source, you might imagine a modern biography of a historical figure or a textbook about an ancient civilization—both are written after the fact by non-participants.

More commonly, a category won't be defined exclusively by contrast, but the contrast will instead supplement the affirmative characteristics of the category that the author provides:

> Postmodern architecture emerged as a reaction against the rigid formalism and perceived elitism of modernism. Instead of pursuing a single, universal style, postmodern design embraces eclecticism, irony, and historical references.

BRIDGE

When you're asked for an example of a category the author explicitly or implicitly defined, your first step is similar to the Interpret Meaning skill: locate the definition, using punctuation and context as guides. The key difference with Imagine Example/Analogy is that you then *apply* that definition to a new example presented in the answer choices. For more on Interpret Meaning, see Chapter 8.

A checklist for an example of postmodernism should include "combines familiar elements in an obviously new or playful way." Crucially, it should also include "avoid characteristics like 'rigid formalism,'" since the category is defined in opposition to modernism.

Analogies: Applying a New Category

Identifying an analogy requires an extra step of abstraction to a new category. The question provides an initial example—a specific individual, situation, or relationship from the passage. Your task is to analyze this example to determine the new category (the abstract structure or principle) it represents. Then, you must find a different example in the answer choices that belongs to that same abstract category.

Consider this passage on the design philosophy of biomimicry:

> Biomimicry is a design philosophy that seeks sustainable solutions to human challenges by emulating nature's time-tested patterns and strategies. The core idea is that the natural world, through billions of years of evolution, has already solved many of the problems we are grappling with. For instance, engineers have designed fan blades that mimic the bumps on a whale's fin to reduce drag and noise, and architects have created self-cooling buildings with ventilation systems modeled after the intricate structure of termite mounds.

To find an analogy for biomimicry, you must first identify the broader, more abstract category it represents. First, consider how biomimicry is defined: it's a process of solving human problems by borrowing designs from the natural world. Next, abstract away specific details like what the problems are ("human") and where the solutions come from ("designs from the natural world"). You're left with the general principle that solutions in one domain can solve problems in other domains, a concept we could shorten to "cross-domain innovation."

Your checklist for this new category might be:

1. A problem exists in one domain (for example, engineering).
2. A solution or principle is identified in a completely different, unrelated domain.
3. That principle is adapted to solve the original problem.

With this checklist, you can now find an analogy—another example of cross-domain innovation that is *not* biomimicry. A strong analogy would be:

> A chef struggling with inefficiency in their restaurant kitchen redesigns the entire workflow based on the principles of a car factory's assembly line.

This is a clear analogy. The chef's solution is not biomimicry (an assembly line is not a natural system), but it is a perfect example of cross-domain innovation: a problem in culinary arts (1) was solved by borrowing a principle from an unrelated domain, manufacturing (2), and adapting it (3).

MCAT EXPERTISE

Because they don't have to fit as literally, analogies can exist on a continuum. If a question asks for the most analogous situation, evaluate each choice against your checklist for the category you abstracted. The correct answer will mirror the core underlying structure more closely than any other option but may not satisfy all criteria completely.

Be careful not to oversimplify. A town upgrading its old bus system to a more efficient one isn't an example of cross-domain innovation (and thus isn't a good analogy for biomimicry) because it's just solving a problem; it fails the criterion of borrowing a solution from a distinct, unrelated domain.

20.2 Question Variations and Examples

The MCAT can present questions that test the Imagine Example/Analogy skill from multiple angles. The core skill remains the same, but you may need to apply it in different ways. Questions can vary in terms of the nature of the correct answer: it can be a new example of a concept, a passage category that matches a new example, or a new example analogous to an existing example (an analogy). Also, some questions ask you to affirm one of these relationships while others ask for the choice that does not match such a relationship.

Element Requested

Questions testing this skill primarily vary based on the element they're asking for, which can be an example, category, or analogy.

Example

Often, the correct answer is a new example of a category from the passage. This common variant involves a given category that was directly or indirectly described in the passage. The question stem will describe the category, while the answer choices will present four different concrete examples, only one of which correctly fits the passage's description.

EXAMPLE QUESTION STEMS

Which of the following best exemplifies a leitmotif (paragraph 2) as described in the passage?

An example of "path dependency" suggested by the passage account is:

Which of the following is a work of "kitsch" art, as described by the author?

According to the passage, a government representative would be exhibiting the most socially responsible behavior by:

If a historian were to take the approach of a university professor as described in the passage, which of the following would be expected?

BRIDGE

Some Imagine Example/Analogy questions that introduce a new person can be challenging to distinguish from Anticipate Response questions (discussed in Chapter 17). The key difference is that the Anticipate Response skill always involves the reaction of the passage author or a person discussed in the passage, while Imagine Analogy/Example questions may ask about the reactions of a new individual.

This variant sometimes introduces a new person in the question stem, as in these last two example stems. The question uses that new individual to create the setting for an example of a concept that was discussed in the passage. Then the choices give specific details or characteristics of the situation as possible examples.

Category

Less commonly, the correct answer is a category from the passage that a new example belongs to, flipping the typical structure. The new example is described in the question stem, and the answer choices consist of different categories. The correct answer describes the category from the passage that best fits the example, on the basis of the new example satisfying its criteria.

EXAMPLE QUESTION STEMS

The act of a pre-recorded phone menu suddenly saying, "We know this is frustrating, but please bear with us," would be classified by the author as an instance of:

Based on information in the passage, the historical development of the QWERTY keyboard, which persists despite more efficient alternatives, is an example of:

Analogy

In this common variant, the question stem will explicitly ask for something that is analogous or similar to an example from the passage. Your task is to find the closest analogy to the idea from the passage.

EXAMPLE QUESTION STEMS

Based on the passage, the literary device of the unreliable narrator is most analogous to:

Which of the following relationships is most similar to the one between a "readymade" object and the artist who designates it as art?

Unlike finding an example, your job is not to find an individual or scenario that fits a definition, but to find one that shares the same underlying logic or structure because it belongs to a common abstract category, as described in the preceding section.

Affirmative or Negative Relationship

While questions testing the Imagine Example/Analogy skill typically ask for the answer choice that establishes an affirmative relationship between examples and/or the categories they belong to, some request the reverse.

Affirmative Relationship

This variant is more common. These questions ask for the answer choice that correctly establishes a relationship between a category and an example, or between two analogous examples from the same category.

EXAMPLE QUESTION STEMS

Which of the following is a work of "kitsch" art, as described by the author?

The act of a pre-recorded phone menu suddenly saying, "We know this is frustrating, but please bear with us," would be classified by the author as an instance of:

Which of the following relationships is most similar to the one between a "readymade" object and the artist who designates it as art?

Negative Relationship

In this less common variant, questions ask for the choice that does not establish an accurate relationship between an example and a category, or between two analogous examples. In these cases, the question stem will use a negative term like NOT or LEAST to ask for the one thing that fails to serve as an example, or for an example that is LEAST analogous to one from the passage.

EXAMPLE QUESTION STEMS

Based on information in the passage, one would expect which of the following people to experience the LEAST amount of freedom?

Which of the following scenarios is NOT in accord with the practice of code-switching, as defined by the author?

The author's description of the dynamic between the individual herder and the commons is LEAST like which of the following situations?

Which of the following is LEAST similar to the principle of a crisis of confidence as described in the passage?

In each of these questions, the three incorrect answer choices will work as examples of a category from the passage, or be analogous to an example from the passage. The correct answer will fail to meet the criteria or contradict a key characteristic.

MCAT EXPERTISE

Some Imagine Example/Analogy question stems include a specific paragraph reference. As with other skills that have this characteristic, the reference enables you to focus more quickly on the part of the passage that is most relevant to answering the question. Be aware, however, that such a reference does not guarantee that the cited paragraph is all you'll need from the passage to reach an answer.

20.3 Applying the Kaplan Method

Step 1: Type the Question

As described in Chapter 6, your first step is to read the question stem and glance at the answer choices to assess the question type and difficulty, which will inform your decision to attack it now or save it for later. Always try to identify the broad skill category of the question as Foundations of Comprehension (surface questions), Reasoning Within the Text (deep questions), or Reasoning Beyond the Text (new info questions). As discussed earlier, this will help you take a strategic approach to answering the question and evaluating the answer choices, even if you cannot precisely identify the specific skill.

Identifying the Skill

The first clue that a question is testing the Imagine Example/Analogy skill is the presence of new information—a scenario not mentioned in the text—located in either the question stem or the answer choices. You can usually identify an Imagine Example/Analogy question by recognizing that the question is asking for an example or analogy of some idea from the passage; less commonly, the question stem will include a new example. Look for key phrases like "best exemplifies," "an example of," "most similar to," "most like" or "most analogous to."

Deciding When to Attack

Imagine Example/Analogy is a Reasoning Beyond the Text skill. These questions are often the most complex and time-consuming on the CARS section because they require you to make a connection between the passage and entirely new information. For this reason, the best strategy is usually to save these questions for *later* in the set. Secure your points on more straightforward questions first, then return to tackle these more complex reasoning tasks.

The one time when you might choose to complete an Imagine Example/Analogy question *now* is when you have a solid understanding of the relevant concept from the passage and the answer choices are not too wordy. Be careful, however, if the concept is discussed in multiple parts of the passage, because identifying nuances between choices may take more time than you anticipate.

MCAT EXPERTISE

On the surface, Imagine Example/Analogy questions can look similar to Predict Outcome/Explanation because they are both "new info" questions. The key difference is that Predict Outcome/Explanation questions generally focus on causal or explanatory relationships: how does one thing lead to another? Imagine Example/Analogy questions focus on the relationships between categories and examples, including analogies as co-examples of a broader abstract category: how are ideas defined and categorized? For more on the Predict Outcome/Explanation skill, see Chapter 18.

Step 2: Rephrase the Stem

After typing the question, your next goal is to translate the test maker's language into a simple, concrete mission for yourself. For this skill, your rephrase should clearly identify the type of correct answer you're looking for (a new example, a passage category, or an analogy) as well as what idea from the passage you're starting with (if any).

To identify the type of correct answer, wording like "instance," "exemplify," or "example" indicates an example or category (it will be a category if the question stem also includes details about a new example), while wording like "analogous," "similar," or "most like" indicates an analogy. If you're looking for a category, the question stem won't tell you what idea from the passage the new example corresponds to because that's actually what you're searching for in the question. Otherwise, the stem will offer a quotation or description of the original idea from the passage, possibly including a paragraph reference.

If you're looking for an example in the correct answer, such as in this question:

> Which of the following scenarios best exemplifies the "tragedy of the commons"?

Then you could rephrase it as:

- Find where the "tragedy of the commons" is defined in the passage and create a mental checklist of criteria as a prediction.
- Evaluate each answer choice against the checklist, selecting the one that satisfies all of the criteria.

Alternatively, you might need to find a category from the passage, as in this question:

> The act of a pre-recorded phone menu suddenly saying, "We know this is frustrating, but please bear with us," would be classified by the author as an instance of:

You might rephrase that this way:

- Look for prominent categories that are defined in the passage, particularly any that seem similar to the passage description. If any are found, evaluate the new example against the criteria for that category.
- If in doubt, use process of elimination by applying the criteria of each answer choice to the new example in the stem, choosing the option for which the new example satisfies all the criteria.

Finally, if you're looking for an analogy like this:

> The design philosophy of biomimicry, as described in the passage, is most analogous to which of the following scenarios?

Rephrase it like this:

- Go back to the passage and see how biomimicry is defined.
- Abstract away surface-level features and other specifics to arrive at a new abstract category with a simple mental checklist of criteria.
- Evaluate each answer choice against the abstract category's checklist, choosing the one that satisfies the criteria perfectly or that satisfies more criteria than any other choice.

Step 3: Investigate Potential Solutions

With your mission clear, you can now turn to the passage to build your prediction. If you're looking for an example or analogy (rather than a category from the passage), then you'll start by locating the original idea from the passage and determining how it's defined. Use a paragraph reference if provided, but if not rely upon the highlights or outline from your distillation to find it.

After you've found the starting idea, look for how the passage defines it, as explained in Section 9.1 above. Once you have a mental checklist of criteria for the concept, you can use that as a prediction if you're dealing with an example.

If you're dealing with an analogy instead, you'll need to abstract away any unessential features to get at the underlying structural characteristics of the passage idea. This will give you criteria for a broader, abstract category that the correct answer will also belong to. This set of criteria for the new abstract category is your prediction when the correct answer is an analogy.

While both examples and analogies end with a prediction in the form of a checklist, questions that ask for a category from the passage are harder to predict. If you don't immediately recognize the new example as belonging to something discussed in the passage and you don't even know where to begin looking, you should instead opt for the process of elimination. Locate in the passage each category described in the answer choices, and then evaluate the new example against its criteria.

Step 4: Match Your Prediction to an Answer Choice

Armed with a prediction (at least when looking for examples and analogies), you can more efficiently assess the answer choices. Answer choices for Imagine Example/Analogy questions can be long, especially when they each describe a complete, new scenario. This is especially likely when the relevant categories have a lot of criteria.

For examples and analogies, systematically apply your mental checklist of criteria to each answer choice. A proper example will satisfy every criterion on the list, meaning any choice that fails in one or more characteristics can immediately be eliminated. However, be careful about certain wordings like "best exemplifies": the "best" here subtly suggests that whether something is an example is on a continuum, which really means that you're looking for an analogy, not a perfect example. In those cases, along with more clearly stated analogies, you'll choose the answer that satisfies the most criteria or the most important criteria, but not necessarily all.

For categories, if you weren't able to arrive at a good prediction, you'll work in reverse, applying the criteria from each answer choice to the new example in the question until you find the perfect fit.

Be on your guard for common traps. For Example questions, a distractor might be a perfect example of a *different concept* mentioned in the passage. For analogy questions, be suspicious of choices that share the *same subject matter* as the passage. A true analogy succeeds by mirroring an underlying structure in a new context, so an option from the same field is often a distractor that mimics the topic without matching the logic.

MCAT EXPERTISE

There are questions in which it is possible to eliminate three choices because they conflict with information in the passage or because they are consistent with a concept that the author specifically contrasts with the concept in the question. Strategic elimination is sometimes easier than recognizing the correct answer, but be careful about time investment.

20.4 Skillbuilder

Use the following shortened passage to practice the Imagine Example/Analogy skill. The reading is scaffolded to reinforce good active reading habits and to let you devote more of your attention to practicing your critical thinking skills. It includes Active Reading Checks with each paragraph to evaluate how well you're uncovering important passage information at every level. Answer both the Active Reading Check and the CARS question that accompanies each paragraph before continuing. You can check your answers on the next page before you move on to paragraph 2, and the same for paragraph 3.

Paragraph 1

The nineteenth-century novel was largely defined by the authority of the omniscient narrator, a god-like voice with unlimited access to the story's world. This narrator could move seamlessly from the public square into the private thoughts of any character, revealing hidden motives and passing moral judgments with unwavering confidence. In the works of authors such as George Eliot and Leo Tolstoy, this narrative convention provided readers with a stable and ordered reality: one in which the world and its inhabitants could be comprehensively known and understood. The narrator acted as a trusted guide whose perspective was not presented as one view among many but as the definitive truth of the fictional universe, reinforcing a sense of social and moral certainty.

Active Reading Check for Paragraph 1

According to paragraph 1, the main purpose of the omniscient narrator in 19th-century novels was to:

- **A.** challenge the reader to adopt the same morals as the characters.
- **B.** create a sense of stability and certainty for the reader.
- **C.** enhance the reader's enjoyment of the novel.

1. Which of the following is most analogous to a 19th-century omniscient narrator as defined in the passage?
   - **A.** A trickster god who leads individuals astray and mocks the results in asides to other gods
   - **B.** A parent who teaches their child to appreciate others' rights and opinions through a story
   - **C.** A reporter who follows a single political figure to communicate thoroughly the observable facts of a situation
   - **D.** A coach who provides unique insight into team members' choices and commentary on their principles

Active Reading Check for Paragraph 1: (B)

(A) The passage states that the omniscient narrator passes "moral judgments," but it never suggests that the goal is for the reader to change or adopt the morals of the characters.

(B) The passage provides direct support for this idea when it states that this narrative style "provided readers with a stable and ordered reality" and was responsible for "reinforcing a sense of social and moral certainty."

(C) While a reader might enjoy this style of narration, the passage does not mention reader enjoyment at all.

Question 1: (D)

Answer Choice Explanations for Question 1

(A) A trickster god who "leads individuals astray" and "mocks" them is the opposite of the "trusted guide" described in the passage who provides "certainty."

(B) Paragraph 1 describes the omniscient narrator's role as presenting a single, "definitive truth" that is "not … one view among many." A parent who teaches appreciation for "others' rights and opinions" is not promoting their teaching as singly definitive.

(C) A reporter who focuses on the "observable facts" of a "single political figure" lacks the "unlimited access to the story's world" that paragraph 1 states as a characteristic of the omniscient narrator.

(D) The coach has special "insight" into their team members; this is similar to the narrator's "unlimited access." Likewise, a coach's "commentary on their principles" is directly analogous to the narrator's role in "passing moral judgments."

Detailed Explanation for Question 1

Skill: This question asks you to understand a concept defined in the passage and then identify a new situation or figure that is most similar to it. Therefore, this question tests the Imagine Example/Analogy skill by asking for an analogy.

Question: The question asks you to find the best analogy for the 19th-century omniscient narrator. To do this, you must first build a clear description of that narrator based on the details in the first paragraph.

Passage: Paragraph 1 describes the omniscient narrator as a "god-like voice with unlimited access to the story's world" who is capable of "revealing hidden motives and passing moral judgments" on any character. The passage also characterizes this figure as "a trusted guide whose perspective was not presented as one view among many but as the definitive truth." Based on this, you should look for an answer choice that describes an individual who has privileged access to a group of people and uses that insight to provide authoritative commentary on their behavior or character. This person will also likely serve as an authority or guide.

Answer: While the god in **(A)** has insight, the fact that he is described as a trickster who leads individuals astray and mocks them means that he is not a trusted guide. The parent in **(B)** can serve as a trusted guide, but this parent is teaching the child to appreciate many views and opinions rather than serving as a guide of definitive truth. The reporter in **(C)** has too limited a view with the focus on a single political figure, and so they are not like an omniscient narrator. The best analogy is a coach who provides unique insight into team members' choices and commentary on their principles, as stated in **(D)**. A coach, like the omniscient narrator, has a privileged position of "unlimited access" to observe their team and serves as a "trusted guide." The coach also offers commentary on the team members' principles, which is parallel to the omniscient narrator "revealing hidden motives."

Paragraph 2

The dawn of the twentieth century, however, heralded a profound shift in literary consciousness, leading to a steady erosion of the omniscient narrator's dominance. The rise of modernism, fueled by psychoanalytic theories and the seismic cultural shocks of events like World War I, cultivated a deep-seated skepticism toward absolute truths and external authorities. In a shattered modern world, no guide could be trusted. Authors began to question whether any single perspective could truly capture the chaotic and subjective nature of reality. Consequently, the "all-knowing" voice of the previous century started to seem not just old-fashioned, but intellectually dishonest. The literary focus pivoted inward, from the social tapestry to the fragmented, complex landscape of individuals' consciousness.

Active Reading Check for Paragraph 2

What phrase from the passage best communicates 20th century authors' view of the omniscient narrator?

A. "seismic cultural shocks"
B. "chaotic and subjective"
C. "intellectually dishonest"

2. The intellectual shift described in paragraph 2 is most analogous to which of the following transitions in another field?

A. In art, the transition from Renaissance painting, which portrayed a single view of a scene, to cubism, which depicts subjects from multiple simultaneous viewpoints
B. In astronomy, the general acceptance of the heliocentric model, which placed the Sun rather than the Earth at the center of the solar system, providing a more accurate model
C. In medicine, the development of the germ theory of disease, which replaced numerous folk explanations with a verifiable scientific cause for illnesses
D. In historiography, the shift from diplomatic history, which focuses on competing viewpoints of world leaders, to social history, which uses the perspectives of everyday people

Active Reading Check for Paragraph 2: (C)

(A) This phrase describes the historical events that caused authors to change their views regarding the omniscient narrator. It refers to the reason for their opinion, but it does not state what the opinion itself was.

(B) This phrase is used to describe 20th-century authors' view of "the nature of reality," not their view of the omniscient narrator. Their perception of reality as chaotic and subjective is what led them to distrust the old narrative style.

(C) The passage states that due to the new skepticism of the era, "the 'all-knowing' voice of the previous century started to seem not just old-fashioned, but intellectually dishonest." This phrase directly communicates 20th-century authors' negative opinion of the omniscient narrator.

Question 2: (A)

Answer Choice Explanations for Question 2

(A) The passage describes a shift from one single, authoritative perspective (the omniscient narrator) to multiple, subjective perspectives (modernism). The transition from single-view Renaissance art to multiple-view cubist art is an appropriate analogy for this change.

(B) The acceptance of the heliocentric model was a transition from one single-view system to a different but still single-view system. It does not reflect the passage's described shift from a single perspective to multiple perspectives.

(C) The development of germ theory represents a move from many varied explanations to a single authoritative one. This is the reverse of the intellectual shift described in the passage, which moved away from a single authority.

(D) This choice describes a transition from one set of multiple perspectives (world leaders) to a different set of multiple perspectives (everyday people). The intellectual shift in the passage begins from a single authoritative viewpoint, not multiple ones.

Detailed Explanation for Question 2

Skill: This question tests your ability to Imagine Example/Analogy. To answer correctly, you must first understand the essential structure of the "intellectual shift" described in the passage. The structure is a key component of an analogy.

Question: The question asks you to find the best analogy for the change in literary thought that occurred in the 20th century. This requires you to break down the shift described in paragraph 2 into its core components. You then have to analyze the four transitions described in the answer choices and determine which one has the most similar structure to identify which is analogous.

Passage: Paragraph 2 explains that literature shifted *away from* the omniscient narrator, who was described in paragraph 1 as a "trusted guide" that presented a "definitive truth." It moved *toward* a modernist approach that was skeptical of "absolute truths and external authorities." These authors "began to question whether any single perspective could truly capture the chaotic and subjective nature of reality." They focused instead on "the fragmented, complex landscape of individuals' consciousness." Therefore, the core structure of the analogy is a transition from a singular perspective to a system of multiple, subjective perspectives.

Answer: The transition from Renaissance painting to Cubism, as described in **(A)**, is the only transition from one perspective to multiple perspectives described in any of the answer choices. Renaissance painting, with its emphasis on linear perspective, "portrayed a single view of a scene," much like the omniscient narrator provided a single, authoritative truth. Cubism, in contrast, "depicts subjects from multiple simultaneous viewpoints," which is directly analogous to the modernist turn from a single perspective toward fragmented, individual points of view. The other choices do not fit this essential singular-to-multiple structure.

Paragraph 3

This evolution is starkly illustrated in the works of modernist pioneers, who championed limited and subjective points of view. William Faulkner's The Sound and the Fury, for example, shatters its narrative into the deeply personal and often contradictory perspectives of three different brothers, forcing the reader to assemble a composite truth from these flawed accounts. Similarly, Virginia Woolf's stream of consciousness technique plunges the reader directly into the flow of her characters' thoughts and sensations. In these works, the reader is no longer a passive recipient of a pre-digested story but an active participant in the construction of meaning. The novel ceases to be a window onto a shared world and becomes instead a reflection of private, often isolated, realities.

Active Reading Check for Paragraph 3

How do the ideas presented in paragraph 3 relate to earlier parts of the passage?

A. Paragraph 3 provides literary examples to illustrate the shift described in paragraph 2.

B. Paragraph 3 presents counterexamples that undermine the ideas described in paragraph 2.

C. Paragraph 3 returns to the topic of 19th-century authors first mentioned in paragraph 1.

3. Which of the following LEAST exemplifies a modernist novel's narrator as described in the passage?

A. A narrator paging through personal letters, diary entries, and newspaper clippings, without already knowing how they relate to each other

B. A narrator whose account of the plot is presented entirely through an unstructured flow of thoughts as they occur to the protagonist

C. A narrator who describes a family's financial ruin along with an assessment of each family member's personal flaws that contributed to their collective downfall

D. A narrator who is a character in the story and openly admits their own biases and confusion, along with their uncertainty of the other characters' true intentions

Active Reading Check for Paragraph 3: (A)

(A) Paragraph 2 describes the theoretical and historical reasons for the shift to modernism. Paragraph 3 opens with the claim that this is "starkly illustrated in the works of modernist pioneers," and then shares the examples of Faulkner and Woolf.

(B) The passage uses the phrase "This evolution is starkly illustrated in the works of modernist pioneers" to introduce the examples in paragraph 3, indicating that they support, rather than undermine, the claims made in paragraph 2.

(C) Paragraph 3 discusses "modernist pioneers," and paragraph 2 states that modernism rose in the 20th century. Therefore, the authors in paragraph 3 are not some of the 19th-century authors who were the focus of paragraph 1.

Question 3: (C)

Answer Choice Explanations for Question 3

(A) This narrator does not have all the answers and is working through fragmented sources that are "limited and subjective points of view." This approach also forces the reader to be an "active participant in the construction of meaning," which is a key trait of modernism as described in paragraph 3.

(B) This narrator uses the "stream of consciousness technique" that the passage explicitly mentions as an example of modernist style writing by Virginia Woolf. This choice can also be described as presenting a "limited and subjective" point of view, so it exemplifies a modernist narrator.

(C) A narrator who can provide an "assessment of each family member's personal flaws" in effect possesses the "unlimited access" and authority to pass "moral judgments" characteristic of the 19th-century omniscient narrator described in paragraph 1. This is the opposite of a limited, subjective modernist narrator.

(D) A narrator who admits to "biases and confusion" and "uncertainty" represents the "limited and subjective points of view" that the passage identifies as a core feature of modernist narration.

Detailed Explanation for Question 3

Skill: This question tests your ability to Imagine Example/Analogy, specifically by requiring you to categorize new examples. You must first use the passage to build a clear definition of a concept—in this case, the "modernist novel's narrator" and then identify examples that directly line up with that concept.

Question: The question asks you to identify the one narrator description that LEAST serves as an example of a modernist narrator as outlined in the passage. This means three of the choices will be good examples of a modernist narrator, while the correct answer will be the outlier that represents a different style. The task is first to identify how the passage defines a modernist narrator.

Passage: Paragraph 2 introduces the modernist trend by describing how authors questioned "whether any single perspective could truly capture the chaotic and subjective nature of reality." The passage goes on to describe the modernist narrator in paragraph 3 as a figure who uses a "limited and subjective" point of view. This style forces the reader to become an "active participant in the construction of meaning." Therefore, examples of modernist narrators should present a limited point of view that requires readers to participate in figuring out the novel rather than taking in a "pre-digested story" that is clearly described for them. The example that is LEAST like a modernist narrator will likely have a less limited perspective or present the story more clearly.

Answer: A narrator who provides an assessment of each family member's personal flaws is not providing a limited or subjective point of view. Instead, this narrator sounds like one who has the kind of "unlimited access to the story's world" and moral authority that the passage attributes to the 19th-century omniscient narrator, so **(C)** is not an example of a modernist narrator. The other three choices clearly fit the modernist mold: **(A)** describes a fragmented and unauthoritative narrative, **(B)** describes the stream of consciousness technique, and **(D)** describes a limited and subjective narrator.

Skill and Strategy Summary

Skill Description

- The **Imagine Example/Analogy** skill involves the coordination of examples and the categories they belong to, including identifying examples and analogies of passage ideas.
    - Imagine Example/Analogy accounts for about 20% of Reasoning Beyond the Text questions.
- Categories given in passages can be defined explicitly or implicitly, but all are in some way defined by a set of characteristics or criteria.
    - An example of a category is something that satisfies all the criteria of that category.
- An analogy is just a different kind of example. An idea from the passage and its analogy will both be examples of a new category—one that you discover by abstracting away the surface-level features of each example, leaving their underlying structure.
    - An analogy won't share all of the features of the original idea, but it shares the same essential or structural characteristics.

Question Variations and Examples

- Imagine Example/Analogy questions can vary in the following ways:
    - **Element Requested**: Questions can ask for a new example of a passage concept, a passage concept that matches a new example, or an example that's analogous to one from the passage.
    - **Affirmative or Negative Relationship**: Questions typically ask for an accurate relationship between an example and a category it belongs to, or two analogous examples of the same concept. Less commonly, they'll ask for the one answer choice that does not establish such a relationship.

Applying the Kaplan Method

- Step 1: Type the Question
    - Recognize the Reasoning Beyond the Text skill category by the presence of new information in the question or choices.
    - Identify the Imagine Example/Analogy skill by wording that mentions examples, analogies, and similar concepts.
    - As new info (Reasoning Beyond the Text) questions, these should usually be saved for *later*.
- Step 2: Rephrase the Stem
    - Include the type of answer that you're looking for (example, category, or analogy), along with the starting idea from the passage (if any).
- Step 3: Investigate Potential Solutions
    - Start by finding the passage idea specified by the question (if any) and looking for its definition.
    - Predict by making a mental checklist of criteria for the category: either a given category for an example, or a new abstract category for an analogy.
- Step 4: Match Your Prediction to an Answer Choice
    - Apply your checklist to the choices, looking for a match that meets all of the essential criteria (example) or more of the criteria than any other choice (analogy).
    - Be on guard against common traps like examples of the wrong concept from the passage or weak analogies that match the subject matter of the passage but not the necessary structure.

CHAPTER 21

REASONING BEYOND THE TEXT PRACTICE

How to Use This Chapter

This practice chapter contains two full MCAT passages and question sets, designed to help you practice answering Reasoning Beyond the Text (RBT) questions using the skills discussed in Chapters 17–20. While RBT questions make up only 40% of the questions you will see on Test Day, the passage sets within this chapter contain *only* RBT questions. Use the strategies discussed in Chapters 1–6 to Read and Distill the passages and answer the associated questions. Then, use the answer explanations at the end of the chapter to review your practice (information on how to review your practice can be found in Chapter 7).

Passage 1 (Questions 1–6)

Fernand Braudel and his fellow *Annales* historians have made significant contributions to historical theory and research, not the least of which is a broad expansion of potential routes of scholastic analysis. In a departure from traditional approaches, the *Annales* historians assume that history cannot be limited to a simple recounting of conscious human actions, but must be understood in the context of forces and material conditions that underlie human behavior. Braudel was the first *Annales* historian to gain widespread support for the idea that history should synthesize data from various social sciences, especially economics, in order to provide a broader view of human societies over time (although Lucien Febvre and Marc Bloch, founders of the *Annales* school, originated this approach).

Braudel conceived of history as the dynamic interaction of three temporalities. The first of these, the *événementielle*, involved short-lived dramatic "events," such as battles, revolutions, and the actions of great individuals, which had preoccupied traditional historians like Thomas Carlyle. *Conjonctures* was Braudel's term for larger cyclical processes that might last up to half a century. He likened *conjonctures* to the tides of the sea, as compared to its breaking waves or deep currents. The *longue durée*, a historical span of great length, was for Braudel the most fascinating of the three temporalities. Here he focused on those aspects of everyday life that might remain relatively unchanged for centuries. What people ate, what they wore, their means and routes of travel—for Braudel, these things create "structures" that define the limits of potential social change for hundreds of years at a time.

Braudel's concept of the *longue durée* extended the perspective of historical physical space as well as time. Until the *Annales* school, historians had generally taken the juridical political unit—the nation-state, duchy, or whatever—as their starting point. Yet, when such enormous timespans are considered, geographical features may well have more significance for human populations than national borders. In his doctoral thesis, a seminal work on the Mediterranean during the reign of Philip II, Braudel treated the geohistory of the entire region as a "structure" that had exerted myriad influences on human lifeways since the first settlements on the shores of the Mediterranean Sea. So, the reader is given such esoteric information as the list of products that came to Spanish shores from North Africa, the seasonal routes followed by Mediterranean sheep and their shepherds, and the cities where the best ship timber could be bought.

Braudel has been faulted for the imprecision of his approach. With his Rabelaisian delight in concrete detail, Braudel vastly extended the realm of relevant phenomena; but this very achievement made it difficult to delimit the boundaries of observation, a task necessary to beginning any social analysis. Indeed, to identify an appropriate scope of work when all options and directions for academic inquiry are available before one's eyes is a nearly impossible task. Further, Braudel and other *Annales* historians minimize the differences among the social sciences. Nevertheless, the many similarly designed studies aimed at both professional and popular audiences indicate that Braudel asked significant questions that traditional historians had overlooked.

1. Reflecting on his history of the Mediterranean in the age of Philip II, Braudel stated, "I could have written it the other way round —beginning with events, then moving on from that spectacular and often misleading pageant to the structural features underlying it, and finally to the bedrock of history." What effect does this statement have on the criticism that his approach was imprecise?

A. It strengthens the criticism by revealing that Braudel himself was uncertain about the best way to organize his historical analysis.

B. It weakens the criticism by explaining how his focus systematically extended from the overarching social trends and structures to the level of specific events and individuals.

C. It weakens the criticism by demonstrating his focus on the concrete details that traditional historians considered to be the "bedrock of history."

D. It strengthens the criticism by admitting that a more traditional, event-based structure would have been more compelling and accurate.

2. Which of the following historical phenomena would the author most likely consider an example of Braudel's *conjonctures*?

A. Julius Caesar's crossing of the Rubicon, which led to a four-year civil war in Rome

B. Populist agitation for land reform and debt relief that destabilized the Roman Republic roughly every 40 to 50 years

C. A gradual shift toward a drier Mediterranean climate that lasted from 250 to 600 CE and impacted food availability and daily life

D. The battle of Carrhae in 53 BCE, in which the Parthians exterminated a large Roman army

3. In the early 17th century, the powerful Italian port city of Genoa, a formerly dominant maritime republic, entered a period of sharp economic decline. Braudel's analysis of this historic downturn would be most likely to emphasize:

A. the implementation of a series of unpopular taxes by the Genoese government that drove wealthy merchants away.

B. a shift in the center of European trade from the Mediterranean Sea region to the coast of the Atlantic Ocean.

C. the military defeat of Genoa's navy at the hands of its primary political rival, the Republic of Venice.

D. a severe outbreak of plague within the city of Genoa that crippled its population and workforce.

4. Which of the following discoveries, if verified, would best support the significance of the *Annales* school's approach to history as described in the passage?
   A. Economists confirm that the specific list of products Braudel cited as coming to Spanish shores from North Africa was accurately recorded in historical ledgers.
   B. A comparative study of multiple civilizations concludes that major societal changes are driven more by singular technological breakthroughs than by long-term societal conditions.
   C. A re-examination of a major revolution shows that its outcome cannot be adequately explained without considering data on long-term dietary changes and minor shifts in local trade routes.
   D. A biography of Thomas Carlyle reveals that his "great individuals" approach to history was primarily shaped by his personal philosophical beliefs rather than empirical research.

5. If the *Annales* school's approach to history fell out of favor and was largely abandoned by the academic community, which of the following outcomes would most likely occur based on the passage discussion?
   A. Important questions about the effects of material conditions on everyday life would be neglected.
   B. Historical research would become more relevant to modern society due to clearer boundaries for analysis.
   C. Popular audiences would lose their interest in studies from all traditional social science disciplines.
   D. The study of short-lived political events would be replaced by a focus on long-term cyclical processes.

6. A new historian produces a study of a coastal region's fishing culture from 1900 to 1950 that synthesizes economic reports on trade, meteorological data, and oral histories. Based on the passage, how would Braudel most likely have responded to this study?
   A. He would have praised the study as an exemplary piece of *Annales* scholarship for its multi-faceted approach.
   B. He would have approved of the methodology but considered the fifty-year timeframe an unfortunate limitation.
   C. He would have questioned the study for the choice to rely on meteorological data rather than geohistory.
   D. He would have criticized the study for focusing too narrowly on human actions revealed from the oral histories.

Passage 2 (Questions 7–12)

If we can establish a stable, unambiguous connection between our words and the concepts they represent, we can build a foundation for objective truth. It was the Swiss linguist Ferdinand de Saussure who formalized this project, proposing a systematic structure of language built on the "linguistic sign." In his model, every sign consists of two parts: the "signifier," which is the word itself (the sound or image of "tree"), and the "signified," which is the mental concept the word evokes (the idea of a tree). Saussure argued that the relationship between these two parts is fundamentally arbitrary—there is no natural reason the letters t-r-e-e must denote a plant with a trunk and leaves.

However, Saussure believed that through social convention these arbitrary links could be fixed, creating a stable and predictable system of meaning. While the word is arbitrary, society agrees on its meaning, allowing for clear communication. This structuralist approach imagines language as a vast, ordered system of signs, where each word, like a piece on a chessboard, has a distinct value and function derived from its relationship to all the other pieces. The ultimate goal of this system is clarity and coherence, a way to map the world of concepts onto a shared, stable network of words. This perspective offered a scientific rigor to linguistics and suggested that meaning, while socially constructed, could ultimately be anchored.

Post-structuralist thinkers, emerging in the mid-twentieth century, challenge this notion of stability head-on. They contend that signifiers do not, in fact, point to stable, external signifieds. Instead, a signifier points only to another signifier. The process of defining a word is illustrative of this view: looking up "truth" in a dictionary leads not to the concept of truth itself, but to other words like "fact," "reality," or "sincerity." To understand these, one must look them up, embarking on an infinite, circular chain of signifiers with no ultimate endpoint or anchor in reality. For post-structuralists, this demonstrates that meaning is not contained within a word but is generated by the endless play of differences between words.

This linguistic insight has profound implications. If language is an unstable, self-referential system, then the concepts it purports to describe—justice, identity, history, truth—are themselves rendered unstable. Post-structuralism argues that language does not simply reflect a pre-existing reality; it actively constructs it. Our understanding of ourselves and our world is therefore a product of "discourse," the web of language, assumptions, and power relations active in a given culture at a given time. As discourse shifts, so too does meaning and our perception of reality. An act of "heroism" in one historical context might be framed as "terrorism" in another, not because the act itself changed, but because the linguistic and cultural framework used to interpret it did.

Herein lies the reason for post-structuralism's far-reaching and controversial influence. While Saussurean structuralism provided a powerful analytical tool for linguistics and anthropology, its impact was largely confined to academic disciplines concerned with classification and systems. Post-structuralism's argument, however, strikes at the very heart of the Western philosophical tradition. By asserting that no meaning is ever final and no truth is absolute, it offers a powerful, if unsettling, tool for deconstructing cherished cultural narratives and questioning the foundations of authority.

7. Which of the following best exemplifies the post-structuralist view of meaning as presented in the passage?
   A. The words "signifier" and "signified" are expressed in different ways across several languages.
   B. All members of a literary club put forth unique interpretations of a fairy tale based on their academic backgrounds.
   C. The relationship between a parent and child shifts dramatically during the course of a novel.
   D. All ten members of a focus group derive the same meaning from the preview of a new situation comedy.

8. Based on the passage's description of post-structuralism, if historians from two rival cultures attempt to write a definitive account of a war they fought, which outcome is most probable?
   A. They would produce two conflicting interpretations, each shaped by their respective cultural usage of terms.
   B. They would debate definitions in order to eventually reveal an impartial account of what occurred during the war.
   C. The historians would conclude that language is an inadequate tool and would abandon the project entirely.
   D. The more powerful culture would successfully impose its version of history as the sole, undisputed record.

9. Which of the following findings, if true, would most WEAKEN the Saussurean model of language as described in the passage?
   A. A linguistic survey is unable to find phonetic similarities between the words used for common objects like "water" and "stone" in historically unrelated languages.
   B. A neurobiological study finds that the human brain is not predisposed to any specific language but develops its linguistic pathways based on environmental exposure.
   C. An analysis of legal documents shows that the interpretation of the term "reasonable" has shifted somewhat over the past century, reflecting changing social norms.
   D. Many languages have similar-sound words for "mama" and "dada," suggesting that these words are based on the phonetic abilities that tend to develop earliest in life.

10. Many fields of study use jargon—specialized terms that are created to have a specific, fixed meaning within that field. How does the existence of jargon affect the claims made in the passage?
   A. It weakens the Saussurean model, because jargon is created purposefully and is not arbitrary.
   B. It strengthens the post-structuralist view, as jargon's meaning is based on other specialized terms.
   C. It supports the Saussurean model, as jargon is used in a consistent manner formed by agreement.
   D. It undermines the post-structuralist view because academic language only has limited uses.

11. Which of the following examples is LEAST analogous to the Saussurean model of language?
   A. In traffic systems, a red octagon is used to signify the command "stop," a meaning that is consistently understood by all drivers.
   B. In medicine, a patient's high body temperature is interpreted as a sign of an underlying infection or illness.
   C. In economics, a rectangular piece of paper with specific markings is assigned a certain value, allowing it to be used as a stable form of currency.
   D. In musical notation, the treble clef symbol at the beginning of a line of music indicates the specific pitches for the notes that follow.

12. A technology firm announces it is developing an AI called "Logos" that can analyze any text and determine its objectively true meaning, with the goal of ending disputes in law and politics. How would the author of the passage most likely view this project?
   A. As a beneficial achievement that successfully creates a stable and predictable system of meaning
   B. As a project of little relevance, since linguistic theory does not impact technological progress
   C. As a philosophically naïve project that ignores the inherent instability and complexity of meaning
   D. As a worrisome tool for social control, given that the power to define terms is a form of authority

Answers and Explanations

Passage 1 (Questions 1–6)

Question 1: (B) – Strengthen/Weaken Argument

Explanation for Question 1

Paragraph 4 indicates that Braudel "has been faulted for the imprecision of his approach." The passage author goes on to acknowledge that Braudel "vastly extended the realm of relevant phenomena" in a way that "made it difficult" to focus analysis into a coherent historical narrative or "identify an appropriate scope of work." The new quote in the question stem indicates that Braudel's method was not unfocused or poorly defined; it was a deliberate, systematic decision to start his analysis with an expansive scope (the *longue durée*) and build up to how those wider systems influenced the level of localized events and influential people (the *événementielle*). The impression created by the pageantry of "spectacular and often misleading" events, according to Braudel, is what often lacks accuracy or precision. He chose instead to build his analysis up from the "bedrock" of a firm foundation to first establish the context in which to interpret the significance of events. **(B)** is the correct answer because Braudel's description of his precise approach directly counters the criticism against him.

Wrong Answer Explanations

(A) The quote does not express uncertainty but rather a firm conviction that his incorporation of the broader context provides a more complete and accurate understanding of the past than the traditional fixation on just the "often misleading" series of events. He is confident that the organization of his multilevel analysis could have been presented from either direction, but his approach, beginning with what he calls the "bedrock," established a firmer grounding before moving on to the spectacle of events, so that his audience would not be misled.

(C) Braudel's "delight in concrete detail" (paragraph 4) refers to "such esoteric information as the list of products that came to Spanish shores from North Africa, the seasonal routes followed by Mediterranean sheep and their shepherds, and the cities where the best ship timber could be bought" (paragraph 3). These "bedrock" specifics are the opposite of what traditional historians focused on, which the passage identifies as the "*événementielle* ... such as battles, revolutions, and the actions of great individuals" (paragraph 2).

(D) Braudel explicitly calls the traditional events-based focus "often misleading," which is the opposite of accurate.

Question 2: (B) – Imagine Example/Analogy

Explanation for Question 2

Paragraph 2 of the passage defines *conjonctures* as "larger cyclical processes that might last up to half a century." The correct answer must fit both of these criteria: it must be a recurring, cyclical phenomenon like "the tides of the sea" (P2), and its timeframe should be around fifty years. The correct answer should develop over a longer time span than examples of *événementielle* but shorter than *longue durée*. **(B)** fits these criteria exactly with a cycle recurring "roughly every 40 to 50 years."

Wrong Answer Explanations

(A) Paragraph 2 lists "revolutions, and the actions of great individuals," as examples of the *événementielle*. Caesar's action and the following war, while significant, represent specific, short-lived dramatic "events," not *conjonctures*.

(C) A phenomenon lasting 350 years is a "historical span of great length" and therefore a clear example of the *longue durée*, not *conjonctures*.

(D) Paragraph 2 lists "battles" as a classic type of short-lived dramatic "event" categorized as *événementielle*, not *conjonctures*.

Question 3: (B) – Predict Outcome/Explanation

Explanation for Question 3

This question asks you to apply Braudel's ideas to a new historical scenario. Paragraph 3 indicates that "Braudel's concept of the *longue durée* extended the perspective of historical physical space as well as time." Traditional historians before the *Annales* school "had generally taken the juridical political unit—the nation-state, duchy, or whatever—as their starting point." Braudel believed that "geographical features may well have more significance for human populations than national borders." **(B)** is the only choice that provides a truly Braudelian, regional, long-term explanation. It frames Genoa's decline as a symptom of a much wider process: the economic marginalization of the entire Mediterranean region. This approach aligns perfectly with Braudel's treatment of "the geohistory of the entire region as a 'structure' that had exerted myriad influences on human lifeways."

Wrong Answer Explanations

(A) This is a classic traditional explanation that focuses on the conscious actions of a single "juridical political unit" (the Genoese government). Braudel argued for looking beyond such localized, political causes.

(C) This is an example of a short-lived, dramatic "event" involving the actions of two nation-states. According to the passage, Braudel's approach deliberately moved away from this type of traditional historical explanation to focus on deeper, long-term structures.

(D) While the plague is a powerful force that could spread beyond political borders, this explanation confines its effects to a single city. A true Braudelian analysis, as described in paragraph 3, would more likely focus on how disease patterns, climate, and trade routes affected the entire Mediterranean region as an interconnected system over an extended period, rather than isolating the event to one political unit of analysis.

Question 4: (C) – Strengthen/Weaken Argument

Explanation for Question 4

This question asks which new finding would best support the significance of the *Annales* school's approach. The passage argues that the school's importance comes from its departure from traditional history to ask "significant questions that traditional historians had overlooked" (paragraph 4). The passage also describes the *Annales* school's focus on the "context of forces and material conditions that underlie human behavior" (paragraph 1) and Braudel's view that "what people ate, what they wore, their means and routes of travel… create 'structures' that define the limits of potential social change" (paragraph 2). To best support the school's significance, a new finding would need to show that these questions and this approach are not just interesting but important to a complete understanding of history. **(C)** takes a classic subject of traditional history—a major revolution—and claims that it cannot be fully understood without using the approach of the *Annales* school (analyzing long-term data on everyday life, like diet and local trade), so **(C)** is correct.

Wrong Answer Explanations

(A) This finding confirms Braudel's accuracy as a researcher on a single detail, but it does not support the broader significance or explanatory power of the *Annales* school's overall approach to history.

(B) The passage states that the *Annales* school assumed that "history cannot be limited to a simple recounting of conscious human actions," and so they promoted "a broader view of human societies over time" (paragraph 1). This finding argues the opposite, suggesting that singular events (technological breakthroughs) are more important, which directly contradicts the core philosophy of the *Annales* school.

(D) While this information, if true, would weaken the credibility of the traditional "great individuals" approach to history, it does nothing to directly support the significance of the *Annales* school's method. The *Annales* approach must be validated on its own merits, not just by pointing out flaws in an alternative, if it is actually significant.

Question 5: (A) – Predict Outcome/Explanation

Explanation for Question 5

This question asks you to predict what would happen if the *Annales* school's approach was abandoned. In paragraph 1, the author states that Braudel and other *Annales* historians "have made significant contributions to historical theory and research, not the least of which is a broad expansion of potential routes of scholastic analysis," which included examination of "forces and material conditions that underlie human behavior." Paragraph 4 concludes with the claim that Braudel "asked significant questions that traditional historians had overlooked," which likely includes questions about those material conditions mentioned in P1—indeed, P3 even offered some examples from Braudel of investigating those conditions. Therefore, if the school's approach were abandoned, the "significant" or "important" questions that were once overlooked would likely become neglected again. **(A)** captures this logical consequence and is correct.

Wrong Answer Explanations

(B) Paragraph 4 does mention the criticism that Braudel made it difficult to delimit (or define) "the boundaries of observation." While it is reasonable to expect that abandoning the *Annales* approach could lead to clearer boundaries, nothing in the passage suggests that this would make history more relevant to modern society. In fact, by calling the *Annales* questions "significant" in the concluding sentence, the author implies they are already relevant.

(C) This is an overgeneralization not supported by the text. The passage mentions in paragraph 4 that some *Annales* studies were aimed at "both professional and popular audiences," but it provides no evidence to suggest that the disappearance of this single historical approach would cause the public to lose interest in all social sciences.

(D) This describes the opposite of the likely outcome. The passage states in paragraph 2 that the *Annales* school and Braudel in particular moved history beyond a focus on short-lived events (*événementielle*) and toward long-term processes (*longue durée*). Therefore, abandoning the *Annales* school would logically lead to a resurgence of the traditional focus on short-lived events, not its replacement.

Question 6: (B) – Anticipate Response

Explanation for Question 6

The hypothetical study employs a method that is central to the *Annales* school as described in paragraph 1: it "synthesize[s] data from various social sciences ... to provide a broader view of human societies." For this reason, Braudel would have approved of the historian's interdisciplinary approach. However, paragraph 2 describes Braudel's concept of history as "the dynamic interaction of three temporalities." The study's 50-year focus places it squarely in the category of studying *conjonctures*. While this is a valid part of his framework, the passage states that the *longue durée*—the study of deep structures over centuries—"was for Braudel the most fascinating of the three temporalities" (paragraph 2). Therefore, Braudel's response would likely be nuanced. He would respect the work as a solid study of *conjonctures* but would ultimately see its timeframe as a missed opportunity to engage in the deeper, more significant analysis of the *longue durée*. Therefore, **(B)** is correct.

Wrong Answer Explanations

(A) This overstates Braudel's likely praise. While he would certainly approve of the study's multi-faceted, interdisciplinary method, the passage indicates that Braudel found the centuries-long focus of the *longue durée* to be "the most fascinating of the three temporalities" (paragraph 2). Because this study's 50-year timeframe does not engage with that level of analysis, he would not praise it as an "exemplary" model of scholarship.

(C) This choice presents a false distinction. Meteorological data, which describes climate and weather patterns, is a crucial component of a region's geography. Braudel, who sought to provide a "broader view of human societies" (paragraph 1), would have welcomed this data as a valuable part of a geohistorical analysis, not questioned it.

(D) It is true that Braudel and the *Annales* historians are described in paragraph 1 as assuming that "history cannot be limited to a simple recounting of conscious human actions," so if the study had focused too narrowly on human actions, then Braudel likely would have criticized it. However, the study described in the question drew on economic reports and meteorological data in addition to oral histories, so Braudel is not likely to claim this is too narrow of a focus.

Passage 2 (Questions 7–12)

Question 7: (B) – Imagine Example/Analogy

Explanation for Question 7

The post-structuralist view of meaning is described in paragraphs 3 and 4. Paragraph 3 describes how attempts to define words are based on our understanding of other words that need to be defined and so, for post-structuralists, "meaning is not contained within a word but is generated by the endless play of differences between words." Paragraph 4 states that our understanding is "a product of 'discourse,' the web of language, assumptions, and power relations active in a given culture at a given time. As discourse shifts, so too does meaning and our perception of reality." Therefore, "no meaning is ever final" (paragraph 5) because it is constructed by the observer's context. A change in one's background, assumptions, or cultural framework—the "discourse" they are exposed to over time—will lead to a change in the meaning they derive from a text or event.

The scenario in **(B)** provides the best example of this principle. The fairy tale is the text, and the "unique interpretations" demonstrate the instability of its meaning. The cause of this instability is the members' differing academic backgrounds, which function as the distinct "discourses" that shape their understanding. This aligns with the post-structuralist argument that meaning is generated by the interpreter, not final or absolute.

Wrong Answer Explanations

(A) Instead of post-structuralism, this example illustrates Saussure's concept of the arbitrary nature of the linguistic sign, as explained in paragraph 1: "there is no natural reason the letters t-r-e-e must denote a plant with a trunk and leaves." Post-structuralism's central argument is about the *instability* of meaning, not its arbitrariness.

(C) This describes a shift in a narrative's plot, not a shift in the fundamental meaning of a concept. Post-structuralism is concerned with how the meaning of a term like "parent" could be constructed differently depending on the cultural discourse, not how a specific character's relationship evolves within a single story.

(D) This scenario directly contradicts the post-structuralist view. It represents a stable, fixed meaning shared by a group, while post-structuralism argues that meaning is never final or absolute.

Question 8: (A) - Predict Outcome/Explanation

Explanation for Question 8

This question asks you to apply the principles of post-structuralism to a real-world scenario. The core of the post-structuralist argument, as described in paragraph 4, is that "language does not simply reflect a pre-existing reality; it actively constructs it. Our understanding of ourselves and our world is therefore a product of 'discourse,' the web of language, assumptions, and power relations active in a given culture at a given time." The passage also provides a direct example of this: "An act of 'heroism' in one historical context might be framed as 'terrorism' in another."

In the scenario, you have two historians from two different—and rival—cultures. According to post-structuralism, they are operating from two different discourses. Therefore, when they attempt to describe the same war, it's most probable that they will construct two different realities. An act one historian calls a "strategic victory," the other might call a "brutal massacre." As a result, they will produce two conflicting but internally coherent accounts, with each version shaped by their culture's distinct language and values. **(A)** captures this likely outcome.

Wrong Answer Explanations

(B) This outcome reflects a traditional or Saussurean belief in a "stable and predictable system of meaning" (paragraph 2) that can be reached through agreement. Post-structuralism, in contrast, argues that "no meaning is ever final and no truth is absolute" (paragraph 5). The idea of a single, impartial account is precisely what the theory rejects.

(C) The passage doesn't suggest that post-structuralism leads to the abandonment of historical work. Instead, it presents it as a "powerful... tool for deconstructing" narratives in paragraph 5. A post-structuralist wouldn't abandon the project; they would analyze why the two accounts are different.

(D) This is not the most direct or probable outcome of the attempt itself. While post-structuralism acknowledges the role of "power relations active in a given culture at a given time" in discourse (paragraph 4), there is no indication that one discourse will completely silence another. Even if one version later becomes the dominant record, post-structuralism would argue it would never truly be undisputed, as the other interpretation would still exist and be available for analysis.

Question 9: (D) - Strengthen/Weaken Argument

Explanation for Question 9

According to the passage, the first premise of Saussure's model presented in paragraph 1 is that the relationship between the "signifier" and the "signified" is "fundamentally arbitrary—there is no natural reason the letters t-r-e-e must denote a plant with a trunk and leaves." The end result described in paragraph 2 is that "through social convention, these arbitrary links could be fixed, creating a stable and predictable system of meaning." This further allows for "clear communication." **(D)** provides a reason for particular words to have a meaning that is *not* fundamentally arbitrary, which would weaken the Saussurean model.

Wrong Answer Explanations

(A) Saussure begins with the idea that the link between a word and its concept is arbitrary. The fact that different cultures independently developed completely different sounds for the same object supports this foundational idea of arbitrariness.

(B) This finding addresses how humans acquire language biologically, confirming that it's a learned process. This is not inconsistent with either Saussure's view (we learn the social conventions) or the post-structuralist view.

(C) This choice is tempting because the meaning of a term has changed slightly, but the choice states that the reason for the shift is a change in social norms. Paragraph 2 states that "Saussure believed that through social convention, these arbitrary links could be fixed, creating a stable and predictable system of meaning." However, if social convention changes, it would not challenge Saussure to say that a word's meaning changes along with the convention.

Question 10: (C) – Strengthen/Weaken Argument

Explanation for Question 10

This question asks you to analyze the real-world phenomenon of jargon and determine its effect on the two competing theories from the passage. Jargon consists of specialized words created by a community to have specific, fixed meanings within a field. This is very similar to the description of Saussure's belief that "through social convention these arbitrary links" between words and meanings "could be fixed, creating a stable and predictable system of meaning" (paragraph 2). Jargon is essentially a deliberate effort to create a small-scale Saussurean language system. Therefore, its existence is strong evidence in support of Saussure's theory of how meaning can be anchored by social agreement. **(C)** is correct.

Wrong Answer Explanations

(A) This choice misinterprets the concept of "arbitrary." Paragraph 1 states that Saussure held that "the relationship between these two parts is fundamentally arbitrary—there is no natural reason the letters t-r-e-e must denote a plant with a trunk and leaves." While the decision to create a term is purposeful, the specific word chosen can still be an arbitrary sound that has no inherent connection to its meaning (for example, "t-o-r-t" in law has no necessary connection to its legal meaning).

(B) The question defines jargon as a specialized term that is created to have a given meaning, which is very different from post-structuralism's view that "meaning is not contained within a word but is generated by the endless play of differences between words" (paragraph 4). If, as the question states, jargon can be assigned a specific, fixed meaning, then it would weaken the post-structuralist view rather than strengthen it.

(D) While the question does state that jargon is a specialized term for a given field, the question of whether academic language has limited uses or broader uses is not considered in the passage by either view.

Question 11: (B) – Imagine Example/Analogy

Explanation for Question 11

This question asks you to find the scenario that is *least* analogous to the Saussurean model of language. The core principles of this model are that the relationship between a "signifier" (the word) and its "signified" (meaning) is "fundamentally arbitrary" and that "through social convention, these arbitrary links could be fixed, creating a stable and predictable system of meaning." **(B)** is correct because it fails on the first and most important principle. A fever is a *natural sign* of illness; its meaning is derived from a direct, causal relationship in biology. It is the opposite of an arbitrary symbol. Because it describes a natural, not conventional, system of meaning, it is the least analogous to Saussure's model of language.

Wrong Answer Explanations

(A) The link between the red octagon and the command to stop is arbitrary (the shape could have been a circle or the color blue) and is made stable by social convention (traffic laws and driver education) to ensure clear communication. It is therefore analogous.

(C) The paper's value is arbitrary (it has no intrinsic worth) and is stabilized by a shared social and governmental agreement. This allows a meaningless object to function as a fixed sign of economic value. Thus, it is analogous.

(D) The symbol is entirely arbitrary—it is a purely conventional choice of symbol. Its meaning is made stable and predictable by the social convention of music theory, which allows musicians worldwide to interpret it in the exact same way. So, it is analogous.

Question 12: (C) – Anticipate Response

Explanation for Question 12

This question asks you to predict the author's reaction to a new scenario based on their perspective as revealed in the passage. The "Logos" AI project aims to reveal the objectively true meaning of a text, which is similar to Saussure's structuralist view that "imagines language as a vast, ordered system of signs, where each word, like a piece on a chessboard, has a distinct value and function derived from its relationship to all the other pieces" (paragraph 2). In contrast, post-structuralism holds that "meaning is not contained within a word but is generated by the endless play of differences between words" (paragraph 3).

In the final paragraph, the author concludes by describing post-structuralism as a "powerful, if unsettling, tool" while claiming that the impact of Saussurean structuralism "was largely confined to academic disciplines." Also, in paragraph 4, the author states that the "linguistic insight" of post-structuralism "has profound implications. If language is an unstable, self-referential system, then the concepts it purports to describe—justice, identity, history, truth—are themselves rendered unstable." Taking these claims from the passage together, the words "powerful" and "profound" indicate that the author believes that post-structuralism has a point worth considering: some of these concepts are unable to be precisely described with language. Given the author's respect for the post-structuralist viewpoint, the author would view the "Logos" project's goal as philosophically misguided. **(C)** is correct.

Wrong Answer Explanations

(A) The goal for "Logos" is closer to the Saussurean goal of "language as a vast, ordered system of signs, where each word, like a piece on a chessboard, has a distinct value and function" (paragraph 2). However, in paragraph 5, the author describes Saussurean structuralism as "largely confined to academic disciplines concerned with classification and systems," so the author would not describe the project as "beneficial" or anticipate its success.

(B) The author concludes the passage by emphasizing the "far-reaching" (paragraph 5) influence of post-structuralism on our understanding of the world and meaning. The author would certainly believe that a project attempting to define objective meaning is connected to these linguistic and philosophical debates, so the author would not dismiss it by saying it has "little relevance."

(D) In paragraph 5, the author does describe post-structuralism as "a powerful, if unsettling, tool for deconstructing cherished cultural narratives and questioning the foundations of authority." However, the unsettling nature seems to be more about questioning difficult ideas. The exertion of social control is not raised in the passage.

UNIT 5

ADDITIONAL PRACTICE

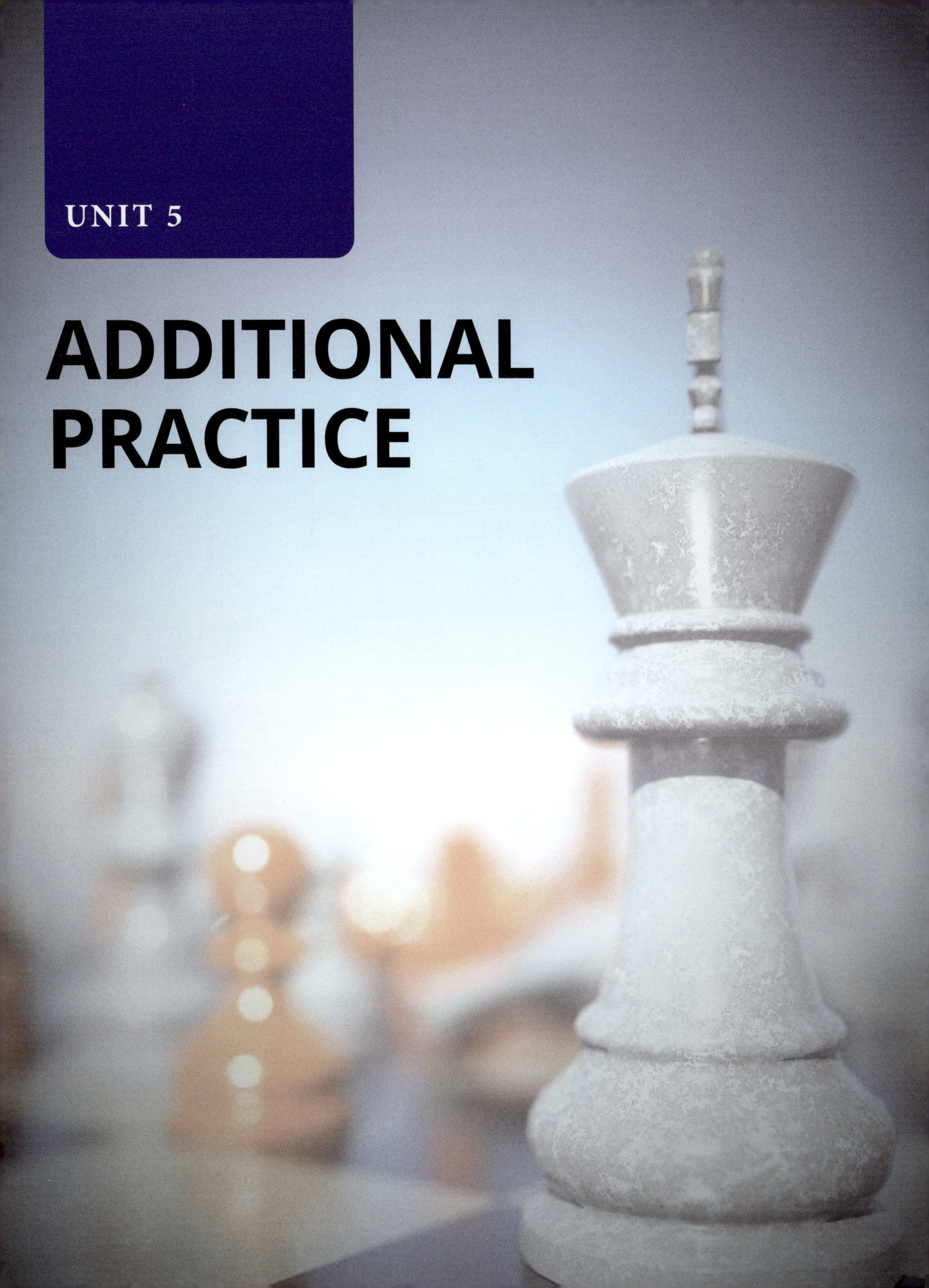

CHAPTER 22

MIXED PRACTICE

How to Use This Chapter

This practice chapter contains three full MCAT passages and question sets, spanning the full range of CARS skills explained in this book and tested on the exam. Students early in their prep should attempt these passages untimed (or time "up" from 0 to see how long it takes you), but if you're looking for a more test-like experience, limit yourself to 10 minutes per passage or 30 minutes if attempting all three passages in one sitting. Use the strategies discussed in Chapters 1–6 to Read and Distill the passages and answer the associated questions. Then, use the answer explanations at the end of the chapter to review your practice (information on how to review your practice can be found in Chapter 7).

Passage 1 (Questions 1–7)

It would be difficult to overstate the complexity of the written Japanese language. The system of writing (or more properly, systems) represents a fusion of almost entirely non-native characters and a spoken language so linguistically isolated that philologists have yet to discover a precursor. The Japanese language lacked any system of writing at all for much of its history. Making up for lost time, though, no fewer than three different systems of writing are now employed.

The first Japanese system of writing was not Japanese. The kanji, a group of logographic Chinese characters, each representing a word or idea, were adopted with minimal change around the seventh century. Few languages are so geographically close yet linguistically dissimilar. As a result, the people of Japan adopted a modified Chinese pronunciation for each kanji (the on-yomi), while retaining the native Japanese spoken word that most closely fit each kanji's meaning (the kun-yomi). In modern Japanese, the on-yomi is used for certain kanji and the kun-yomi for others, with compound words often involving both. Further adding complication, the Chinese language contains many words in which variations in tone alone indicate drastically different meanings. The adaptation of these words to Japanese pronunciation led to a number of homophones that has, without hyperbole, been called "embarrassing" and "alarming" by scholars of the language.

The hiragana syllabary was developed in the eighth century by court women, who were not permitted to study kanji because they were deemed unfit to master its complexities. In response, they developed a simplified, flowing form of the kanji that represented all the sounds in spoken Japanese. Hiragana is phonetic rather than logographic and is therefore far more accessible to a foreign learner than the kanji. Because Japanese is an open language, syllables typically don't end with consonants. Hiragana is therefore not strictly an alphabet. Katakana came about around the same time as hiragana, also as an attempt to simplify the kanji. The sparse, angular characters correspond fairly closely to the hiragana and, as befitting their origin among Buddhist monks, have a look generally considered more masculine than hiragana, which was originally called onnade, or "women's hand." The katakana have essentially become the print counterparts of the "cursive" hiragana.

With so many systems jostling for position, each used more or less independently of the other, it would not be unreasonable to anticipate that a national movement toward systematization of the language would settle on a single one. A national movement was in fact started after World War II: a radical idea encouraging the use of all three systems together. A glance at any Tokyo newspaper will reveal kanji used to represent most standard actions and ideas, hiragana to indicate grammatical inflections and tenses, and katakana to represent adopted non-native and technical words, as well as to indicate emphasis. The use of the three systems has become sufficiently standardized in this way that deviations often lend a piece of writing strong connotations. A piece written entirely in katakana, for example, may be disconcerting to a modern reader and may have a vaguely pre–World War II military air to it, much as a piece written all in capital letters with telegraph punctuation might in English. While such a complex system has made the language's learning curve high for native and non-native speakers alike, it has also contributed to a stunning richness of expression such that any list of the world's great works of art a hundred years from now will have to be written in a combination of kanji, hiragana, and katakana.

1. The author mentions Chinese kanji (paragraph 2) primarily for what reason?
- **A.** To argue that the large number of homophones in Japanese is due to its closeness to Chinese
- **B.** To illustrate that the presence of homophones in a language can be considered embarrassing
- **C.** To show it as a precursor to the Japanese method of writing that caused some linguistic quirks
- **D.** To provide evidence for the fact that the meanings of homophones are often dependent on variations in tone

2. The author's primary purpose in the passage is to:
- **A.** argue that the Japanese language is extremely complex.
- **B.** describe the origins of the complexity of written Japanese.
- **C.** propose a simplification in how Japanese is written.
- **D.** trace the origins of one particular logographic writing system.

3. Based on information in the passage, which of the following pieces of Japanese literature would probably NOT be written entirely in katakana?
- **A.** A modern Japanese novel
- **B.** A list of adopted foreign words
- **C.** An eleventh-century Buddhist text
- **D.** An early twentieth-century general's log

4. The author's description implies that open languages generally contain:
- **A.** borrowed systems of writing.
- **B.** intrinsic acceptance of change.
- **C.** syllables that end in vowels.
- **D.** few consonant sounds.

5. It can be inferred from the passage that the Buddhist monks who developed katakana:
- **A.** were predominantly male.
- **B.** used hiragana as a model.
- **C.** couldn't master the complexities of kanji.
- **D.** were involved with the military.

6. Which of the following is a claim the author makes without providing evidence, explanation, or example?
   - **A.** The hiragana system was primarily developed by court women.
   - **B.** Deviations from standard written Japanese can embody strong connotations.
   - **C.** The logographic kanji system of writing originated in China.
   - **D.** The katakana are essentially counterparts of the "cursive" hiragana.

7. Suppose that the Vietnamese language, which uses tonal variations to distinguish word meanings, was adopted as the basis for a writing system by a neighboring culture whose spoken language lacks tones. The passage author would most likely expect that the neighboring culture's:
   - **A.** writing system would contain an unusually large number of homophones.
   - **B.** language would retain Vietnamese pronunciations but assign new meanings to the words.
   - **C.** women would develop a simplified, phonetic script.
   - **D.** system of writing would indicate grammatical inflections and tenses.

Passage 2 (Questions 8–13)

Peter Gay's book, *The Education of the Senses*, reexamines Victorian bourgeois attitudes about sensuality and sexuality in an attempt to discredit the pervasive and negative view of the Victorian bourgeois as repressed and repressive people whose outwardly prim public appearances often hypocritically masked inner lascivious thoughts and private behaviors. One of the most interesting facets of Gay's study is his treatment of the necessary, yet at the time largely taboo, subject of birth control during the latter part of the nineteenth century.

Gay points out that the very process of giving birth was dangerous to both baby and mother—many infants did not survive being born, and many others perished within their first five years, while most women suffered greatly during the birth, and a not inconsiderable number of them died as well. It is no wonder that women often approached the child-bearing process with trepidation even though they believed that producing offspring was a woman's ultimate fulfillment. Advice or assistance from the medical profession—whether licensed doctors or less formally trained midwives—was sorely lacking and inconsistent, hardly capable of reassuring the expectant parents about the safety of either mother or baby.

In fact, the medical profession itself was often responsible for promulgating myths and rumors about the dangers of some forms of birth control, regardless of the fact that so many women and children died each year due to complications of pregnancy or birth. Some medical, religious, and social experts did acknowledge that the continual cycle of childbearing was not only detrimental to the health of the mother, but also could take a toll on the quality of life of the family as a whole because multiple children increased the financial burden and responsibility of the father. Furthermore, women were often caught in this cycle of pregnancy and childbirth well into their late 40s, greatly increasing the health risks and mortality rate of mothers and children alike. It seemed appropriate and even necessary, then, to make efforts to limit the number of offspring in order to benefit the family unit and thus the greater good of society itself.

Nonetheless, open discussion of birth control methods, both natural and device-assisted, was rare, even between doctor and patient. Most information was quietly passed between women by word of mouth, which inevitably led to a great deal of unchecked misinformation that was, at times, deadly. Gay maintains that a primary motivation for this reticence was deeply ingrained in the Victorian bourgeois mindset that emphasized the value of family and traditional roles and thus encouraged women to be productive—in the very literal, procreative sense. Though concerned husbands certainly did sometimes take steps to ensure that their wives and families were not jeopardized by an overabundance of offspring, widespread efforts to limit family size were not firmly rooted in society until the advent of a strong women's movement, which did not make many real and meaningful strides toward changing public attitudes and behaviors until the early twentieth century. Thus, Victorian bourgeois women were obliged to fulfill their societal role as childbearers despite very real fears about the toll this could take on their health and on the well-being of their family.

8. Which of the following is NOT suggested by the author as a reason underlying many Victorian women's failure to use birth control?

- **A.** Rather than offering birth control options, many doctors at most only suggested limiting the number of pregnancies.
- **B.** Cultural pressures related to their role within the family meant that women were expected to continue having children.
- **C.** It could be difficult for women to rely on the accuracy of information about the safety of birth control methods.
- **D.** Many medical authorities were themselves not well informed of effective techniques for preventing pregnancy.

9. Which of the following, if true, would most seriously weaken Gay's argument that deeply ingrained social attitudes were responsible for the lack of open discussion about birth control?

- **A.** The majority of Victorian women were satisfied with their role as wives and mothers.
- **B.** Bourgeois Victorian families often hired nannies to undertake child-rearing duties.
- **C.** Many middle-class Victorians believed that the ideal family consisted of three children.
- **D.** Most Victorian physicians knew that family planning would improve women's overall health.

10. According to the passage, which of the following was commonly associated with the birth of children during the Victorian era?

- **I.** Death of the child
- **II.** Added financial pressure
- **III.** Greater social status

- **A.** I only
- **B.** I and II only
- **C.** I and III only
- **D.** II and III only

11. Which of the following statements is most consistent with Gay's arguments as presented in the passage?

- **A.** Understanding the psychological basis for social actions can help to explain apparently contradictory behavioral patterns.
- **B.** Examination of sociohistorical context offers the historian little useful information about the prevailing attitudes of the Victorian bourgeois.
- **C.** Social historians can best analyze past cultures by applying modern theories to the work of earlier critics.
- **D.** Critics should not attempt to rework prior studies of social class because they cannot properly understand the historical context of their predecessors.

12. How would the author most likely react to the observation that most of the passage depicts Gay representing Victorian bourgeois attitudes as both repressed and repressive?

- **A.** The representation is accurate and is a fitting microcosm for Gay's view of Victorian bourgeois society in general.
- **B.** The representation of Victorian bourgeois attitudes focuses primarily on birth control, which is only one facet of a larger topic.
- **C.** The representation of Victorian bourgeois attitudes is meant to serve primarily as a contrast to those of other social classes.
- **D.** The representation presents a biased and perhaps deliberately distorted vision of Victorian bourgeois attitudes toward childbearing.

13. Which of the following does the passage cite as an important factor directly contributing to the high danger associated with Victorian childbirth?

- **A.** Misleading information about the risks of childbirth
- **B.** Unsanitary conditions in birthing rooms
- **C.** Successive cycles of pregnancy and childbirth
- **D.** The lack of a strong women's movement

Passage 3 (Questions 14–20)

At the end of the first decade of this century, a literary genre dedicated to history emerged in France. Anticipated in 2006 by Jonathan Littell's novel, *Les Bienveillantes*, a wave of novels dedicated to the relatively recent past swept throughout the country. The topics covered included the Algerian War, the Shoah, the Second World War, and the Great War. Recollection of these momentous events has been largely taken over by literary fiction that has shown itself to be very effective in reproducing historical knowledge of facts and, moreover, in providing depth and meaning to the past. This recourse to narrative—and to so-called "competent" narrative—is not only a challenge to the traditional productions of historians; it is also supported by the Aristotelian claim that views literary fiction, because of its universality, as superior to history.

This literary fiction has carved out a specific space for itself, filling that no man's land that lies between memory and history: the protagonists of these recent historical landscapes were disappearing and some of the archives were not yet accessible to historians. "Who bears witness for the witness?"—a reworked quotation from Paul Celan that Yannick Haenel puts in the title of his novel—is a real program embraced by a good number of writers of this period. Historians rightly see it as a challenge on their own ground, and they smell defeat.

Faced with the loss of hegemony over the narratives of the past, historians have reacted in two ways: one is to publicly question and confront the value of literature and its role in the transmission of history; the other is to experiment. The upshot of this experimentation is that one can find not only a few changes in the presentation of historical works, such as the minimization or even elimination of formal tools such as footnotes, but also more substantial ones, such as the abandonment of scientific objectivity in favor of a subjectivity that makes the authority of the historian the main criterion of validation. These are just two examples of an ongoing transformation of contemporary historiography as it aims to situate itself on a terrain close to, if not identical to, that of literary creation.

Ivan Jablonka, an academic who writes under his own name as a historian and used to write fiction under a pseudonym, is probably the clearest embodiment of this tendency, which he makes explicit in one of his latest works. Jablonka seeks to re-establish the dialogue between the social sciences and a wider audience through the recomposition of different genres in a new category—that of the "literature of reality," which includes history, literature, memoirs, and testimonies. According to Jablonka, this is one tool among many to better achieve the goals that social scientists set for themselves. It also represents a new freedom for historians.

The features of this new freedom, however, raise questions about the means by which the historical discourse is scientifically validated. That history must be dusted off is a fact. The literary posture of historians, however, goes well beyond the narrative resources they choose to deploy. The knowledge of the world produced by literature and that produced by history are not identical—the two mobilize different resources. The destruction, by historians, of the frontier between history and literature engenders a loss, not a gain. We lose appreciation of a critical approach that requires a dispassionate relationship to sources, and we no longer compel the reader to develop an interpretation that is more intellectual than empathetic.

14. The author's position on some historians' embrace of a literary approach is that:
    A. a new freedom for historians is beneficial for communicating history to readers.
    B. merging history with literature negatively impacts the quality of scholarly investigations.
    C. the blending of history with literature in a new "literature of reality" is a valuable tactic.
    D. goals set by social scientists are fundamentally incompatible with the goals of novelists.

15. The "no man's land" that the passage author mentions in paragraph 2 is:
    A. a desolate battlefield region between opposing armies in the Great War.
    B. events for which there are neither surviving witnesses nor accessible historical records.
    C. the period of history before the arrival of human civilization at a particular location.
    D. an Aristotelian claim regarding the superiority of literature to history.

16. Suppose that most writers of historical fiction engage in extensive research into their novel's historical setting before writing. Is this information relevant to any of the ideas in the passage?
    A. No; it has no relevance to the discussion of literature dedicated to recent history.
    B. Yes; it strengthens the Aristotelian claim that literary fiction is superior because of its universality.
    C. Yes; it strengthens the claim that literary fiction has shown itself to be effective at preserving knowledge.
    D. Yes; it weakens the claim that historians rightly see such fiction as a challenge to their own work.

17. The passage implies that Jablonka would be most likely to agree with which one of the following statements about social scientists?
    A. Memoirs are more likely to contain bias and should be avoided by social scientists.
    B. Social scientists should seek to increase freedom in other scholarly pursuits as well.
    C. The "literature of reality" is the best way to truly reach social scientists' goals.
    D. Social scientists have lost some of the connection to their desired audience.

18. Which of the following passage statements best expresses the author's conclusion regarding the transformation in contemporary historiography that is discussed in the passage?
    A. "Faced with the loss of hegemony over the narratives of the past, historians have reacted in two ways."
    B. "The destruction of the frontier between history and literature by historians engenders a loss, not a gain."
    C. "That history must be dusted off is a fact."
    D. "Historians rightly see it as a challenge on their own ground, and they smell defeat."

19. Why does the author most likely refer to "formal tools such as footnotes" (paragraph 3)?
    A. To provide an example of ways that historians are altering their works to be more similar to literature
    B. To disparage what the author sees as a highly detrimental aspect of historians' experimentation
    C. To describe a way in which historians establish their authority in order to validate their works
    D. To promote an appropriate means by which historical works can be independently verified

20. Suppose a historian publishes a book in which each chapter begins with a letter written by a historical figure and continues with an imaginative account of what it was like to live through the events described in the letter. How would the author likely view such a work?
    A. As a misguided work that falls short in the impartial analysis of sources
    B. As a praiseworthy example of the new genre "literature of reality"
    C. As unnecessary, given the success already achieved by historical fiction
    D. As an admirable challenge to the productions of historical fiction writers

Answers and Explanations

Passage 1 (Questions 1–7)

Question 1: (C) – Describe Purpose

Explanation for Question 1

According to paragraph 2, "The kanji, a group of logographic Chinese characters, each representing a word or idea, were adopted with minimal change around the seventh century." The author goes on to explain that the resulting adaptation of Chinese words with variations in tone to Japanese resulted in lots of homophones, so many that this has "been called 'embarrassing' and 'alarming' by scholars of the language." Thus, the adoption of kanji as an early form of Japanese writing had some rather odd, unanticipated effects on the Japanese language. **(C)** fits this prediction perfectly.

Wrong Answer Explanations

(A) The author does not say that the Japanese language is "close" to the Chinese language—quite the opposite! Although China and Japan are *physically* near each other, the author points out, "Few languages are so… linguistically dissimilar."

(B) Nothing in paragraph 2 implies that the mere *presence* of homophones can be embarrassing, only that an excess of homophones can be embarrassing.

(D) This supposed "fact" is false: it was the *loss* of "variations in tone" that led to the formation of homophones in Japanese. If two words are pronounced differently, they are not homophones.

Question 2: (B) – Describe Purpose

Explanation for Question 2

The first paragraph of the passage makes the point that the Japanese language is complex. Paragraph 2 examines the origins of the Japanese written language, and paragraphs 3 and 4 discuss how it evolved into three systems of writing that are interrelated in complicated ways. The only option that cites both the origins and the complexity of the Japanese language is **(B)**, and it is the correct choice.

Wrong Answer Explanations

(A) This is wrong both because the author is neutral and does not make any strong arguments, and because it completely neglects the passage's goal of tracing the history of written Japanese.

(C) Although a reader might conclude that it would be easier if written Japanese were simplified, the author makes no such proposal—or proposals of any kind—in this passage.

(D) Kanji is the only logographic writing system the author discusses, and its origins (in China) are mentioned only in a single phrase in paragraph 2. That's too narrow to be the passage's purpose.

Question 3: (A) – Imagine Example/Analogy

Explanation for Question 3

The katakana writing system is introduced in paragraph 3, which states that it was developed sometime around the eighth century by Buddhist monks to simplify the kanji. Paragraph 4 goes on to describe a synthesis, beginning "after World War II" and now relatively universal, that combines all three writing systems (including katakana). Within this modern fusion, the author notes that katakana is used primarily to "represent adopted non-native and technical words, as well as to indicate emphasis." Thus, any long, multifaceted contemporary work, such as a "modern novel," should include kanji and hiragana as well as katakana. The correct choice is **(A)**.

Wrong Answer Explanations

(B) According to paragraph 4, katakana are used nowadays to represent "adopted non-native and technical words." A list of foreign words, therefore, would be expected to be written entirely in katakana.

(C) According to paragraph 3, katakana originated "among Buddhist monks" "around the same time" as hiragana, which the author says were developed "in the eighth century." Thus, it would not be surprising for an eleventh-century text written by Buddhist monks to be rendered in katakana.

(D) Paragraph 4 states that "A piece written entirely in katakana, for example, may be disconcerting to a modern reader and may have a vaguely pre–World War II military air to it." This suggests that an "early twentieth-century general's log" would most likely be written in katakana.

Question 4: (C) – Paraphrase Detail

Explanation for Question 4

The fourth sentence of paragraph 3 states that "Because Japanese is an open language, syllables typically don't end with consonants." If syllables in open languages don't end in consonants, they must end in vowels. **(C)** is the correct answer.

Wrong Answer Explanations

(A) Although this happens to be true of the Japanese language, there is nothing in the passage to indicate that it is true of "open languages" in general.

(B) Although this is a common meaning of the word "open," it does not fit into the context of the author's discussion of Japanese.

(D) Although the passage states that Japanese syllables typically don't *end* with consonants, this does not imply that there are few consonants in them overall.

Question 5: (A) – Paraphrase Detail

Explanation for Question 5

Paragraph 3 discusses the development of the katakana, stating that their "sparse, angular characters correspond fairly closely to the hiragana and, as *befitting their origin* among Buddhist monks, have a look *generally considered more masculine* than hiragana." The italicized portions of that sentence—especially the use of the word "befitting," clearly implies that the Buddhist monks who developed katakana were men. Furthermore, the author also notes that hiragana was developed by women and was known as "women's hand," and sets up a contrast between katakana and hiragana on this basis of gender. The katakana system was definitely developed by men, and **(A)** is correct.

Wrong Answer Explanations

(B) Although this is possible, there is nothing that actually indicates what model the monks who developed katakana used. All the passage says is that "Katakana came about around the same time as hiragana."

(C) There is no support in the passage for this. Although it does say that the women who developed hiragana were "*considered* unfit to master the complexities of kanji." It does not say that those women were *actually* unable to master kanji's complexities; neither does the author say anything remotely similar regarding the monks who developed katakana.

(D) Although the author points out that katakana is seen by modern readers as possessing a "vaguely . . . military air" (paragraph 4), there is nothing in the passage to suggest that the monks who developed katakana over a thousand years ago were involved with the military.

Question 6: (C) – Evaluate Reasoning

Explanation for Question 6

The claim that kanji originated in China appears, in passing, in paragraph 2, which states, "The kanji, a group of logographic Chinese characters, each representing a word or idea, were adopted with minimal change around the seventh century." There is no evidence presented for this claim, and no other reference in the passage to how or where the kanji were developed. The correct answer is **(C)**.

Wrong Answer Explanations

(A) Paragraph 3 discusses the development of hiragana by court women, explaining that these women "were not permitted to study kanji because they were deemed unfit to master its complexities. In response, they developed a simplified, flowing form." The paragraph goes on to expand on this even further.

(B) This claim from paragraph 4 is supported by the following illustration: "A piece written entirely in katakana, for example, may be disconcerting to a modern reader and may have a vaguely pre–World War II military air to it."

(D) This claim from paragraph 3 is supported and amplified by the sentence that immediately precedes it, which states that katakana's "sparse, angular characters correspond fairly closely to the hiragana."

Question 7: (A) – Predict Outcome/Explanation

Explanation for Question 7

Paragraph 2 explains that, because the Chinese language uses tonal variations to create different meanings and

Japanese pronunciation does not, the adaptation of Chinese characters into Japanese "led to a number of homophones that has, without hyperbole, been called 'embarrassing' and 'alarming' by scholars of the language." The scenario described in the question is directly analogous to this process, so a similar linguistic outcome with many homophones is likely. **(A)** is correct.

Wrong Answer Explanations

(B) This is the opposite of the process described in the passage. Paragraph 2 states that when adopting Chinese kanji, the Japanese "adopted a modified Chinese pronunciation for each kanji (the on-yomi), while retaining the native Japanese spoken word that most closely fit each kanji's meaning (the kun-yomi)." Therefore, they changed the pronunciation but kept the meaning, not the other way around.

(C) This choice alludes to the origin of the hiragana script, which according to the passage was not a linguistic outcome of adopting a tonal writing system, but instead was dictated by specific beliefs about women in that period of Japanese history. Since there is no indication that the neighboring culture discussed in the question stem would have a similar attitude toward women, there is no reason to expect the development of a simplified script as occurred in Japan.

(D) According to paragraph 2, the kanji were adapted from a culture in China whose spoken language used variations in tone to signify different meanings, so the scenario in the question stem is comparable to how this system was adopted in Japan. Since paragraph 4 states that the hiragana script, not kanji, is used for "grammatical inflections and tenses," the result described in this choice is not connected to the question stem.

Passage 2 (Questions 8–13)

Question 8: (D) – Evaluate Reasoning

Explanation for Question 8

Paragraph 2 contains language directly supporting **(A)**, while paragraph 4 supports both **(B)** and **(C)**. However, the closest that the passage comes to suggesting that **(D)** is true is the statement that "the medical profession itself was often responsible for promulgating myths and rumors about the *dangers* of *some* forms of birth control." Just because doctors might have been misinformed about the dangers of some forms of birth control, however, they weren't necessarily misinformed about "*effective* methods of preventing pregnancy," which is what **(D)** maintains. Safety and effectiveness are two different things (hence the phrase "safe *and* effective"). Since it is not supported by the passage, **(D)** is the correct choice.

Wrong Answer Explanations

(A) This is directly supported by the following statement from paragraph 2: "Advice or assistance from the medical profession—whether licensed doctors or less formally trained midwives—was sorely lacking and inconsistent."

(B) According to paragraph 4, "the Victorian bourgeois mindset ... emphasized the value of family and ... encouraged women to be productive—in the very literal, procreative sense."

(C) According to paragraph 4, discussions of birth control were subject to "a great deal of unchecked misinformation that was, at times, deadly." Moreover, according to paragraph 3, "the medical profession itself was often responsible for promulgating myths and rumors about the dangers of some forms of birth control."

Question 9: (C) – Strengthen/Weaken Argument

Explanation for Question 9

According to the passage, Gay argues that deeply ingrained social attitudes were responsible for the lack of open discussion of birth control. Paragraph 2 states that people "believed that producing offspring was a woman's ultimate fulfillment." Paragraph 4 builds on this by saying that "Gay maintains ... a primary motivation" for the reluctance to discuss birth control "was deeply ingrained in the Victorian bourgeois mindset that emphasized the value of family and traditional roles and thus encouraged women to be productive—in the very literal, procreative sense." As a result of these attitudes, women were caught in a "continual cycle of childbearing" and "widespread efforts to limit family size were not firmly rooted in society until the advent of a strong women's movement, which did not make many real and meaningful strides toward changing public attitudes and behaviors until the early twentieth century." If, in contrast to this picture, Victorians believed that an ideal family contained only three children, there would have been strong social pressures to limit family size, undermining Gay's thesis about why birth control wasn't openly discussed. **(C)** is the right answer.

Wrong Answer Explanations

(A) This is completely consistent with Gay' argument, reflecting the claim that Victorian women "believed that producing offspring was a woman's ultimate fulfillment."

(B) Because they provide additional logistical support, hired nannies would have allowed families to raise more children than they would have been able to raise without nannies. Thus, it is consistent with Gay's argument.

(D) If doctors actually knew that family planning was beneficial, and yet still did not discuss it openly, the argument that prevailing social attitudes were responsible for preventing such discussions would be supported, not undermined, because it would remove an alternative explanation (that the doctors were ignorant of family planning's benefits) for the lack of discussion.

Question 10: (B) – Paraphrase Detail

Explanation for Question 10

Paragraph 2 states that "many infants did not survive being born, and many others perished within their first five years," so Item I is true. Paragraph 3 states that "multiple children increased the financial burden" on families, so Item II is also true. Although the passage argues that there were social pressures to have more children, there is nothing to suggest that having children conferred increased social status upon a family. So, Item III is unsupported. **(B)**, "I and II only," is the correct choice.

Roman Numeral Explanations

(I) True. The death of the child was unfortunately a common occurrence with Victorian-era births, according to paragraph 2: "many infants did not survive being born."

(II) True. Additional financial pressure on the family is associated with birth in the Victorian era, as described in paragraph 3: "multiple children increased the financial burden."

(III) False. The passage never suggests that births commonly conferred status benefits to parents in the Victorian era, despite the fact that there was social pressure to have more children, as explained in the last paragraph.

Question 11: (A) – Recognize Opinion

Explanation for Question 11

The first paragraph of the passage says that Gay "reexamines Victorian bourgeois attitudes about sensuality and sexuality in an attempt to discredit the pervasive and negative view of the Victorian bourgeois as repressed and repressive people whose outwardly prim public appearances often hypocritically masked inner lascivious thoughts and private behaviors." This provides direct support for the idea that psychological analyses can be used to understand "apparently contradictory behavioral patterns." The correct answer is **(A)**.

Wrong Answer Explanations

(B) Based on the passage, Gay clearly uses "sociohistorical context" to help understand the "prevailing attitudes of the Victorian bourgeois." This directly contradicts the claim in this answer choice that such context provides "little useful information."

(C) This claim is arguably out of scope of the passage, as Gay does not apply modern theories to the work of earlier *critics*. Even if Gay actually did that, however, there is certainly no support for the claim in the answer choice, that this is the "best" way to proceed.

(D) The first paragraph implies that Gay does indeed "rework prior studies" using "sociohistorical context." This is not consistent with the claim in the answer choice that critics "should not attempt" to do such things.

Question 12: (B) – Anticipate Response

Explanation for Question 12

The first paragraph of the passage states that Gay's book attempts "to discredit the pervasive and negative view of the Victorian bourgeois as repressed and repressive people." Nevertheless, Gay's discussion of birth control, as it's depicted in the passage, does seem to represent the Victorian bourgeois as somewhat "repressed and repressive." How would the author most likely react to this apparent contradiction? Paragraph 1 also states that the discussion of birth control is only "one of the ... facets of Gay's study." By saying this, the author is implying that Gay's study has other facets as well, in which he, by implication, must engage in his project to discredit the negative stereotypes of the Victorian bourgeois as repressed and repressive hypocrites. The only answer choice consistent with this analysis is **(B)**, which is correct.

Wrong Answer Explanations

(A) Far from being a "fitting microcosm for Gay's view," the picture of the Victorian bourgeois as "repressed and repressive" represents the vision that Gay is attempting to "discredit."

(C) There is no reference, either explicit or implied, to other social classes anywhere in the passage.

(D) Nothing in the passage suggests that the author does not accept the vision of Victorian attitudes presented in Gay's book.

Question 13: (C) – Paraphrase Detail

Explanation for Question 13

Paragraph 3 acknowledges that many women died in childbirth, and that "the continual cycle of childbearing was ... detrimental to the health of the mother." Furthermore, "Women were often caught in this cycle of pregnancy and childbirth well into their late 40s, greatly increasing the health risks and mortality rate of mothers and children alike." The correct choice is **(C)**.

Wrong Answer Explanations

(A) Although the passage extensively discusses misinformation about birth control, it does not suggest that people were misinformed about the dangers of childbirth itself. On the contrary, paragraph 2 states that because of this danger, "women often approached the child-bearing process with trepidation."

(B) Although unsanitary conditions in birthing rooms may well have contributed to the dangers of childbirth, this is not discussed at all in the passage.

(D) Although paragraph 4 suggests that the advent of a strong women's movement allowed women a greater likelihood of *avoiding* the dangers of childbirth, it cannot be said that the lack of a women's movement contributed "directly" to those dangers themselves, as required by the question stem.

Passage 3 (Questions 14–20)

Question 14: (B) – Recognize Opinion

Explanation for Question 14

The author is openly critical of historians who blur the line between history and literature. This position is most clearly expressed in the last paragraph, which states that the destruction of the frontier between history and literature results in "a loss, not a gain." The author elaborates that this is the loss of "appreciation of a critical approach that requires a dispassionate relationship to the sources." In other words, by incorporating a literary approach, these historians are damaging their scholarly relationship with source materials. **(B)** is correct.

Wrong Answer Explanations

(A) The author states at the beginning of the last paragraph that the new freedom raises questions, devoting most of the paragraph to describing its drawbacks rather than its advantages—the author does not think this freedom has been beneficial for "communicating history."

(C) Jablonka, as described in paragraph 4, advocates that historians embrace a literary approach and create a "literature of reality." The author's position, however, is contained in paragraph 5—this approach results in "a loss, not a gain."

(D) The idea that the goals of social scientists are "fundamentally incompatible" with the goals of novelists is an extreme claim that the author never makes.

Question 15: (B) – Interpret Meaning

Explanation for Question 15

Paragraph 2 refers to the "no man's land that lies between memory and history," and speaks of a time when "the protagonists of ... recent historical landscapes were disappearing and some of the archives were not yet accessible to historians." The colon that separates these two statements indicates that the second phrase is supposed to explain what the phrase "no man's land" refers to. In other words, the phrase "no man's land" refers to the time period that lies between the disappearance of the protagonists ("memory") who directly participated in events and the lack of access to archives ("history") that have yet to become available—the time period in which neither human nor archive sources are available. **(B)** is correct.

Wrong Answer Explanations

(A) The phrase "no man's land" is commonly used to refer to the terrain situated between opposing armies, particularly in the Great War (World War I). But, in talking about "the no man's land *that lies between memory and history*" the author is clearly using the phrase metaphorically rather than literally and is not describing a physical area.

(C) Nowhere in the passage does the author discuss history before the advent of human civilization.

(D) The "Aristotelian claim that views literary fiction, because of its universality, as superior to history," is mentioned in paragraph 1. The discussion in paragraph 2 that cites a "no man's land" is completely unrelated to this.

Question 16: (C) – Strengthen/Weaken Argument

Explanation for Question 16

The first paragraph introduces writers of historical fiction and claims that their "literary fiction ... has shown itself to be very effective in reproducing historical knowledge of facts." If most writers of historical fiction engaged in extensive research into their subject before beginning to write, this claim from the passage would be strengthened, making **(C)** correct.

Wrong Answer Explanations

(A) The hypothetical information in the question stem concerns writers of historical fiction, so it definitely has relevance to literature about history, which is discussed extensively in the passage.

(B) Whether or not writers of historical fiction do extensive research about their subjects has nothing to do with the claim that "literary fiction" (not historical fiction) is superior to history because of its "universality."

(D) If anything, the hypothetical information in the question stem would *support* the claim that historians "rightly" view historical fiction as a challenge to their own work, not weaken that claim.

Question 17: (D) – Make Deduction

Explanation for Question 17

Jablonka is described in paragraph 4 as both an academic historian and a fiction writer who is seeking "to re-establish the dialogue between the social sciences and a wider audience." If someone is trying to "re-establish" a connection, then some of that connection must have been lost at some point. In this case, the connection is one between social scientists and "a wider audience." Since Jablonka is himself a social scientist and wants to re-establish the connection, the "wider audience" he is trying to connect with must also be a "desired audience." The correct choice is **(D)**.

Wrong Answer Explanations

(A) Paragraph 4 mentions memoirs as one of the genres that Jablonka includes in the "literature of reality" category, so Jablonka would not recommend that social scientists avoid them.

(B) The passage never directly provides Jablonka's opinion about the increase of freedom in pursuits *other* than history, so this statement is unsupported.

(C) Jablonka's view is that the "literature of reality" is "one tool among many to better achieve the goals" of social scientists. The passage provides no evidence that he believes it is "the best" tool.

Question 18: (B) – Summarize Text

Explanation for Question 18

The "transformation of contemporary historiography" from the question stem is described at the end of paragraph 3 as consisting primarily of history aiming to be more like literature. The author's disapproval of this approach is expressed most strongly in the final paragraph, in which the author states that the "knowledge of the world produced by literature and that produced by history are not identical." Blurring the line between the two disciplines, the author contends, is a mistake. This conclusion is most succinctly summarized in the statement that "The destruction of the frontier between history and literature by historians engenders a loss, not a gain." The following sentence, which begins "We lose appreciation of a critical approach ..." is merely expanding on this point. The correct answer is **(B)**.

Wrong Answer Explanations

(A) This statement serves to introduce historians' responses to literature. Rather than representing the author's conclusion regarding the "transformation in contemporary historiography," it provides background information about what motivated that transformation.

(C) The author uses this statement to concede that some changes to history are necessary, but it is only a preface to the author's criticism, in the next sentence, of the actions that historians have actually taken.

(D) This statement expresses the author's opinion that historians are right to feel threatened by recent historical fiction, rather than expressing the author's reaction to the "transformation in contemporary historiography."

Question 19: (A) – Describe Purpose

Explanation for Question 19

In paragraph 3, the author mentions the "minimization or even elimination of formal tools such as footnotes" as an example of the "changes in the presentation of historical works." After bringing up other examples, the author goes on to say that, together, these changes represent an "interesting transformation of contemporary historiography that aims to situate itself on a terrain close to, if not identical with, that of literary creation." To paraphrase, the omission of footnotes is one way that historians are making their works more like literature, making **(A)** correct.

Wrong Answer Explanations

(B) The author describes the elimination of footnotes as one of "a few formal changes," and follows it with a mention of "more substantial ones." Thus, compared to other changes cited in the paragraph, the author thinks that the omission of footnotes is a minor issue rather than "highly detrimental." Moreover, the mere mention of this relatively neutral fact could not, by itself, serve to "disparage" anything.

(C) Although footnotes, as often used, may in part function to help establish the authority of a historical text, the author's mention of the omission of footnotes from some recent historical texts is intended merely as an example of a shift in contemporary historiography.

(D) Although footnotes can be used to check the sources for a text, the author does not mention them to promote their use, but rather as an example of a shift in contemporary historiography. Moreover, it would be very unusual to promote the use of footnotes by speaking—in passing—of their exclusion from some texts.

Question 20: (A) – Anticipate Response

Explanation for Question 20

In paragraph 5, the author contends that literature and history produce different types of knowledge and use different resources. They go on to describe the "literary posture" of some historians as involving the "loss" of a "critical approach that requires a dispassionate relationship to the sources," after which "we no longer compel the reader to draw an interpretation that is more intellectual than empathetic." The hypothetical work by the historian in the question stem is described as consisting of "imaginative account[s] of what it was like to live through the events" described in letters by historical figures. This sounds a lot like what the author is talking about when they say that some historians are essentially imitating literature: Rather than a dispassionate reliance on historical sources, the historian in the stem is relying on imagination, and rather than trying to reconstruct what actually happened, they are concerned with imagining the subjective experience of events. The passage author would undoubtedly respond by thinking of this as a perfect example of the kind of "literary" history they believe is problematic. **(A)** is correct.

Wrong Answer Explanations

(B) It is Jablonka, not the author, who according to the passage promotes the "literature of reality." The author, in contrast, is at best skeptical of this "genre."

(C) In the first two paragraphs, the author does note the success of recent historical fiction. Rather than rendering a response from historians "unnecessary," though, the author believes that this success means "history must be dusted off." On the other hand, the author would not approve of the way this hypothetical historian did so.

(D) Paragraph 2 states that historians are right to view recent historical fiction as "a challenge on their own ground." However, the author does not praise historians who respond in the way described in the question stem (essentially imitating literature) and states that "The destruction of the frontier between history and literature by historians engenders a loss, not a gain."

APPENDIX

THE MCAT INTERFACE

In This Chapter

Interface Shortcuts 370
Selecting an Answer 370
Navigating the Test 371
Section Interface 371
Navigator Window 372
Timer and Question Progress 374
Leveraging Interface Features. 374
Highlight Function 374
Strikethrough Function 375
Question Flagging 376
Changing Color Scheme. 376
Zoom Function 376
The Periodic Table. 376
Conclusion. 377
Skill and Strategy Summary 378

LEARNING OBJECTIVES

After this appendix, you will be able to:

- Recognize how to use the MCAT test interface, including keyboard shortcuts
- Navigate between passages and questions during testing and review
- Leverage your interface knowledge to increase efficiency when tackling MCAT passages and questions

"10 blade," "forceps," "suction"—if you've ever had the opportunity to observe a surgery or just marathon your favorite medical drama, you've likely heard these tools called for by a surgeon or an actor playing a surgeon. Even if Hollywood's portrayal of these events can be exaggerated, the truth remains that the tools of a surgeon are vital for a successful surgery. To this end, surgeons must not only be experts in their anatomical and procedural knowledge, but also experts on the tools at their disposal and their capabilities. In this way, the MCAT is much like surgery. Not only does the MCAT require science knowledge and critical reasoning, but also a thorough understanding of the tools provided on Test Day. Two of these tools, the note booklet that lets you build outlines and the interface tool that lets you highlight passages, are discussed in depth in Chapter 5 of this book. One other important tool that's essential both for CARS and the science sections is the MCAT testing interface, and that is the subject of this appendix.

MCAT EXPERTISE

Despite being a computer-based test, the MCAT is usually taken with a note booklet and wet-erase marker provided by the testing center. A typical booklet contains 9 white laminated pages, each 8" by 14" in size. You can exchange your booklet for a new one if you run out of space, but we recommend you do so only between sections to maximize testing time. See Chapter 5 for how to use this booklet to build outlines for CARS passages.

Interface Shortcuts

The MCAT has been administered as a computer-based test (CBT) since 2007. In the years since, many adjustments have been made to the CBT interface, with the latest changes (as of the writing of this book) occurring in January 2025.

Inputting commands on the MCAT can be done two ways. One input method is via on-screen buttons using the mouse, and the second is via keyboard-based shortcuts, also known as hotkeys (see Table A.1). As a general rule, the use of hotkeys is more efficient than on-screen controls, so it is recommended that test takers become comfortable with the hotkey system for the MCAT prior to Test Day. If you find yourself using a function only once or twice per section, then the keyboard shortcut may not be worth incorporating into your Test Day habits.

Shortcut	Function	Shortcut (Section Review)	Function (Section Review)
Alt + N	Advance to Next/Answer No	Alt + E	End Review of Section/ Exam
Alt + P	Return to Previous	Alt + W	Return to Section Review
Alt + V	Open Navigation	Alt + A	Review All Questions
Alt +C or Esc	Close Navigation		
Alt + H	Highlight/Remove Highlight	Alt + I	Review Incomplete
Alt + S	Strikethrough/Remove Strikethrough	Alt + R	Review Flagged
Alt + T	Open Periodic Table	Alt + Y	Answer Yes
ESC	Close Periodic Table	Alt + O	Answer OK/Open Section Review Instructions
Alt + F	Flag for Review		
Ctrl + +	Zoom in		
Ctrl + -	Zoom out		
Ctrl + 0	Restore default zoom		

Table A.1 Keyboard Shortcuts

Selecting an Answer

Perhaps the most important feature on Test Day is the ability to select an answer. This can be done in two ways. First, you can select an answer by clicking on the answer choice (either the letter or the answer). Alternatively, pressing the A, B, C, or D key on the keyboard selects the corresponding answer choice. Upon selecting an answer, the circle beside the answer choice will fill in. To deselect an answer choice, select the same answer choice again or select a different answer choice.

Navigating the Test

Compared to a pencil-and-paper exam, where you can glance at upcoming questions or even flip pages back and forth, the computer-based MCAT may seem like an unnecessary nuisance. In reality, the navigation tools available on the MCAT provide time-saving opportunities.

Section Interface

The section interface is the main interface you will use on Test Day (Figure A.1), displaying both a passage and one associated question. On Test Day you will use
this interface both to analyze passages and to answer questions. The features of this interface allow efficient navigation between questions and passages as you work through the section.

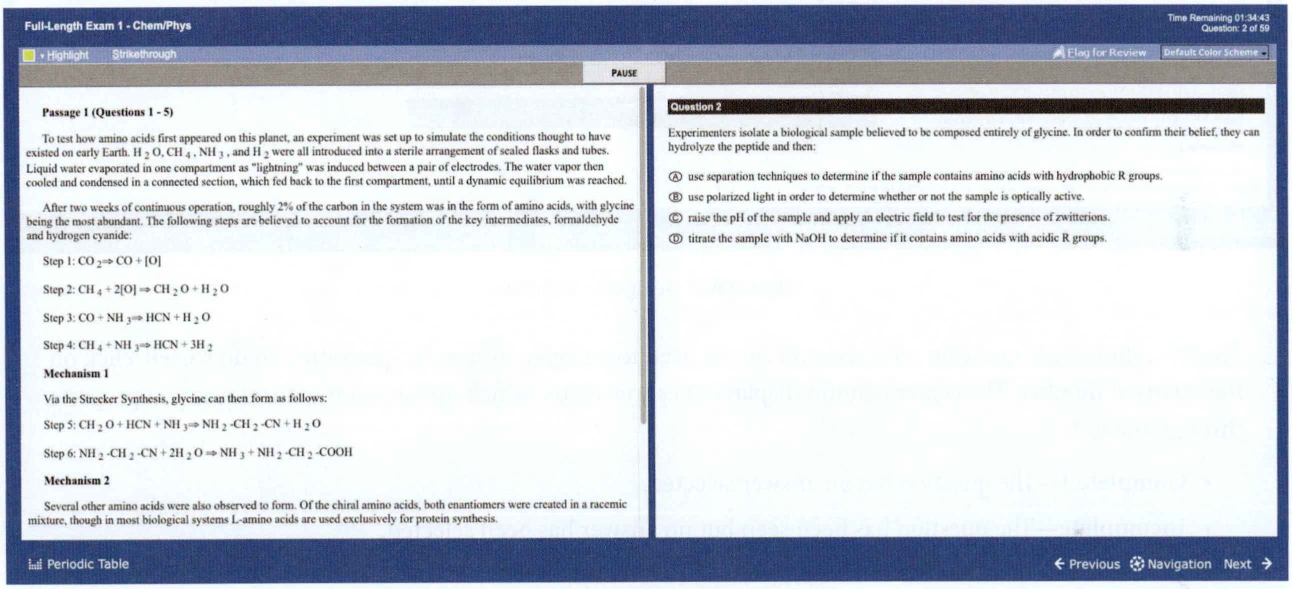

Figure A.1 Section Interface

To navigate the section, use the three on-screen buttons at the bottom right of the screen, or their associated hotkeys:

- **Next** (Alt + N) brings up the next question.
- **Previous** (Alt + P) brings up the previous question.
- **Navigation** (Alt + V) brings up the Navigator window.

Navigator Window

The Navigator window lists the questions, displays question status, and displays flagged status (Figure A.2).

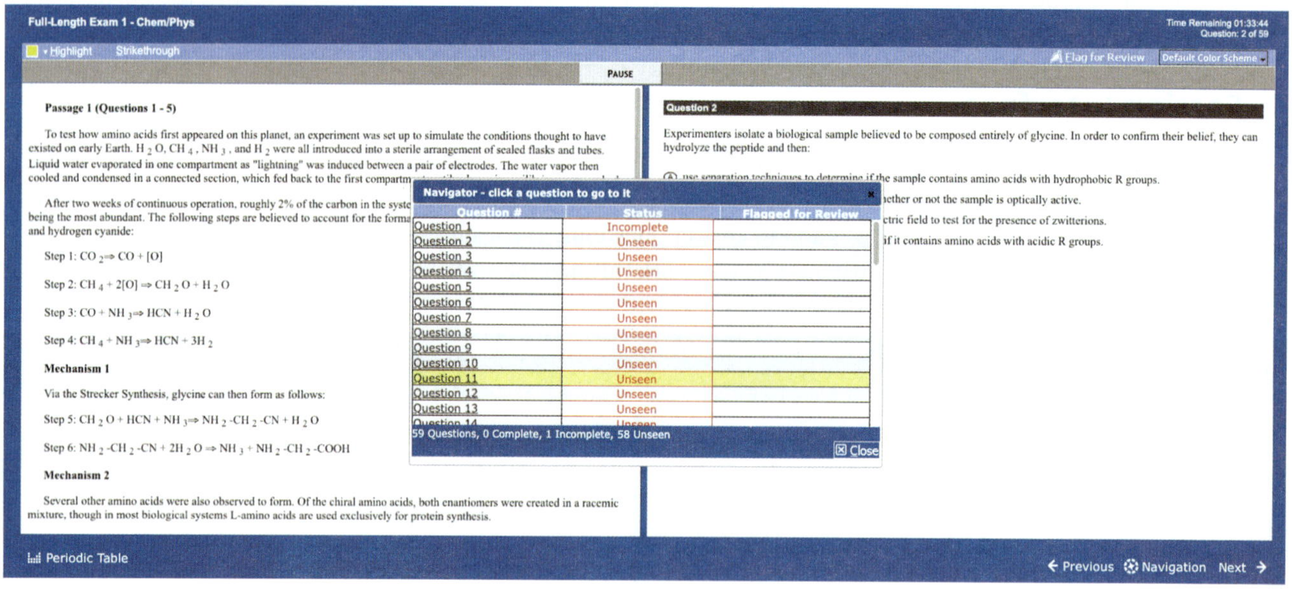

Figure A.2 Navigator Window

The left column lists question numbers and can be used to navigate to specific questions. To do so, left-click on the question number. The center column displays question status, which updates automatically as you progress through the test:

- **Completed**—The question has an answer selected.
- **Incomplete**—The question has been seen but no answer has been selected.
- **Unseen**—The question has not been seen.

In the right column, the question's flagged status is shown. As you take the exam, you can flag a question to remind you to return to it at the end of the section. We'll expand upon this strategy below

The Navigator window itself can be moved by clicking and dragging the top bar and resized by clicking and dragging the borders. To close the navigation window without jumping to a different question, click **Close** or press ESC or Alt + C.

With the ability to jump to any question in the section, the Navigator window can allow a savvy MCAT tester to skip difficult passages (saving them for last) and quickly return to them near the end of the section. To skip a passage, note the title of a passage, such as "Passage 1 (Questions 1–5)," then use the Navigator window to bring up the first question of the next passage (e.g., Question 6).

Returning to any previously seen passage, including passages skipped due to their difficulty, requires a bit of foresight. Consider reserving a space in your notes booklet for passage navigation, a place where you can jot down each passage number and the number of the first question associated with each passage (e.g., "P6: Q31"). When you wish to return to a skipped passage, simply bring up the Navigator window and click on the first question of the passage (e.g., Question 31).

Section Review Tool

Transition from the general section interface (seen above) to the Section Review interface (Figure A.3) occurs when the section is finished (more specifically, when the **Next** button is clicked on the last question of the section). When you reach this screen, you can click **Instructions** (Alt + O) to access directions on using the interface. The purpose of the Section Review interface is to allow the tester to return to any lingering questions and to ensure no questions remain unanswered. Toward this end, the Section Review provides three ways to review the section.

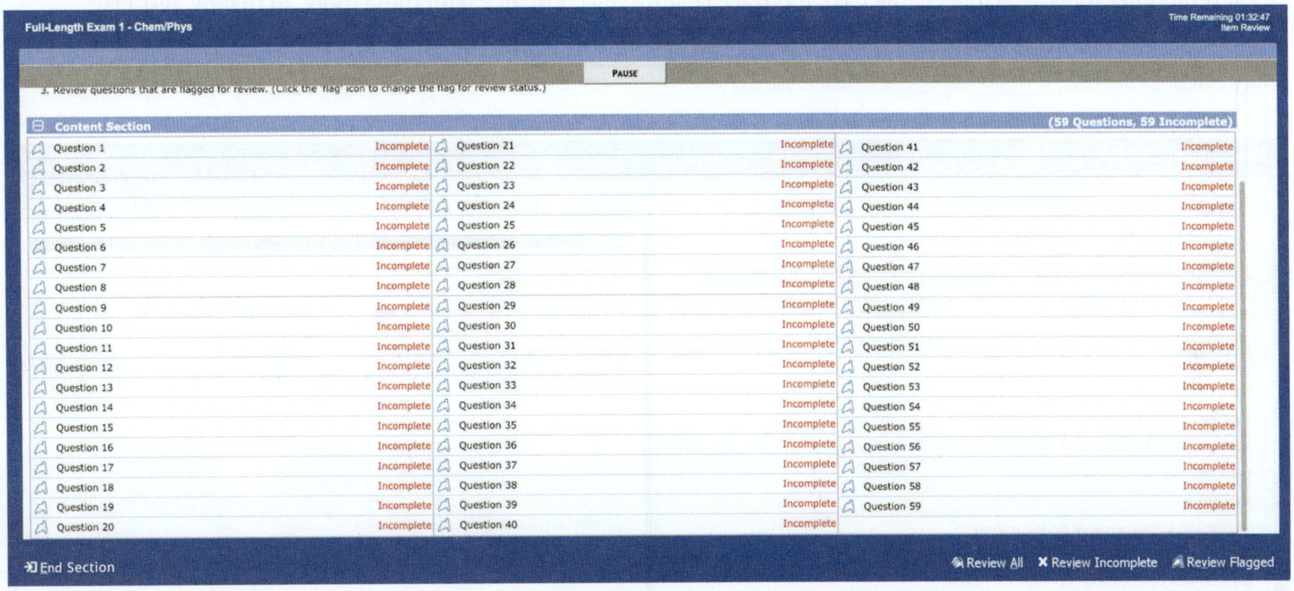

Figure A.3 Section Review

1. **Review All (Alt + A)**—brings up Question 1 and allows for navigation to every question with the next/previous buttons.
2. **Review Incomplete (Alt + I)**—allows for review of incomplete questions only. The next and previous button only navigate to incomplete questions, skipping completed questions.
3. **Review Flagged (Alt + R)**—allows for review of flagged questions only. The next/previous buttons will only navigate to flagged questions, skipping non-flagged questions.

Similar to the Navigator window, Section Review allows you to review individual questions by clicking the question number on the screen. When viewing questions through the Section Review interface, the **Navigation** button is replaced with the **Review Section** button (Alt + V), which returns to the Section Review screen.

Most testers will have limited time remaining when they enter the Section Review interface, so it's important to use its functions strategically. We recommend using the **Review Incomplete** function to ensure no questions remain unanswered and then **Review Flagged** to return to those questions you've marked for further review. To end the section, click the **End Review** (Alt + E) button at the bottom right of the screen.

Timer and Question Progress

The time remaining and question progress are displayed at the top right of all interfaces within a section of the MCAT. Although these items can be hidden by left-clicking on them, it is highly recommended to keep both visible—they are important tools for managing your section pacing.

Leveraging Interface Features

In addition to the tools available to navigate throughout the sections of the MCAT, the testmaker has made several other tools available via the CBT interface (Figure A.4). Practice with these tools, so that by Test Day you can efficiently highlight text, strike out text, flag questions, change the color zoom in and out, and call up the periodic table in the science sections.

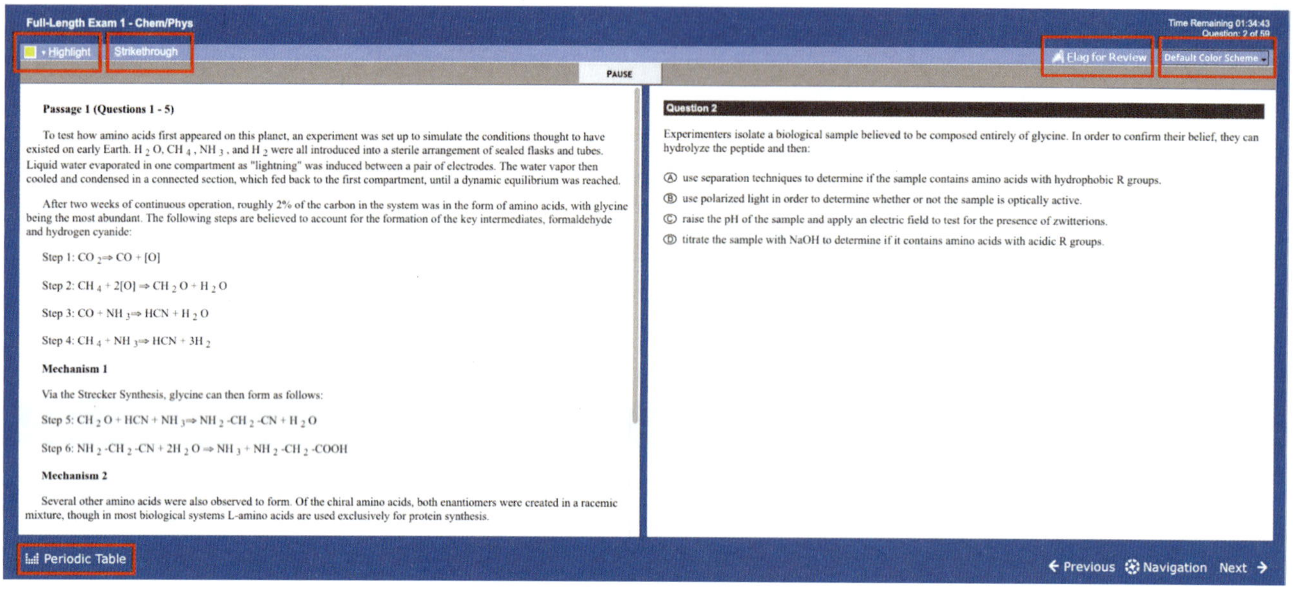

Figure A.4 Interface Tools

Highlight Function

Much like its everyday counterpart, the highlight function highlights text. As of 2025, there are two color options for highlighting, yellow and blue. Strategically, highlighting text should stress the text's importance. To highlight text:

1. Ensure the **Highlight** option is selected in the top left corner, indicated by a yellow or blue box (yellow is the default highlight color).
2. Use the cursor to left-click and hold while dragging over the desired text.
3. Press Alt + H or alternatively left-click the **Highlight** button in the top left of the screen.

You can also change the highlighting color or even erase existing highlighting. Unfortunately, this process is somewhat cumbersome. To change the color of your highlighter or to remove highlighting from text:

1. Left-click the box beside the word "Highlight" in the top left corner and then select **Remove Highlight** to erase highlighting, or the yellow or blue box to change your highlighter color.
2. Left-click and hold while dragging over the highlighted text using the cursor.
3. Press Alt + H or left-click the **Highlight** button.

When highlighting, we highly recommend using the hotkey, Alt + H, rather than clicking the highlight button. In addition, due to the cumbersome nature of switching between the highlighting and remove highlighting modes, use the highlight tool carefully to avoid ever needing to use the remove highlight function. And if you do highlight something you didn't intend to, consider just leaving it on screen unless you're sure it would distract you. Finally, be cautious about trying to use two colors for highlighting since switching colors involves the same cumbersome process as erasing.

Highlighting in Passages

If you choose to highlight within the passage, we recommend that you do so sparingly to avoid creating more work for yourself when referring back to the passage later. In general, "less is more" when it comes to highlighting. In the sciences, it can be useful to highlight key terms or given values within passages.

BRIDGE

See Chapter 5 for a systematic way to highlight passages strategically.

Highlighting in Questions

Highlighting in question stems should be used as needed. To clarify, many students will find highlighting question stems unnecessary, while others may find highlighting helps them avoid careless mistakes. For example, if you find yourself often overlooking meaning-shifting words and phrases like "NOT" and "least supported," you can highlight them to help you remember what kind of correct answer you need. Highlighting in the answer choices, although possible, is not recommended.

Strikethrough Function

The strikethrough function crosses out selected text, ~~as seen here~~. Typically, this is used to indicate that the crossed out text is not important. To strikethrough text:

1. Left-click and hold while dragging over the desired text using the cursor.
2. Press Alt + S or alternatively left-click the **Strikethrough** button in the top left of the screen.

To remove strikethrough from text, click and drag to select *only* the strikethrough text, then press Alt + S. If non-strikethrough text is accidentally selected along with the strikethrough text, then the Alt + S function will strikethrough *all* selected text.

Strikethrough in Passages

Generally speaking, a limited use of the Strikethrough tool during passage reading is best. Although it is no secret that each passage on the MCAT has its own amount of "fluff" (irrelevant) text, the Strikethrough tool should be used sparingly, since it's often more efficient to simply read past the fluff than to stop and strikethrough the text. It can be difficult to determine when text is actually irrelevant in CARS passages, so we recommend using the Strikethrough tool more on passages in the science sections (where it is easier to determine when material won't be targeted by questions) than in CARS.

Strikethrough in Questions

Like highlighting, the Strikethrough tool should be used as needed in questions. Most testers find little value using the Strikethrough tool in the question stem, but find it useful to eliminate answer choices. The key here is to keep use of the tool purpose driven; do not strikethrough answer choices simply because they are wrong, as these extra seconds add up over a section! Rather, aim to use the Strikethrough tool in a way that reduces your chance of error. For instance, let's say you begin working on a question, then ultimately choose to triage it. Before moving on to the next question, first use Strikethrough on any choices you managed to eliminate. When you return to the triaged question later, those eliminated choices will remain crossed out, even if you don't remember why!

Question Flagging

The **Flag** (Alt + F) function allows testers to flag a specific question, usually to remind them to return to it at the end of the section. Flagged questions can be seen at a glance in the Navigator window and the Section Review screen. To flag a specific question, click the flag icon at the top right corner or use the hotkey Alt + F. Once flagged, the flag icon will turn yellow.

In order to make the most of this function, it's important to use it sparingly. Remember, the MCAT is a timed test: if there is extra time at the end of a section, it is best spent reviewing questions you could feasibly answer. In other words, do not flag every difficult question or every question that you guess on; rather, flag only those questions that you know you could answer correctly if you just devoted some extra time to them.

MCAT EXPERTISE

The Flag function loses much of its usefulness in the CARS section. CARS questions are completely passage based and therefore best answered shortly after analyzing the passage. Thus, you should aim to answer every question in a CARS passage before moving on to the next one, and save the Flag function for the science sections.

Changing Color Scheme

As of 2025, the AAMC offers three options for the interface's color scheme. The default color scheme is black text on a white background, but you can use the drop-down menu in the upper right to switch to black text on a salmon (orange/pink) background, or white text on a black background, similar to the "dark mode" used in some apps.

Zoom Function

The AAMC interface allows you to zoom in or out on your screen to adjust the size of text and graphics on screen. This functionality is only available through keyboard shortcuts that are similar to those found on most web browsers and applications, using the control key along with the +, -, and 0 keys. Use Ctrl + + to zoom in on content. Use Ctrl + - to zoom out on content. In order to return to the default zoom, use Ctrl + 0. Adjusted zoom views will persist between passages and questions until changed by the test taker.

The Periodic Table

The periodic table of elements is made available in both the Chem/Phys and Bio/Biochem sections of the MCAT and provides for each element its symbol, atomic number, and atomic weight. To bring up the periodic table, left-click the **Periodic Table** (Alt + T) button at the bottom left. This will bring up a centered window displaying the periodic table (Figure A.5). Similar to the Navigator window discussed previously, the Periodic Table window can be manipulated by clicking and dragging the top bar and window borders. To close the periodic table, left-click **Close** (Alt + C).

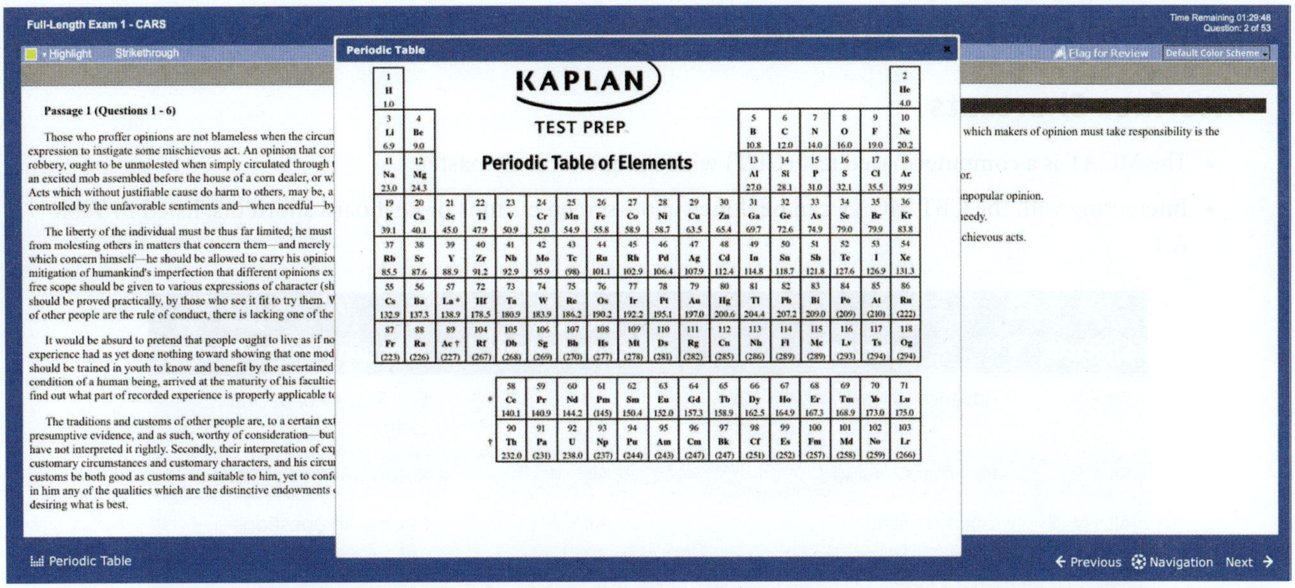

Figure A.5 Periodic Table

Strategically, the periodic table should be used only when needed. Keep in mind that the periodic table always displays the same information and that bringing it up obscures the view of the question and passage. Thus, you should use the periodic table only when seeking a specific piece of information, such as an element's group or an element's atomic weight. When opening up the periodic table, you should know exactly what you are looking for.

Conclusion

Well done! You've taken your first step toward mastering the computerized tools, that allow for smooth navigation of the interface on Test Day. Now you're ready to practice with them! If you're learning how to swim, it's not enough to read a book about different swim strokes; you're better off finding a shallow body of water where you can practice those strokes safely. So too with these CBT tools: to truly master them, practice using them whenever you use a test-like MCAT interface.

During your practice, you will likely find some tools are more useful to you than others, and you might even find yourself disregarding some of the recommendations in this chapter. This is perfectly acceptable: the tools are yours to make use of (or not) based on your preferences. The key is to ask yourself, before your test-taking habits become too entrenched, "Is my usage of the tools helping or hurting?" As long as it helps you, you're using the tools in the right way for you.

Skill and Strategy Summary

Interface Shortcuts

- The MCAT is a computer-based test (CBT) with unique tools to master.
- Interacting with the CBT MCAT can be done via on-screen buttons or keyboard shortcuts, listed in Table A.1.

Shortcut	Function	Shortcut (Section Review)	Function (Section Review)
Alt + N	Advance to Next/Answer No	Alt + E	End Review of Section/ Exam
Alt + P	Return to Previous	Alt + W	Return to Section Review
Alt + V	Open Navigation	Alt + A	Review All Questions
Alt +C or Esc	Close Navigation		
Alt + H	Highlight/Remove Highlight	Alt + I	Review Incomplete
Alt + S	Strikethrough/Remove Strikethrough	Alt + R	Review Flagged
Alt + T	Open Periodic Table	Alt + Y	Answer Yes
ESC	Close Periodic Table	Alt + O	Answer OK/Open Section Review Instructions
Alt + F	Flag for Review		
Ctrl + +	Zoom in		
Ctrl + -	Zoom out		
Ctrl + 0	Restore default zoom		

Table A.1 Keyboard Shortcuts

Navigating the Test

- Section Interface displays the passage and associated questions one at a time. Use the buttons listed below to navigate the section.
  - **Next** brings up next question.
  - **Previous** brings up previous question.
  - **Navigation** brings up the Navigator window, which displays the status of all questions at a glance and allows the tester to jump to any specific question.
- Use the Navigator window like an expert.
  - Jot down in your note booklet the passage number and first question number for each passage (e.g., “P6: Q31”).
  - When you wish to return to a skipped passage, simply bring up the Navigator window and click on the first question of the passage (e.g., Question 31).

- The Section Review interface shares most of the functions of the Navigator interface, but allows for targeted review of questions, including:
  - **Review Incomplete** allows for review of incomplete questions only.
  - **Review Flagged** allows for review of flagged questions only.
  - Use the Review Incomplete function first, then the Review Flagged before ending your section (Alt + E).
- Timer and Question Progression functions are located at the top right of the screen and should be kept visible to assist in your pacing.

Leveraging Interface Features

- Highlight keywords or phrases, as needed.
  - Use the cursor to select text and the keyboard shortcut, Alt + H, to highlight text.
  - Reserve highlighting for important terms or phrases, while avoiding the need to remove highlighting.
  - Highlight key phrases in question stems that have been missed on previous questions.
  - The less text that is highlighted, the more effective it is.
  - You can choose to highlight in yellow or in blue, but you should usually stick to one color because switching is a slow process in the interface.
- Strikethrough irrelevant text, as needed.
  - Use the cursor to select text and then the keyboard shortcut, Alt + S, to strikethrough text.
  - Strikethrough should be used for wrong answer choices, in particular when a question may be returned to later.
  - Strikethrough with purpose! Do not simply strikethrough wrong answers because they are wrong; this will use too much time.
- Flag questions that you want to return to at the end of the section.
  - Be conservative in your question flagging because there will be limited time at the end of the section.
  - You can navigate through only flagged items from the Section Review interface.
- You can change the color scheme by selecting a new scheme from the drop-down menu at the upper right.
  - Choose between the default (black text on a white background), black on salmon, and white on black.
- The periodic table is available in the Chem/Phys and Bio/Biochem sections.
  - The periodic table contains an element symbol, atomic number, and atomic weight for each element.
  - When using the periodic table, you should know what you are looking for. Do not use the periodic table for inspiration.
- Adjust the size of text and graphics by zooming in (Ctrl + +) or out (Ctrl + -) on the test interface.
  - Restore the default zoom settings by pressing Ctrl + 0.

GLOSSARY

AAMC question type–The three official CARS question categories used by the Association of American Medical Colleges (AAMC), the maker of the MCAT. According to the AAMC, 30% of CARS questions test the Foundations of Comprehension, 30% test Reasoning Within the Text, and 40% test Reasoning Beyond the Text.

Active reading–The process of reading a CARS passage at all three levels: content, architecture, and perspective. It is the most effective way to read a passage and best prepares you to answer the questions.

Active reading checks–Multiple-choice exercises included in Skillbuilders. They are designed to test your fundamental understanding of the key information in each paragraph of the passage, and ask basic questions about the content and structure of the text.

Amplifying keywords–Words or phrases, also known as Amplifiers, that indicate a stronger or more extreme opinion. They are often adjectives or adverbs that accompany a Positive or Negative keyword, such as very, really, quite, primarily, especially, obviously, foremost, and always. Other common examples include verbs like need, must, should, and ought, and phrases such as in fact, above all, and it is clear that.

Analogy–A relationship between two ideas in CARS passages or questions that are both examples of the same broader category. Two ideas connected by this kind of relationship typically have significant differences, and superficially they often seem to have very little in common. But on a deeper level, they both involve a similar structure.

Anticipate Response–One of eleven question skills identified by Kaplan: it involves identifying what the author or someone else would feel/say/do about a new situation based on its similarities to passage ideas. This skill falls under the AAMC question type Reasoning Beyond The Text, so it is tested by new info questions.

Apparent difficulty–A judgment about how hard or time-consuming a question will be to answer, which may override any triaging decision based on type alone.

Architecture–The middle level of reading CARS passages. It involves how the passage is organized and the logical and conceptual connections between ideas in the text.

Arguments–Logical structures made up of two parts: a conclusion, some claim that the author or someone else wants you to believe, and evidence, the reason(s) for accepting the conclusion. Arguments are a one-way relationship, since the evidence supports the conclusion, but not vice versa.

Assumption–A statement that isn't written in the argument, but that needs to be true in order for the logic of the argument to work. It's a missing piece of evidence, often one that connects the existing evidence more strongly to the conclusion. CARS questions that ask for assumptions test the Make Deduction skill.

Author keywords–Words or phrases that reveal opinions in the passage, usually the passage author's. They include language that expresses the tone of someone's beliefs (Positive and Negative keywords) or the intensity level of those beliefs (Amplifying and Limiting keywords).

Category–An idea or concept in a CARS passage or question that is broad enough to have various specific examples that correspond to it. Your understanding of the relationship between categories and examples is tested by Imagine Example/Analogy questions.

Cause and effect–A logical relationship in CARS passages where one event appears to lead to another. It is a central concept for Predict Outcome/Explanation questions, and Evaluate Reasoning questions will sometimes ask about cause and effect relationships that are directly discussed in the passage.

Cause keywords–Words or phrases that indicate the passage is about to mention something that led to another event or phenomenon. Common examples include caused by, due to, and as a result of.

Chatting–The skill of "asking the author" targeted questions that you use the passage to answer. A major part of active reading. Intended to reveal information about the passage's architecture and the author's perspective.

Choose–The second step of the PCRD Method for CARS Passages. Based on your initial impression of a passage from the Preview step, determine whether you should attempt it now or come back to it later.

Chunk borders–Keywords that typically mark the end of a chunk or a start of a new one, including Contrast and Conclusion keywords.

Chunk glue–Keywords that connect sentences that are typically part of the same chunk, including Continuity and Evidence keywords.

Chunking–The skill of breaking down a passage and its paragraphs into smaller pieces. Each chunk serves a separate function. A major part of active reading, so dividing paragraphs this way reveals the architecture, or logical and conceptual structure, of the passage.

Conclusion–The main point of an argument presented in the passage by the author or someone else. It is supported by evidence.

Conclusion keywords–Words or phrases that appear before conclusions in an argument. They indicate that a particular claim is supported by evidence somewhere else in the passage. Common examples include therefore, thus, then, so, argue for, argue that, and conclude.

Connection keywords–Words or phrases that reveal specific kinds of relationships between ideas. Most fall into one of two subtypes: Continuity or Contrast.

Content–The surface level of reading CARS passages, which addresses what the author directly talks about.

Continuity keywords–Words or phrases that signal that the author will continue to discuss the same kind of ideas, including those that convey a continuous sequence of events. They belong to the broader category of Connection keywords. Common examples include and, also, moreover, furthermore, first, second, third, next, and pronouns such as this, that, these, and those. Like Contrast keywords, Continuity keywords serve as transitions between sentences.

Contrast keywords–Words or phrases that indicate the passage is about to discuss something new or different than what it was addressing previously. They signal disagreement, the passage of time, or contrasting comparisons. Common examples include but, however, on the other hand, yet, and although. Like Continuity keywords, Contrast keywords serve as transitions between sentences.

Counterarguments–Logical structures that function like arguments in reverse, providing reasons to reject a claim rather than to accept a claim. The target is the claim the author or someone else wants you to doubt, while counterpoints are reasons for you to doubt the target.

Counterpoint–A claim in the passage that is designed to disprove a target claim as part of a counterargument. Counterpoint keywords often appear before a counterpoint, and sometimes a counterpoint is also introduced by Contrast keywords like however or despite.

Counterpoint keywords–Words or phrases that appear before claims used as justification for a counterargument; that is, they appear before reasons that the passage provides to doubt a target claim. Common examples include challenged by, undermined by, called into question by, objects that, and counters that.

Deep questions–Questions that involve the Reasoning Within the Text skill category, since they typically are more complex than Foundations of Comprehension questions and answering them involves a more elaborate process.

Deduction–A statement that is not included directly in the passage, but that must be true (or is extremely likely to be true) based on the information in the text. Also known as an inference or implication. The correct answer to a Make Deduction question will always be a somewhat complex deduction, while very direct deductions are tested by Paraphrase Detail questions.

Describe Purpose–One of eleven question skills identified by Kaplan: it involves identifying why the author wrote the passage or a part of it. This skill falls under the AAMC question type Reasoning Within The Text, so it is tested by deep questions.

Dictionary definition trap–A wrong answer pathology that is unique to questions testing the Interpret Meaning skill ,where incorrect choices simply reproduce the most common definition of the quoted text, especially when dealing with words that have widely-known, common meanings.

Distill–The fourth and final step of the PCRD Method for CARS Passages, which involves preparing yourself for the questions by building a mental model of the passage (distillation) through outlining or highlighting.

Distortion (Dist)–One of the four wrong answer pathologies for CARS questions. These answer choices reference ideas from the passage, but twist them in some way that doesn't match the author's intentions. A Distortion is often an extreme answer choice, one that is tempting because it matches the author's general attitudes but goes a little (or much) further than the passage justifies. Less commonly, a Distortion answer choice might misrepresent a relationship described in the passage, such as by portraying a correlation as cause and effect.

Educated guess–A strategy for identifying the correct answer to a CARS question during the Match step of the TRIM Method for CARS Questions. It is used when a prediction is not useful and the process of elimination only partially succeeds. If you are unable to make further progress after eliminating one or two incorrect choices, you should select your best guess from the remaining choices. Every choice you have confidently eliminated increases your chances of a successful guess.

Effect keywords–Words or phrases that indicate the passage is about to mention an event or phenomenon that was caused by something else described in the passage. Common examples include consequently, leading to, and resulting in.

Elaborative interrogation–A technique used as a part of active reading, which is often just referred to as interrogation. It involves having a conversation with the author, asking them "how" and "why" questions that you answer with the text, transforming the process of reading the passage into more of an interactive dialogue.

Evaluate Reasoning–One of eleven question skills identified by Kaplan: it involves characterizing logical connections between ideas in the passage. This skill falls under the AAMC question type Reasoning Within The Text, so it is tested by deep questions.

Evidence–The information that justifies the conclusion in an argument presented by the author or someone else.

Evidence keywords–Words or phrases that appear before a piece of evidence in an argument. They indicate that a particular claim supports a conclusion somewhere else in the passage. Common examples include because, since, if, why, the reason is, on account of, is justified by, after all, for example, and for instance.

Example–A specific idea or entity in a CARS passage or question that can be interpreted as belonging to a broader category. Your understanding of the relationship between examples and categories is tested by Imagine Example/Analogy questions.

Explanation–One part of a cause and effect relationship in CARS passages or questions. It is the likely (or certain) reason for a particular effect, identified through reasoning based on the text. Predict Outcome/Explanation questions often ask for an explanation of events described in the passage or question stem.

Extreme–A very common type of incorrect answer choice that exaggerates attitudes or claims presented in the passage. It falls under the Distortion wrong answer pathology. Strong opinions and radical proposals are relatively rare in CARS passages, so watch out for language like all, every, only, or never in the choices: these are often a sign of extreme answers.

Factual claim–A statement that is theoretically either objectively true or false. It does not matter whether anyone actually knows whether it is true or false.

Faulty Use of Detail (FUD)–One of the four wrong answer pathologies for CARS questions. These choices accurately reflect ideas or claims from the passage, but do so in a way that is not relevant to what the question asks for. The answer choice might be too general when a question requires a detail or too specific when a question requires a summary, or it might just focus on the wrong details.

Foundations of Comprehension (FOC)–One of the three AAMC question types. Questions that fall under this category are called surface questions since they address the basic meaning of the passage. Skills tested by Foundations of Comprehension questions include Interpret Meaning, Recognize Opinion, Paraphrase Detail, and Summarize Text.

Highlighting–One of the two major approaches to the Distill step of the Kaplan PCRD Method. It involves distilling in the author's words by using the built-in highlighting tool in the MCAT user interface to mark the most important terms in each paragraph. Glancing at these highlights gives a sense of the general structure of the passage and provides information needed to answer various questions.

How I'll Fix It (HIFI)–A list that serves as an action plan for how to correct the errors you're making on CARS questions, and which is based on your Why I Missed It (WIMI) spreadsheet. While it's possible to develop a HIFI plan for each question you answer incorrectly in practice, it's more efficient to use the patterns you've generated in review to select common misses and prioritize which corrections to work on first.

Humanities–One of the two passage types in the CARS section, the other being social sciences. Passages in this category typically involve less scientific topics that are based more heavily on opinion.

Hybrid highlighting–An approach to highlighting that includes all three levels of CARS reading: content, architecture, and perspective (or what, how, and why).

Imagine Example/Analogy–One of eleven question skills identified by Kaplan: it involves identifying new examples of categories defined in the passage or analogies of passage concepts. This skill falls under the AAMC question type Reasoning Beyond The Text, so it is tested by new info questions.

Interpret Meaning–One of eleven question skills identified by Kaplan: it involves using context to determine what a word/phrase from the passage is intended to communicate. This skill falls under the AAMC question type Foundations of Comprehension, so it is tested by surface questions.

Investigate–The third step of the TRIM Method for CARS Questions. It involves executing the plan from the Rephrase step and typically ends when you have a prediction of the correct answer in your own words. It may also involve pivoting if your initial Rephrase of the question wasn't helpful.

Kaplan Method for CARS Passages–The four-step strategy for navigating the CARS section as efficiently as possible. Its steps are abbreviated as PCRD: Preview, Choose, Read, and Distill.

Kaplan Method for CARS Questions–A four-step strategy designed to leverage the understanding of the passage provided by the PCRD method and answer questions as efficiently as possible. Its steps are abbreviated as TRIM: Type, Rephrase, Investigate, and Match.

Keywords–Words and short phrases that point to the major ideas in a passage, revealing its structure and its author's intentions. Focusing on keywords facilitates the process of elaborative interrogation and enhances the understanding of even the most difficult passages.

Limiting keywords–Words or phrases, also known as Limiters, that indicate a weaker or more qualified opinion. They narrow a claim or tone down its strength. They are often adjectives or adverbs attached to Positive or Negative keywords, such as somewhat, moderately, and largely. They include verbs that deal with possibility like can, could, may, might, and is possible. Other common examples include here, at times, in some cases, in this instance, to some extent, in a manner of speaking, and in some sense.

Logic keywords–Words or phrases that reveal relationships within arguments (Conclusion and Evidence keywords) or counterarguments (Counterpoint and Target keywords). Each of these relationships has two variations of keywords for each distinct part of a one-way connection.

Main idea–The author's thesis (the specific, central claim that the author makes about the topic of the passage) or the passage's major theme (the idea that connects all the paragraphs together). Identifying the main idea is a good backup plan if determining the overall goal is too challenging.

Make Deduction–One of eleven question skills identified by Kaplan: it involves inferring a claim that follows from multiple parts of the passage, such as an assumption in an argument. This skill falls under the AAMC question type Reasoning Within The Text, so it is tested by deep questions.

Match–The fourth and final step of the TRIM Method for CARS Questions. Ideally, it involves looking for an answer choice that reflects the same idea as your prediction, although the exact wording will almost always be different. If it was not possible to make a specific prediction, then the correct answer should be located through the process of elimination.

Negative keywords–Words or phrases that indicate disapproval of a topic, idea, or claim. Common examples include nouns such as disaster, farce, and limitation; verbs such as miss, fail, and confuse; adjectives such as problematic, so-called, and deceptive; and adverbs such as questionably, merely, and purportedly.

New info questions–Questions that involve the Reasoning Beyond the Text skill category, so called because they introduce new information in the question stem, answer choices, or both.

Opinion–A subjective statement that could never be proven true or false, because it cannot be "fact-checked": typically a value judgement or another matter of personal preference. Statements about what "should" be done are almost always opinions. The Recognize Opinion skill tests your ability to locate these types of statements as they are stated or implied in CARS passages.

Opposite (Opp)–One of the four wrong answer pathologies for CARS questions. These answer choices contradict the passage or its author in some way. Despite being the reverse of what a correct answer would suggest, they can be very tricky to recognize when the contradiction is caused by a single word like not (or even just part of a word, like the prefix un- or the suffix -less).

Out of Scope (OS)–One of the four wrong answer pathologies for CARS questions. An Out of Scope answer choice typically sounds reasonable but relies on outside information, claims that seem plausibly connected to the question but that aren't stated or implied in the passage. In this sense, Out of Scope choices are the reverse of Faulty Use of Detail (ideas or claims that are included in the passage but irrelevant to the question).

Outcome–One part of a cause and effect relationship in CARS passages or questions. It is the likely (or certain) result of a particular cause, identified through reasoning based on the text. Predict Outcome/Explanation questions often ask for an outcome of events described in the passage or question stem.

Outlining–One of the two major approaches to the Distill step of the Kaplan PCRD Method. It involves distilling in your own words by producing written notes in the booklet or other note-taking device provided on Test Day. These notes should make up a paragraph-by-paragraph outline of the passage, which will help to identify the relevant paragraph to research when answering the questions. In some cases the outline can answer a question directly and avoid the need to reread the passage.

Outside information–Claims or ideas that are not directly discussed or implied to be true in the passage, but that seem plausibly connected to that passage or a particular question. Outside information is not a valid way to justify answer choices, since you can't use real-life facts to answer any CARS question (unlike the other sections of the MCAT). Many wrong answer choices are tempting only when combined with outside information, so limiting yourself to facts from the passage can significantly improve your accuracy.

Overall goal–The author's purpose for writing the passage, expressed in your own words. Identifying this goal is the best way to grasp the big picture.

Paradox–A logical relationship between two parts of a CARS passage that seem to directly conflict with each other, so that they cannot both be true at once. Evaluate Reasoning questions will sometimes ask about paradoxes.

Paraphrase Detail–One of eleven question skills identified by Kaplan: it involves recognizing a specific piece of information that is stated or strongly implied at one location in the passage. This skill falls under the AAMC question type Foundations of Comprehension, so it is tested by surface questions.

PCRD–An abbreviation for the four steps of the Kaplan Method for CARS Passages: Preview, Choose, Read, and Distill.

Perspective–The deepest level of reading CARS passages. It captures the author's attitudes, intentions, and opinions, including why the passage was written.

Positive keywords–Words or phrases that indicate that someone approves of a topic, idea, or claim. Common examples include nouns such as victory, asset, and competence; verbs such as excel, succeed, and know; adjectives such as compelling, impressive, and elegant; and adverbs such as skillfully, reasonably, and fortunately.

Post-phrasing–The process of reviewing why incorrect answers are wrong and why correct answers are right. This is a different approach from WIMI and HIFI in that it's a much more in-depth and elaborate technique, with the goal of proactively reviewing questions by dissecting them step-by-step.

Predict Outcome/Explanation–One of eleven question skills identified by Kaplan: it involves applying causal reasoning or another connection from the passage to a new situation. This skill falls under the AAMC question type Reasoning Beyond The Text, so it is tested by new info questions.

Preview–The first step of the PCRD Method for CARS Passages. It describes your initial encounter with a CARS passage, when you should spend 10–15 seconds examining it and getting a sense of its topic and difficulty level.

Process of elimination–A strategy for identifying the correct answer to a CARS question during the Match step of the TRIM Method for CARS Questions. Use this approach when it's not possible to make a specific prediction, or when no answer choice matches your prediction. It requires you to Investigate each answer choice to determine whether it accurately answers the question. Search your distillation and the passage itself for information that eliminates wrong choices, and stop if you can find direct support for one answer. If this approach fails, make an educated guess instead.

Question skills–The specific critical thinking skills that are evaluated in CARS questions. Kaplan has identified eleven such skills, and each question tests exactly one of them. The question skills Interpret Meaning, Recognize Opinion, Paraphrase Detail, and Summarize Text fall under the AAMC category of Foundations of Comprehension. The question skills Describe Purpose, Evaluate Reasoning, and Make Deduction fall under the AAMC category of Reasoning Within the Text. The question skills Anticipate Response, Predict Outcome/Explanation, Strengthen/Weaken Argument and Imagine Example/Analogy fall under the AAMC category of Reasoning Beyond the Text. You should use skills primarily as diagnostic tools: they feature prominently in much of the feedback that Kaplan provides with our CARS practice materials.

Rarest concept–The phrase or idea in a CARS question stem that has the least significant role in the passage. It is usually the main clue about the part(s) of the passage you should return to during the Investigate step of the TRIM Method for CARS Questions. For many questions, the rarest concept is mentioned at only one or two points in the text, so focusing on it can save a lot of time.

Read–The third step of the PCRD Method for CARS Passages. It involves reading passages actively, through the process of elaborative interrogation.

Reasoning Beyond the Text (RBT)–One of the three AAMC question types. Questions that fall into this category are called new info questions since they always involve ideas that aren't directly mentioned in the passage. Skills tested by Reasoning Beyond the Text questions include Anticipate Response, Predict Outcome/Explanation, Strengthen/Weaken Argument, and Imagine Example/Analogy.

Reasoning Within the Text (RWT)–One of the three AAMC question types. Questions that fall into this category are called deep questions since they involve analyzing arguments, evaluating evidence, and understanding the relationships between different passage ideas. Skills tested by Reasoning Within the Text questions include Describe Purpose, Evaluate Reasoning, and Make Deduction.

Recognize Opinion–One of eleven question skills identified by Kaplan: it involves identifying what the author or someone else feels about a passage idea based on word choice or other context clues. This skill falls under the AAMC question type Foundations of Comprehension, so it is tested by surface questions.

Rephrase–The second step of the TRIM Method for CARS Questions. It involves developing a plan to answer the question by translating the question stem into a specific, simple task (sometimes two or three tasks for tougher questions).

Scattered questions–CARS questions that use words like "NOT" or "LEAST" in the question stem, as well as those that use Roman numerals containing multiple details. They often need to be approached with a more time-consuming process of elimination, requiring you to find three or four specific details in the passage instead of just one. Thus, they are often best saved for once you've addressed the other questions associated with the current passage.

Social sciences–One of the two passage types in the CARS section, the other being humanities. Passages in this category are typically based more on factual claims rather than opinion, and are more scientific in their approach.

Strengthen/Weaken Argument–One of eleven question skills identified by Kaplan: it involves characterizing the logical relationship between a new claim and arguments from the passage. This skill falls under the AAMC question type Reasoning Beyond The Text, so it is tested by new info questions.

Summarize Text–One of eleven question skills identified by Kaplan: it involves articulating the main idea of the passage or of a part of it. This skill falls under the AAMC question type Foundations of Comprehension, so it is tested by surface questions.

Surface questions–Questions that involve the Foundations of Comprehension skill category, since the majority of them involve paraphrasing stated details or other straightforward tasks.

Target–A claim in the passage that is attacked by one or more counterpoints as part of a counterargument designed to disprove the target.

Target keywords–Words or phrases that appear before claims that are disputed or attacked by a counterargument in the passage. Examples include challenges, undermines, calls into question, objects to, critiques, criticizes, argues against, rejects, and doubts.

Topic–The subject matter of the passage, that is, what the passage is about. The topic is typically only a few words at most and addresses the ideas discussed in a paragraph or passage. It is less detailed than the main idea, and is only of limited usefulness in answering Summarize Text questions.

Traffic light system–A metaphor used to classify keywords based on how much attention they should demand. Green lights (Continuity and Evidence keywords) indicate more of the same or supporting details, so they're usually less important if you already understand what you're reading. Yellow lights (Contrast, Cause and Effect, and Author keywords) indicate that you should slow down to make sure you understand exactly what these keywords indicate before moving on. Red lights (Conclusion, Counterpoint, and Target keywords) indicate that you should slow down to ensure your understanding and seriously consider including these particular details in your distillation of the passage.

Triage–the process of evaluating passages or questions as you begin reading them. In order to maximize your score, the most challenging passages should be saved for the end of the section, and the most challenging questions should be saved until after you've answered the other questions connected to the current passage.

TRIM–An abbreviation for the four steps of the Kaplan Method for CARS Questions: Type, Rephrase, Investigate, and Match.

Type–The first step of the TRIM Method for CARS Questions. Its main goal is making a triage decision to attack the question now or later. Later means after completing all the now questions for that passage, but before moving on to any other passages. This approach ensures that you are as prepared as possible to tackle the most difficult questions, after you've already refined your understanding of the text by answering the other questions. Triage decisions for questions should be based on the AAMC question type and the apparent difficulty.

Why I Missed It (WIMI)–A spreadsheet built up from tracking each CARS question you review and recording specific metrics that will help you to diagnose your practice and find opportunities for improvement. Treat it as a "patient chart" for your CARS skills. While you can choose the individual metrics that are most important for you to track, common ones include the question skill, the AAMC question type, the wrong answer pathology, and the time spent on that particular question.

Wild guess–Picking a CARS answer choice entirely at random. This is an absolute last resort, recommended only when you're totally stumped or almost completely out of time. But a wild guess has a 25% chance of getting you credit for answering the question correctly, and there is no downside since the MCAT treats incorrect answers the same as questions left blank.

Word charge–A representation of the strength and direction of an opinion in a passage. It is conveyed by one or more Author keywords.

Wrong answer pathologies–The four most common recurring logical patterns that make CARS answer choices incorrect. They each represent a different kind of disconnect between the choice and the passage: Faulty Use of Detail (FUD), Out of Scope (OS), Opposite (Opp), and Distortion (Dist).

INDEX

A

AAMC. *See* Association of American Medical Colleges
AAMC question types
  in CARS section, 5–8
  HIFI action plan for errors with, 100*t*
  identifying, for post-phrasing, 102
  identifying, in TRIM Method (*See* Type the question step of TRIM Method [Type step])
  question skills within, 75–78, 79*f*
  triaging questions based on, 69–72, 90
  See also Foundations of Comprehension (FOC) questions; Reasoning Beyond the Text (RBT) questions; Reasoning Within the Text (RWT) questions
Abbreviations, in outlines, 45, 47
Absence
  Evaluate Reasoning questions on absence of support, 218–222
  Imagine Example/Analogy questions on absence of relationship, 329–330, 339
  Paraphrase Detail questions on absent details, 151–153
  Strengthen/Weaken Argument questions on absence of relationship, 311, 321
Action plan(s)
  for fixing errors (*See* How I'll Fix It [HIFI] technique)
  pivoting to a new, 73–74, 239
  reminding yourself about, 102
  rephrasing question stems as, 72–73 (*See also* Rephrase the stem step of TRIM Method [Rephrase step])
Active reading
  defined, 32, 41
  elaborative interrogation in, 34–35
  identifying logical connections with, 214
  passive vs., 32–35, 41
  reasons for engaging in, 34
  without outlining or highlighting, 56
  worked example, 32–33
  See also Architecture level of active reading (Level 2); Content level of active reading (Level 1); Perspective level of active reading (Level 3)
Active Reading Checks
  Anticipate Response Skillbuilder, 275–280
  defined, 7, 8
  Describe Purpose Skillbuilder, 201–206
  Evaluate Reasoning Skillbuilder, 223–228
  Imagine Example/Analogy Skillbuilder, 333–338
  Interpret Meaning Skillbuilder, 117–122
  Make Deduction Skillbuilder, 243–248
  Paraphrase Detail Skillbuilder, 155–160
  Predict Outcome/Explanation Skillbuilder, 293–298
  Recognize Opinion Skillbuilder, 135–140
  in Skillbuilding phase, 94
  Strengthen/Weaken Argument Skillbuilder, 315–320
  Summarize Text Skillbuilder, 172–177
Affirmative characteristics, category definitions composed of, 326–327
Affirmative relationships
  Imagine Example/Analogy questions about, 329–330, 339
  Strengthen/Weaken Argument questions about, 311, 321
Amplifying keywords (Amplifiers)
  with Conclusion keywords, 54
  defined, 26, 29
  in Evaluate Reasoning tests, 214–215
  examples of, 28*t*
  functional outlines and, 47, 48, 59
  functions of, 26, 129
  identifying indirect opinions with, 128, 129
  as signals of importance, 54, 60
  in Summarize Text tests, 165
  in word charge model, 26, 27
Analogies
  applying a new category to make, 325, 327
  continuum of fit for, 327
  coordinating examples and categories to find, 324
  in Predict Outcome/Explanation tests, 285–286, 290, 291
  in Strengthen/Weaken Argument tests, 307–308, 313
  tests requesting, 329, 331–333, 339
  See also Imagine Example/Analogy (skill)
Answer choice(s)
  clues about response within, 267
  comparing, 75
  containing stated vs. implied information, 152, 161
  directness of, 131–132, 141
  justification in, 269–270, 281
  length of, 113, 123, 134, 287, 332–333
  as logical elements that strengthen or weaken, 308
  matching predictions to (*See* Match your prediction to an answer choice step of TRIM Method [Match step])
  misunderstanding, 99, 101*t*
  new information appearing in questions and, 288–289, 310
  new information appearing only in, 288, 307, 310
  reading, before making predictions, 134, 171
  selecting, in CBT MCAT, 370, 370*t*
  swapping or debating, 99, 101*t*
  using Strikethrough function on, 376
  verbs in, 194, 198, 200
Answer choice explanations
  Anticipate Response questions, 276, 278, 280, 348, 351, 365–366, 368
  Describe Purpose questions, 202, 204, 206, 256–259, 362, 368
  Evaluate Reasoning questions, 224, 226, 228, 257–260, 363, 364
  FOC question practice set, 184–188
  Imagine Example/Analogy questions, 334, 336, 338, 346, 348–351, 362–363
  Interpret Meaning questions, 118, 120, 122, 185, 187, 366–367
  Make Deduction questions, 244, 246, 248, 256, 257, 259–260, 367
  mixed practice set, 362–368
  Paraphrase Detail questions, 156, 158, 160, 184–187, 363, 365, 366
  Predict Outcome/Explanation questions, 294, 296, 298, 346–349, 363–364
  RBT question practice set, 346–351
  Recognize Opinion questions, 136, 138, 140, 186–188, 365, 366
  RWT question practice set, 256–260
  Strengthen/Weaken Argument questions, 316, 318, 320, 346, 347, 349–350, 364–365, 367
  Summarize Text questions, 173, 175, 177, 184–185, 187, 367–368
  TRIM practice question set, 84–89
Anticipate Response (skill), 91, 263–282
  applying Kaplan TRIM Method to, 87, 270–274, 281–282
  author opinions in tests of, 25
  characteristics of questions on, 264–265

described, 78, 263–265, 281
in diagnostic test result delivery, 264
everyday use of, with friends, 274
example question stems, 268–270
finding clues about the responder, 265–266
finding clues about the situation and response, 266–267
frequency of questions testing, 78, 263
identity of responder in tests of, 268, 281
Imagine Example/Analogy questions vs. tests of, 328
justification in answer choices for, 269–270, 281
keywords in tests of, 25
and other RBT skills, 78
practice questions and answers, 343, 345, 348, 351, 359, 361, 365–366, 368
requests for responses vs. situations in tests of, 268–269, 281
sample question, 264, 265
Skillbuilder for, 274–280
Apparent difficulty
passage triage based on, 10–12, 11*f*, 15
question triage based on, 70–72, 90
Applications, one-way connection of principles and, 286
Architecture level of active reading (Level 2), 32, 41, 45
chunking to uncover, 35–37, 41
highlighting at, 51, 54
question skills focusing on, 77
RWT questions focusing on, 70, 90
worked example, 33
Arguments
analyzing components of, 211–216
assumptions in, 235–236, 240
counterarguments and, 23–24, 214–215
defined, 210
evidence and conclusion in, 22–23, 29, 213–214, 235, 304
focusing on relationships in, 213–214
identifying problems in, 215, 219
incomplete, 215
keyword use in, 211–213
one-way relationships in, 22, 286
predicting missing piece of, 307–308, 313–314
premises and propositions in, 304
questions on identifying relationships in, 217–218
recognizing, in blocks of text, 213
strength of, 235
uncovering assumptions in, 235–236, 240
See also Strengthen/Weaken Argument (skill)
Association of American Medical Colleges (AAMC)
CARS passage disciplines, 5*t*
on CARS section scores, 4
categories of skills tested by (*See* AAMC question types)
computer-based MCAT interface from (*See* MCAT testing interface)
justification for correct answers from, 73
topic sentences in excerpts from, 14
wrong answer traps designed by, 75
Assumptions
finding missing piece of argument to identify, 240
Make Deduction questions about necessary, 237
reinforcing or contradicting, 308
testing validity of, 236
uncovering, 235–236, 240
Author(s)
opinions of, 25, 126–127, 130
paraphrasing details in statements not by, 148
recognizing opinions of people who are not, 127, 130–131
as responder, 266, 268, 271–273
responders who are not, 268, 272, 273
Author keywords
in chatting technique, 38
defined, 25, 29
examples of, 28*t*
in hybrid highlighting, 51–53, 74
identifying indirect opinions with, 128, 129, 131, 272
outlining and strong feelings indicated by, 46
at perspective level of reading, 33, 52
in quick highlighting, 55
in Recognize Opinion tests, 128, 133–135
in Rephrase step of TRIM Method, 72, 73
in Summarize Text tests, 165, 166, 170
tone indicated by, 100*t*
in traffic light system, 19
types of, 25–28
word charge/emotional polarity of, 26, 26*f*, 27
See also Amplifying keywords (Amplifiers); Limiting keywords (Limiters); Negative keywords; Positive keywords

B

Because, as keyword, 20, 23, 211, 212, 285
"Big picture" of passage
in Distill step, 14–16
failing to see, 99, 101*t*
Brevity
of highlights, 50
of outline, 45

C

CARS section. *See* Critical Analysis and Reasoning Skills section
Categories
applying, to examples, 325–327
defining, 325–327
with explicit definitions, 325
fitting Anticipate Response situations into, 266–267, 273, 274
Imagine Example/Analogy questions about, 328–329, 331–333, 339
in Imagine Example/Analogy skill use, 324–325
with implicit definitions, 326–327
new, in analogies, 325, 327
recognizing examples as part of, 324
Causality, chain of, 20, 20*f*
Cause–effect relationships
in Evaluate Reasoning tests, 216–218
identifying, 217–218
keywords denoting, 20–22, 285
locating elements of, 217
logical connections in, 216
as one-way relationships, 20
in Predict Outcome/Explanation tests, 286
Cause keywords
defined, 20, 29
examples of, 21*t*, 285
functional outlines and, 47
identifying cause–effect relationships with, 216
in Predict Outcome/Explanation tests, 285, 289, 290, 299
similarities between Logic and, 22, 23
in traffic light system, 19–21, 285
Chatting technique, 37–42
answering sample RBT question with, 40
asking questions in conversation and, 35
in Evaluate Reasoning tests, 212
practice passage, 58
worked example, 38–40
Choose step (PCRD Method), 10–12, 15
Chunk borders, 35, 41
Chunk glue, 35, 41
Chunking technique, 35–37, 41
answering sample RBT question with, 40
identifying pauses in conversation and, 34–35
keywords used in, 35–37
practice passage, 58–60
worked example, 36–37
Chunks, defined, 35, 41
Claims
answer choices as strengthened or weakened, 309
changing scope of, 307
combining, in Make Deduction tests, 234–235
factual, 127–129, 214, 219
identifying source of, 305–306
in Strengthen/Weaken Argument tests, 305–307, 309
Cognitive endurance, 97–98, 100, 101*t*
Colons, as keywords, 19, 109
Color
changing CBT MCAT color scheme, 376, 379
changing highlighting, 50–51
Commas, as keywords, 109
Completed question status, 372
Computer-based MCAT, interface for. *See* MCAT testing interface

Conclusion keywords
- as chunk borders, 35
- defined, 23, 29
- differentiating Evidence keywords from, 23
- in Evaluate Reasoning tests, 211–213
- examples of, 25*t*
- and functional outlines, 48
- functions of, 37, 54
- in hybrid highlighting, 54
- in Strengthen/Weaken Argument tests, 303
- in traffic light system, 19, 24

Conclusions
- in arguments, 22–23, 29, 213–214, 235, 304
- defined, 210
- identifying, in Evaluate Reasoning tests, 217
- identifying, in Make Deduction tests, 240
- identifying, in Strengthen/Weaken Argument, 304, 306–308
- keywords to identify, 211–212
- one-way connection of evidence and, 22, 286
- in passage distillation, 19, 24
- support needed by, 213–214
- tonal clues to identify, 214

Concrete examples, for Strengthen/Weaken Argument tests, 307–308

Conditional language, 305, 309

Confirmation bias, 302

Connection keywords
- in chatting technique, 38
- defined, 18, 29
- in Evaluate Reasoning tests, 218, 221
- examples of, 21, 21*t*
- identifying one-way connections with, 285
- overlooked, 100*t*
- in Predict Outcome/Explanation tests, 285, 289, 299
- types of, 18–21
- *See also* Cause keywords; Continuity keywords; Contrast keywords; Effect keywords

Content level of active reading (Level 1), 32, 41
- chat questions for, 38
- FOC questions focusing on, 33, 70, 90
- highlighting at, 51–54
- outlining at (*See* Content outlines)
- worked example, 33

Content outlines, 65
- in high-pressure situations, 49, 55
- for Summarize Text questions, 166
- worked examples, 46–48

Context clues
- in Interpret Meaning tests, 109–110
- in Make Deduction tests, 239

Continuity keywords, 18–19
- in chatting technique, 39, 60
- as chunk glue, 35–37, 39, 58
- defined, 18, 29
- in Evaluate Reasoning tests, 214
- examples of, 18, 21*t*
- in Interpret Meaning tests, 109–110, 115
- in Make Deduction tests, 233
- in Paraphrase Detail tests, 147
- quick highlighting and, 55
- in traffic light system, 19

Contradictions
- identifying, 217–218
- reconciling, 234

Contrast, implicit definitions provided by, 326

Contrast keywords
- architecture and, 33
- in chatting technique, 39
- as chunk borders, 35, 36, 39, 58, 60, 61
- in counterarguments, 214–215
- defined, 19, 29
- with Evidence keywords, 212
- examples of, 21*t*
- functional outlines and, 48
- function of, 13
- in Interpret Meaning tests, 110
- introducing counterpoints with, 24
- in quick highlighting, 55
- in traffic light system, 19

Correct answers
- AAMC's justification for, 73
- categories of, in Describe Purpose tests, 200
- characteristics of, 80–81, 92
- new information provided in, 289
- in post-phrasing, 102–103

Counterarguments
- arguments and, 23–24, 214–215
- counterpoints and targets in, 23–24, 29, 214–215, 304
- identifying relationships in, 217–218
- one-way relationships in, 23
- in passage distillation, 19, 24
- predicting missing piece of, 307–308, 313–314

Counterpoint keywords
- defined, 24, 29
- in Evaluate Reasoning tests, 214–215
- examples of, 25*t*
- functional outlines and, 48
- in hybrid highlighting, 54
- in traffic light system, 19, 24

Counterpoints
- in counterarguments, 23–24, 29, 214–215, 304
- identifying, 304, 306–308
- as weakeners of targets, 304

Critical Analysis and Reasoning Skills (CARS) section
- basic facts about, 4*t*
- deep analytical reading for, 4
- difficulty of, 4, 8
- format, 4–5, 8
- preparing for, 7–8
- question categories/types, 5–8
- science sections of MCAT vs., 8
- strategies for improvement on, 93–104
- *See also specific skills and skill types by name*

D

Dashes, as keywords, 19, 109

Deductions (implications)
- defined, 232
- nature of, 236–237, 249
- *See also* Inferences; Make Deduction (skill)

Deep analytical reading, 3–4, 34

Deep questions, 6, 8, 71, 90, 233
- *See also* Reasoning Within the Text (RWT) questions

Definitions
- of categories, 325–327
- Interpret Meaning question clues about, 112–113, 123

Denial test strategy, for Make Deduction questions, 240

Describe Purpose (skill), 91, 191–207
- applying Kaplan TRIM Method to, 197–201, 207
- described, 77, 191–193, 207
- direct quotations in questions, 196–197, 207
- in evaluation of patient's self-assessment, 192
- example question stems, 195–197
- frequency of questions testing, 77, 191
- functional outlines to answer questions, 46, 49
- keywords in tests of, 194
- location clues in questions, 196, 207
- and other RWT skills, 77
- passage elements in questions, 195, 207
- positive or negative phrasing of questions, 197, 207
- practice questions and answers, 253, 255–259, 356, 361, 362, 368
- qualifying language in tests of, 194
- rephrasing questions that test, 85
- sample question, 192–193
- Skillbuilder for, 201–206
- Summarize Text questions vs. tests of, 169
- understanding purpose of passage, 193
- understanding role of specific elements, 194

Detail(s)
- Describe Purpose questions about, 195, 199
- description of, 148–149, 161
- functions of, in CARS passages, 194
- number of details requested, 150–151, 161
- presence of, in passages, 151–152, 161
- *See also* Paraphrase Detail (skill)

Detailed explanations of Skillbuilder questions and answers
- Anticipate Response, 276, 278, 280
- Describe Purpose, 202, 204, 206
- Evaluate Reasoning, 224, 226, 228–229
- Imagine Example/Analogy, 334, 336, 338
- Interpret Meaning, 118, 120, 122
- Make Deduction, 244, 246, 248
- Paraphrase Detail, 156, 158, 160
- Predict Outcome/Explanation, 294, 296, 298
- Recognize Opinion, 136, 138, 140
- Strengthen/Weaken Argument, 316, 318, 320
- Summarize Text, 173, 175, 177

Diagnosis and Troubleshooting phase (Phase 2) of CARS Prep, 95, 104

Dictionary definition trap, 79, 108, 115, 123
Difficulty, triaging based on. *See* Apparent difficulty
Direction of reasoning, in Predict Outcome/Explanation questions, 286–287, 299
Direct opinions, 132
Direct quotations, 196–197, 207
Dist. *See* Distortion wrong answer
Distill step (PCRD Method), 12–15
  choosing tool for, 55–56
  described, 12, 16
  determining central point of passage and, 165–167
  highlighting in, 14, 16, 43, 44, 50–65
  outlining in, 14, 16, 43–49, 55–65
  with practice passage, 57–62
  progressing from Read step to, 45, 50
  purpose of entire passage in, 193
  reflecting on big picture in, 14–15
Distortion (Dist.) wrong answer, 80, 81, 92
  HIFI action plan for, 101
  for Paraphrase Detail questions, 154, 162
  in practice set, 86
  for Predict Outcome/Explanation questions, 291, 299
  for Recognize Opinion questions, 135, 141
  recording, on WIMI spreadsheet, 99
  for Strengthen/Weaken Argument questions, 304, 306, 314, 321

E

Educated guesses, 75, 91, 221, 240
Effect keywords
  defined, 20, 29
  examples of, 21*t*, 285
  identifying cause–effect relationships with, 216
  in Predict Outcome/Explanation tests, 285, 289, 290, 299
  similarities between Logic and, 22, 23
  in traffic light system, 19–21
Elaborative interrogation, 31–42
  chatting technique in, 37–42, 212
  chunking technique in, 35–37, 41
  defined, 13, 16, 41
  to make clinical diagnoses, 31–32
  and passive vs. active reading, 32–35, 41
  in Read step, 13
  for Strengthen/Weaken Argument tests, 303
Emotional polarity, of keywords, 26
  See also Word charge model
Entire passage, questions spanning
  Anticipate Response, 266
  Describe Purpose, 169, 193, 195, 199
  Evaluate Reasoning, 219, 221
  Interpret Meaning, 112
  Recognize Opinion, 169
  Recognize Opinion questions on, 130, 134
  Summarize Text, 167, 169, 170
Evaluate Reasoning (skill), 91, 209–230
  analyzing components of arguments, 211–216
  analyzing logical relationships, 21, 216
  applying Kaplan TRIM Method to, 84, 219–222, 230
  by assessing support, 218–219, 230
  described, 77, 209–211, 230
  by describing passage structure, 219, 230
  by determining connections, 217–218, 230
  example question stems, 217–219
  by finding requested roles, 216–217, 230
  frequency of questions testing, 77, 209
  by identifying problem, 219, 230
  keywords in tests of, 24, 211
  and other RWT skills, 77
  practice questions and answers, 253, 255, 257–260, 357, 359, 363, 364
  sample question, 210–211
  Skillbuilder for, 222–229
  Strengthen/Weaken Argument questions vs. tests of, 305
  in treatment plan assessment, 210
Evidence
  in arguments, 22–23, 29, 213–214, 235, 304
  defined, 210
  identifying, in Evaluate Reasoning tests, 216–217
  identifying, in Make Deduction tests, 240
  identifying, in Strengthen/Weaken Argument tests, 304, 306–308
  in incomplete arguments, 215
  keywords to identify, 211–212
  one-way connection of conclusion and, 22, 286
  as provider of support, 213–214
  as strengthener of conclusion, 304
  tonal clues to identify, 214
Evidence keywords
  in chatting technique, 39
  as chunk glue, 35, 36
  defined, 23, 29
  differentiating Conclusion keywords from, 23
  in Evaluate Reasoning tests, 211, 212
  examples of, 20, 23, 25*t*
  in quick highlighting, 55
  in traffic light system, 19, 24
Examples
  applying a given category to, 325–327
  clinical skill of recognizing, 324
  implicit category definitions provided by, 326
  questions requesting, 328, 331, 332, 339
  in Strengthen/Weaken Argument tests, 307–308
  See also Imagine Example/Analogy (skill)
Expert analysis
  chatting, 39–40
  chunking, 36–37
  outlining and highlighting, 58–64
Explanations
  following one-way connections to, 285
  investigating potential, 291
  in Make Deduction tests, 232–235
  one-way connection of phenomena and, 286
  reasoning backward to arrive at, 284, 287
  in Skillbuilder activities (*See* Answer choice explanations; Detailed explanations of Skillbuilder questions and answers)
  See also Predict Outcome/Explanation (skill)
Explicit definitions, of categories, 325
Extreme positions, wrong answers that reflect, 80, 81

F

Factual claims (facts)
  distinguishing opinions from, 127–129, 219
  tone of evidence and, 214
False
  factual statements that are, 128
  treating assumptions as, 236
Faulty Use of Detail (FUD) wrong answers, 79–80, 92
  for Anticipate Response questions, 274, 282
  for Describe Purpose questions, 200–201, 207
  for Evaluate Reasoning questions, 222, 230
  HIFI action plan for, 101
  for Paraphrase Detail questions, 154, 162
  in practice set, 87
  recording, on WIMI spreadsheet, 99
  for Strengthen/Weaken Argument questions, 314, 321
  for Summarize Text questions, 171, 178
50/50 errors, 99, 101*t*
Flag function (CBT MCAT), 370*f*, 376, 379
Flagged questions, 370*t*, 372, 373, 376, 379
Focus fade, 100, 101*t*
Foundations of Comprehension (FOC) questions
  answers and explanations for practice set, 184–188
  characteristics of, 5–6
  Interpret Meaning, 76, 107–123
  key/component skills tested by, 6, 76–77, 79*f*
  Paraphrase Detail, 77, 143–162
  as part of RBT questions, 266
  practice passages and question sets, 86, 88, 179–183
  Recognize Opinion, 76, 125–141
  Summarize Text, 77, 163–177
  as surface questions, 6, 8, 70, 90, 114
  using content to answer, 33, 70, 90
FUD wrong answers. *See* Faulty Use of Detail wrong answers
Full definitions, questions with, 112
Functional outlines
  choosing to use, 56
  content of, 45–46

defined, 45, 65
in high-pressure situations, 49
practice passage, 58–62
in Summarize Text tests, 166–167
worked examples, 46–48

G

Guesses
educated, 75, 91, 221, 240
wild, 75, 91, 240
Guided descriptions of details, questions with, 149

H

HIFI technique. *See* How I'll Fix It technique
Highlighting, 50–55, 65
to answer practice question, 64
in case presentation, 43, 44
choosing between outlining and, 55–56, 65
in Distill step of PCRD Method, 14, 16
electing not to use, 56
errors with, 100, 101*t*
in high-pressure environments, 55
hybrid approach to, 51–52
keyboard shortcuts for adding/removing, 370*t*
for practice passage, 57–64
removing, 50–51, 370*t*
specializing in, 56
tips on, 50–51
use cases for, 55
when pivoting to a new plan, 74
worked examples, 52–54
Highlight tool (CBT MCAT), 14, 50, 370*t*, 374–375, 379
High-pressure situations
content outlines in, 49
quick highlighting in, 55
Hotkeys. *See* Keyboard shortcuts
How does this connect to what you were saying before? question, 37, 39, 41
How I'll Fix It (HIFI) technique, 100–102, 100*t* –101*t*, 104
Humanities disciplines, passages from, 5, 5*t*, 8
Hybrid highlighting strategy, 51, 65
choosing to use, 55, 56
in high-pressure environments, 55
levels of information in, 51–52
practice passage, 58–63
worked example, 52–54
Hypothetical language, 305, 309

I

Identity of responder, in questions, 268, 281
If true, RBT questions containing phrase, 81
Imagine Example/Analogy (skill), 91, 323–339
affirmative vs. negative relationship questions, 329–330, 339
applying given category to examples, 325–327
applying Kaplan TRIM Method to, 330–333, 339
applying new category in analogies, 327
in clinical diagnosis process, 324
described, 78, 323–325, 339
element requested in questions, 328–329, 339
example question stems, 328–330
frequency of questions testing, 78, 323
and other RBT skills, 78
practice questions and answers, 342, 345, 346, 348–351, 356, 362–363
sample question, 324
similarities between Anticipate Response and, 267
Skillbuilder for, 333–338
Implications. *See* Deductions
Implicit definitions, categories with, 326–327
Implied information, in answer choices, 152, 161
Improvement, strategies for
HIFI technique, 100–102, 104
post-phrasing, 102–104
reviewing CARS errors, 98–104
structured practice with CARS passages and questions, 94–98, 104
surgical debriefing, 93–94
WIMI technique, 98–100, 104
Incomplete arguments, 215
Incomplete questions, 370*t*, 372, 373
Inconsistent statements, 151–152
Indirect inferences, 236–237
Indirect opinions
answer choices containing, 131–132
identifying, 128–129, 272
Inferences
defined, 232
Make Deduction questions about, 152, 236–237
Paraphrase Detail answers containing, 152, 161
in Paraphrase Detail vs. Make Deduction skills, 232
See also Deductions (implications)
Interpret Meaning (skill), 91, 107–123
answer choice length for, 113, 123
applying Kaplan TRIM Method to, 88, 113–115, 123
context clue locations for tests, 109–110
definition clues in questions, 112–113, 123
described, 76, 107–109, 123
dictionary definition trap with, 79, 108, 115, 123
in differential diagnosis, 108
example question stems, 111–113
frequency of questions testing, 76, 107
Imagine Example/Analogy questions vs. tests of, 326
location clues in questions, 111–112, 123
and other FOC skills, 76
practice questions and answers, 181, 183, 185, 187, 361, 366–367
quote length in questions, 111, 123
sample question, 108–109
Skillbuilder for, 115–122
Interrogating passages. *See* Elaborative interrogation
Investigate potential solutions step of TRIM Method (Investigate step), 73–74, 90, 91
Anticipate Response questions, 272–274
Describe Purpose questions, 200
Evaluate Reasoning questions, 221
Imagine Example/Analogy questions, 332
Interpret Meaning questions, 115
Make Deduction questions, 239, 240
with no or limited prediction possible, 74
Paraphrase Detail questions, 154
pivoting to a new action plan, 73–74
practice question set, 84–89
Predict Outcome/Explanation questions, 291
Recognize Opinion questions, 134
Strengthen/Weaken Argument questions, 313–314
Summarize Text questions, 170
Irrelevant answers, 306

J

Justification
in answer choices for Anticipate Response tests, 269–270, 281
for correct answers, by AAMC, 73
in post-phrasing, 102–103

K

Kaplan Method for CARS Passages (PCRD Method), 9–16, 10*f*
Choose step, 10–12, 15
described, 9
Distill step, 12–16, 45, 50, 193 (*See also* Highlighting; Outlining)
practicing with, 15 (*See also* Practice passages, questions, and answers)
Preview step, 10–11, 15
Read step, 12, 13, 16, 45, 50 (*See also* Elaborative interrogation; Keywords)
for RWT questions, 6
surgical plan analogy for, 9
TRIM Method and, 68
Kaplan Method for CARS Questions (TRIM Method), 68–75, 69*f*
answers and explanations for practice set, 84–89
Anticipate Response questions, 87, 270–274, 281–282
Describe Purpose questions, 197–201, 207
Evaluate Reasoning questions, 84, 219–222, 230
Imagine Example/Analogy questions, 330–333, 339
Interpret Meaning questions, 88, 113–115, 123
Investigate step overview, 73–74, 90, 91
Make Deduction questions, 238–241, 249
Match step overview, 74–75, 90
medical reasoning and, 68
Paraphrase Detail questions, 152–155, 161–162
PCRD Method and, 68
post-phrasing and, 103–104
practice question set, 81–83
Predict Outcome/Explanation questions, 89, 289–291, 299

Recognize Opinion questions, 132–135, 141
Rephrase step overview, 72–73, 90
Strengthen/Weaken Argument questions, 84, 312–314, 321
Summarize Text questions, 86, 169–171, 178
Type step overview, 69–72, 90
Keyboard shortcuts (CBT MCAT), 370, 370*t*, 378
Flag function, 370*f*, 376
Highlight tool, 50, 370*f*, 374, 375
periodic table use, 370*f*, 376
Section interface navigation, 370*f*, 371
Section Review interface, 370*f*, 373
Zoom function, 370*f*, 376
Keywords, 17–29
in active reading, 32
answers to chat questions revealed by, 38
in Anticipate Response tests, 25
in arguments, 211–213
in chunking technique, 35–37
defined, 18, 28
denoting cause–effect relationships, 20–22, 285
in Describe Purpose tests, 194
in Evaluate Reasoning tests, 24, 211
identifying conclusions with, 211–212
identifying evidence with, 211–212
in Make Deduction tests, 24, 233
in Match step of TRIM Method, 74
overlooking, 99, 100*t*
in Read step of TRIM Method, 13, 16–29
in Recognize Opinion tests, 25
relevance of, in clinical rotation, 17–18
in Strengthen/Weaken Argument tests, 24, 312
traffic light system for, 19, 20, 24, 28
See also specific types

L

Labels, for outline, 44
Limiting keywords (Limiters)
in chatting technique, 39
defined, 26–27, 29
describing viewpoints of others with, 39
in Distortion wrong answers, 135
examples of, 28*t*
functions of, 26–27, 129
identifying indirect opinions with, 128, 129
at perspective level of reading, 33
in Predict Outcome/Explanation questions, 289
in word charge model, 26, 27
Location clues
in Describe Purpose questions, 196, 199, 207
in Interpret Meaning questions, 111–112, 123
in Make Deduction questions, 237–238, 249
in Paraphrase Detail questions, 149–150, 161
passage-wide references, 112
questions without, 112, 131, 150, 196, 199, 237, 311–312
in Recognize Opinion questions, 131, 141
in Strengthen/Weaken Argument questions, 311–312, 321
See also Paragraph references
Location of new information
answer choices, 288, 307, 310
correct answers, 289
in Predict Outcome/Explanation questions, 287–289, 299
question stems, 288, 305, 309–310, 313, 328
question stems and answer choices, 288–289, 310
in Strengthen/Weaken Argument questions, 309–310, 321
Logical relationships
active reading to identify, 214
analyzing, 21, 216
in arguments, 213–214, 235
cause–effect, 20–22, 216–218, 285, 286
changing scope of claim in, 307
combining claims with, 234–235
contradictions, 217–218, 234
in counterarguments, 214–215
in Evaluate Reasoning tests, 216–218, 220–221, 230
finding requested element of, 216–217, 230, 308–309, 321
identifying, 217–218, 220–221, 230
in incomplete arguments, 215
keywords for identifying elements of, 23
one-way, 20, 22, 23
paradoxes, 216–219, 234
predicting role of missing piece in, 307, 313–314
recognizing, 306–307
rephrasing, 313
in Strengthen/Weaken Argument tests, 304–309, 313–314, 321
with unspecified direction of impact, 307
Logic keywords
in chatting technique, 38
in chunking technique, 35
defined, 22, 29
in Evaluate Reasoning tests, 210, 212, 218, 221
Evaluate Reasoning tests without, 213
examples of, 25*t*
function of, 13
identifying logical element indicated by, 23
overlooked, 100*t*
in Summarize Text tests, 165, 170
in traffic light system, 24
types of, 22–25
See also Conclusion keywords; Counterpoint keywords; Evidence keywords; Target keywords

M

Main idea
identifying purpose and, 193
from passage distillation, 165–167
stating, 14–16
in Strengthen/Weaken Argument tests, 305–306
in Summarize Text tests, 49, 77, 170
topic of passage vs., 166
Make Deduction (skill), 91, 231–249
applying the Kaplan TRIM Method to, 238–241, 249
combining claims, 234–235
described, 77, 231–233, 249
in diagnoses based on medical training, 232
example question stems, 237, 238
frequency of questions testing, 77, 231
inferences in tests of, 152, 236–237
Interpret Meaning questions vs. tests of, 114
keywords in tests of, 24, 233
location clues in questions, 237–238, 249
nature of deduction in questions, 236–237, 249
and other RWT skills, 77
Paraphrase Detail questions vs. tests of, 153
practice questions and answers, 253, 255–257, 259–260, 361, 367
Recognize Opinion questions vs. tests of, 133
sample question, 232–233
Skillbuilder for, 241, 243–248
uncovering assumptions, 235–236
Match your prediction to an answer choice step of TRIM Method (Match step), 74–75, 90
Anticipate Response questions, 274
avoiding wrong answer pathologies in, 80
Describe Purpose questions, 200–201
Evaluate Reasoning questions, 221–222
Imagine Example/Analogy questions, 332–333
Interpret Meaning questions, 115
keyword use in, 74
Make Deduction questions, 241
Paraphrase Detail questions, 154–155
practice question set, 84–89
Predict Outcome/Explanation questions, 291
Recognize Opinion questions, 134–135
Strengthen/Weaken Argument questions, 314
Summarize Text questions, 171
MCAT testing interface, 369–379
accessing periodic table, 376–377, 377*f*, 379
answer selection, 370
changing color scheme, 376, 379
Flag function, 370*f*, 376, 379
Highlight tool, 14, 50, 370*t*, 374–375, 379
keyboard shortcuts, 50, 370, 370*t*, 378
leveraging features of, 374–377, 374*f*, 379
navigation tools, 371–374, 378–379

Navigator window, 370*t*, 372, 372*f*, 378
Question Progression function, 374, 379
Section interface, 371, 371*f*, 378
Section Review interface, 370*f*, 373, 373*f*, 379
Strikethrough tool, 370*t*, 375–376, 379
surgical tool analogy for, 369
Timer function, 374, 379
Zoom tool, 370*t*, 376, 379
Meaning, interpreting. *See* Interpret Meaning (skill)
Memory reinforcement
highlights for, 52, 56
outline for, 45, 46, 56
Mental fatigue, 100, 101*t*
Mistaken Identity errors, 99, 100*t*
Mixed practice
answers and explanations for practice set, 362–368
practice passages and question sets, 355–361
Must not, as keyword phrase, 27

N

Navigation aids
in CBT MCAT interface, 371–374, 378–379
highlights as, 52
outlines as, 46
Navigation function (Section interface), 373, 378
Navigator window (CBT MCAT), 370*t*, 372, 372*f*, 378
Necessary assumptions, questions about, 237
Negative keywords
Amplifiers or Limiters used with, 26–27
in chatting, 39, 60
defined, 26, 29
examples of, 28*t*
and functional outlines, 48
identifying indirect opinions with, 128, 129
in word charge model, 26, 27
Negative phrasing
Describe Purpose questions with, 197, 207
Evaluate Reasoning questions with, 218–222
Imagine Example/Analogy questions with, 329–330, 339
Make Deduction questions with, 238
Paraphrase Detail questions with, 151–153
process of elimination for questions with, 151–152, 311
in scattered questions, 70, 80, 311
Strengthen/Weaken Argument questions with, 311, 321
word charge and, 27
Never, as keyword, 27
New information
in answer choices only, 288, 307, 310
answers that characterize impact of, 309
in both question stems and answer choices, 288–289, 310
in correct answers to RBT questions, 289
in Imagine Example/Analogy tests, 330
language introducing, 305, 309
new info questions, 7, 8, 71, 90 (*See also* Reasoning Beyond the Text [RBT] questions)
in Out of Scope wrong answers, 289
in Predict Outcome/Explanation tests, 287–289, 299
in question stems only, 288, 305, 309–310, 313, 328
in Strengthen/Weaken Argument tests, 309–310, 321
Next function (Section interface), 373, 378
No, keyboard shortcut for answering, 370*t*
Not, as keyword, 27, 80
Note booklet, MCAT, 44, 370
Number of details requested, by questions, 150–151, 161
Number of questions, as factor in choice, 12, 15

O

OK, keyboard shortcut for answering, 370*t*
One-way connections (unidirectional relationships)
for cause and effect, 20
for counterpoint and target, 23
for evidence and conclusion, 22, 286
following, 285–286
following, to outcome or explanation, 285–286
identifying, 285, 290, 291
for phenomenon and explanation, 286
in Predict Outcome/Explanation tests, 284
for principle and applications, 286
wrong answers due to reversing, 20
Open-ended question stems
Paraphrase Detail, 149, 152, 153
Summarize Text, 168
Opinions
author's, 25, 126–127, 130
author's purpose and, 194
defined, 128
direct, 132
factual claims vs., 127–129, 219
indirect, 128–129, 131–132, 272
not from author, 127, 130–131
source of, 130–131, 133, 141
tone of conclusions and, 214
See also Recognize Opinion (skill)
Opposite (Opp.) wrong answer, 80, 92
for Anticipate Response questions, 274, 282
for Evaluate Reasoning questions, 222
HIFI action plan for, 101
for Paraphrase Detail questions, 155
in practice set, 84, 85, 87, 89
for Predict Outcome/Explanation questions, 291, 299
recording, on WIMI spreadsheet, 99
for Strengthen/Weaken Argument questions, 304, 314, 321
OS wrong answer. *See* Out of Scope wrong answer
Outcomes
following one-way connections to, 285–286
investigating potential, 291
reasoning forward to arrive at, 284, 286–287
See also Predict Outcome/Explanation (skill)
Outlining, 45*f*, 64–65
to answer practice question, 64
in case presentation, 43–44
choosing between highlighting and, 55–56, 65
content outlines, 46–49, 55, 65, 166
defined, 44
in Distill step of PCRD Method, 14, 16
electing to stop, 56
errors in use of, 100, 101*t*
functional outlines, 45–49, 56, 58–62, 65, 166–167
in high-pressure environments, 49
practice passage, 57–64
specializing in, 56
tips for, 44–45
use cases for, 56
worked examples, 46–49
Out of Scope (OS) wrong answer, 80, 92
for Anticipate Response questions, 274, 282
HIFI action plan for, 101
new information in, 289
in practice set, 88
recording, on WIMI spreadsheet, 99
Outside information, answers that rely on, 13, 234, 273
Overall goal
in Describe Purpose tests, 193, 194
in Distill step of PCRD Method, 14–16
in hybrid highlighting, 51, 62
in outlining, 45, 48–49, 62
in Summarize Text tests, 170
Oversimplification, in Imagine Example/Analogy tests, 327

P

Pacing
errors due to issues with, 100, 101*t*
on Test Day, 10, 96–97
Paradoxes
defined, 216
identifying, 217–219
resolving, 234
Paragraph(s)
evaluating reasoning in a single, 170
interpreting meaning from context clues in surrounding, 110
length of, as factor in passage choice, 12, 15
summary of a single, 168, 170
Paragraph references
in Describe Purpose questions, 196
in Evaluate Reasoning questions, 221
in Imagine Example/Analogy

questions, 330
in Interpret Meaning questions, 111–112
in Make Deduction questions, 238
questions without, 112, 131, 150, 196, 237, 311–312
in Recognize Opinion questions, 111–112
in Strengthen/Weaken Argument questions, 306, 312
Paraphrase Detail (skill), 91, 143–162
answer choices containing stated vs. implied information, 152, 161
applying Kaplan TRIM Method to, 152–155, 161–162
causal relationships in questions on, 21
described, 77, 143–145, 161
description of detail in questions, 148–149, 161
in diagnosis based on patient history, 144
example question stems, 149–152
frequency of questions testing, 77, 143
Interpret Meaning questions vs. tests of, 114
isolating relevant information, 146–147
location clues in questions, 149–150, 161
Make Deduction questions vs. tests of, 232, 233, 236, 238, 239
number of details requested in questions, 150–151, 161
and other FOC skills, 77
paraphrasing effectively for, 147–148
practice questions and answers, 181, 183–187, 356, 359, 363, 365, 366
presence or absence of details in passage, 151–153, 161
Recognize Opinion questions vs. tests of, 133
sample question, 144–145
searching for rarest concept, 145–146
Skillbuilder for, 155–160
Paraphrasing
effective, 147–148
in Predict Outcome/Explanation question stems, 288
in Strengthen/Weaken Argument question stems, 306, 308
Parentheses, as keywords, 19, 109
Partial definitions, questions containing, 112
Partial details, questions containing, 148–149
Passage(s)
Describe Purpose questions about specific elements of, 195, 207
describing structure of, 219, 230
elaborative interrogation of, 31–42
evaluation of, on WIMI spreadsheet, 99, 104
highlighting within, 375
jumping between, 96
length of, as factor in triage decisions, 12, 15
questions about purpose of segments from, 195
questions about statements absent from/inconsistent with, 151–152
skipping, in Navigator window, 372
strikethrough in, 375
understanding role of specific elements of, 194
word choice differences between question stems and, 147
See also Entire passage, questions spanning; Kaplan Method for CARS Passages (PCRD Method); Practice passages, questions, and answers
Passage distillation
conclusion in, 19, 24
converting, to main idea, 165–167
counterarguments in, 19, 24
predicting missing pieces in argument by referring to, 313–314
reading, before beginning questions, 45, 50
Passive reading
active vs., 32–35, 41
defined, 32, 41
errors in sample questions due to, 34, 40
PCRD Method. *See* Kaplan Method for CARS Passages
Periodic table of elements, accessing, 370*t*, 376–377, 377*f*, 379
Perspective level of active reading (Level 3), 32, 41
chatting to reveal, 37–42
in Describe Purpose tests, 200–201
as focus of functional outline, 45
highlighting at, 52–54
question skills focusing on, 77
RWT questions focusing on, 70, 90
worked example, 33
Perspectives, misattributing, 99, 100*t*
Pivoting, to a new action plan, 73–74, 239
Positive keywords
Amplifiers or Limiters used with, 26
defined, 26, 29
examples of, 28*t*
identifying indirect opinions with, 128, 129
in Summarize Text tests, 166
in word charge model, 26, 27
Positive phrasing
about characteristics for implicit definitions of categories, 326–327
of Describe Purpose questions, 197, 207
for Evaluate Reasoning questions on support, 218–219
of Imagine Example/Analogy questions about relationships, 329–330, 339
for Paraphrase Detail questions, 151–152
of Strengthen/Weaken Argument questions about relationships, 311, 321
Possibility, Limiters to indicate, 27
Post-phrasing, 102–104
Practice passages, questions, and answers
Anticipate Response, 343, 345, 348, 351, 359, 361, 365–366, 368
Describe Purpose, 253, 255–259, 356, 361, 362, 368
Evaluate Reasoning, 253, 255, 257–260, 357, 359, 363, 364
Foundations of Comprehension questions, 179–188
highlighting approach, 57–64
Imagine Example/Analogy, 342, 345, 346, 348–351, 356, 362–363
Interpret Meaning, 181, 183, 185, 187, 361, 366–367
Make Deduction, 253, 255–257, 259–260, 361, 367
mixed practice, 355–368
outlining approach, 57–64
Paraphrase Detail, 181, 183–187, 356, 359, 363, 365, 366
Predict Outcome/Explanation, 342, 343, 345–349, 357, 363–364
Reading Beyond the Text questions, 341–351
Reading Within the Text questions, 251–260
Recognize Opinion, 181, 183, 186–188, 359, 361, 365, 366
Strengthen/Weaken Argument, 342, 343, 345–347, 349–350, 359, 361, 364–365, 367
Summarize Text, 181, 183–185, 187, 361, 367–368
TRIM Method use, 81–89
See also Skillbuilder activities; Worked examples
Predictions
about type of missing logical elements, 307–308
Describe Purpose, 200
generality in, for Strengthen/Weaken Argument, 307
matching, to answer choice (*See* Match your prediction to an answer choice step of TRIM Method [Match step])
in post-phrasing, 102
reading answer choices before making, 134, 171
as result of Investigate step, 73, 91
situations with limited or no possible, 74, 91
Predict Outcome/Explanation (skill), 91, 283–299
Anticipate Response questions vs. tests of, 270–271
applying Kaplan TRIM Method to, 89, 289–291, 299
in clinical reasoning involving cause and effect, 284
described, 78, 283, 284, 299
direction of reasoning in questions, 286–287, 299
example question stems, 287–289
following one-way connections, 285–286
frequency of questions testing, 78, 283
identifying one-way connections, 285
Imagine Example/Analogy questions vs. tests of, 331
new information in questions/answers, 287–289, 299
and other RBT skills, 78

practice questions and answers, 342, 343, 345–349, 357, 363–364
sample question, 284
Skillbuilder for, 291, 293–298
testing cause–effect relationships with, 20, 21
Premises, in arguments, 304
Presence of support, questions on, 218–219
Present details, paraphrasing, 151–152
Preview step (PCRD Method), 10–11, 15
Previous function (Section interface), 373, 378
Principle, one-way connection of applications and, 286
Problem identification, in Evaluate Reasoning tests, 215, 219, 230
Process of elimination
for Anticipate Response questions, 274
based on overall goal, 49
choosing between two answers in, 99, 101*t*
for Describe Purpose questions, 200
educated guesses after, 75
efficiency of prediction matching vs., 75
for Evaluate Reasoning questions, 222
for Imagine Example/Analogy questions, 333
for Make Deduction questions, 239–241
for Paraphrase Detail questions, 155
for questions with unspecified direction of impact, 307
for scattered questions, 70, 151–152, 311
when prediction is limited or not possible, 74, 91
Propositions, in arguments, 304
Punctuation marks, as Continuity keywords, 19, 109
Purpose, describing. *See* Describe Purpose (skill)

Q

Qualifying language, in questions, 194
Question and answer evaluation, on WIMI spreadsheet, 99, 104
Question details, on WIMI spreadsheet, 98, 104
Question Progression function (CBT MCAT), 374, 379
Question skills
AAMC question types and, 75–78, 79*f*
defined, 76
FOC category, 6, 76–77, 91, 107–188
HIFI action plan for errors with, 100*t*
identifying, in Type step of TRIM, 72, 76, 113, 133, 153, 169, 198, 220, 238, 270–271, 289, 312, 330
keywords for tests of specific, 24, 25
RBT category, 7, 77–78, 91, 283–351
RWT category, 6, 77, 91, 191–260
in Skillbuilding phase of CARS Prep, 94–95
targeted practice with, 76
Question stems
Anticipate Response, 265–270
Describe Purpose, 195–197
Evaluate Reasoning, 217–219
highlighting in, 375
Imagine Example/Analogy, 328–330
information given in, 168–169, 178
Interpret Meaning, 111–113
length of rephrase vs., 170
Make Deduction, 237, 238
misunderstanding, 99, 101*t*
new information appearing in answers and, 288–289, 310
new information appearing only in, 288, 305, 309–310, 313, 328
Paraphrase Detail, 149–152
paraphrasing, in post-phrasing, 102
Predict Outcome/Explanation, 285, 287–289
Recognize Opinion, 129–132
rephrasing, in Kaplan Method (*See* Rephrase the stem step of TRIM Method [Rephrase step])
Strengthen/Weaken Argument, 308–312
strikethrough in, 376
Summarize Text, 167–169, 178
word choice differences between passages and, 147
Question types. *See* AAMC question types
Quotation marks, as keywords, 19
Quotations
Describe Purpose questions with direct, 196–197, 207
in Interpret Meaning questions, 109–111
length of, in questions, 111, 123
word choice in questions that do not use, 147

R

Rarest concept, searching for
to locate relevant text, 145–147, 154
to optimize speed and accuracy of answer, 146
in Paraphrase Detail test, 145–146, 153
in Recognize Opinion test, 134
RBT questions. *See* Reasoning Beyond the Text questions
Read step (PCRD Method)
described, 12, 16
elaborative interrogation in, 13, 16, 31–42
keywords in, 13, 16–29
with practice passage, 57–62
progressing to Distill step from, 45, 50
Reasoning
in backward direction, to explanation, 284, 287
direction of, in questions, 286–287, 299
evaluating (*See* Evaluate Reasoning [skill])
in forward direction, to outcome, 284, 286–287
Reasoning Beyond the Text (RBT) questions, 90
answers and explanations for practice set, 346–351
Anticipate Response, 78, 263–282
characteristics of, 6
chunking and chatting to answer, 40
FOC questions as part of, 266
Imagine Example/Analogy, 78, 323–339
key/component skills tested by, 7, 77–78, 79*f*
as new info questions, 7, 8, 71
new information in answers to, 289
practice passages and question sets, 341–345
in practice set, 84, 87–89
Predict Outcome/Explanation, 78, 283–299
Strengthen/Weaken Argument, 78, 301–321
Reasoning Within the Text (RWT) questions
answers and explanations for practice set, 256–260
on architecture, 70, 90
characteristics of, 6
as deep questions, 6, 8, 71, 90
Describe Purpose, 77, 191–207
Evaluate Reasoning, 77, 209–230
key/component skills tested by, 6, 77, 79*f*
Make Deduction, 77, 231–249
on perspective, 70, 90
practice passages and question sets, 251–255
in practice set, 85
Recognize Opinion (skill), 91, 125–141
answer choice directness for, 131–132, 141
applying Kaplan TRIM Method to, 132–135, 141
in assessment of patient behavior during interview, 126
author opinions in tests of, 25
described, 76, 125–127, 141
distinguishing opinions from facts, 127–128
example question stems, 129–132
frequency of questions testing, 76, 125
identifying indirect opinions, 128–129
keywords in tests of, 25
location clues in questions, 131, 141
and other FOC skills, 76
Paraphrase Detail questions vs. tests of, 153
practice questions and answers, 181, 183, 186–188, 359, 361, 365, 366
sample question, 126, 127
scope of subject in questions, 129–130, 141
similarities of Anticipate Response and, 266
Skillbuilder for, 135–140

source of opinion in questions, 130–131, 141
strategies for Describe Purpose questions and tests of, 194
Summarize Text questions vs. tests of, 169
Relative relationships, 20, 22, 23
Relevant information, isolating, for Paraphrase Detail questions, 146–147
Rephrase the stem step of TRIM Method (Rephrase step), 72–73, 90
Anticipate Response questions, 87, 271–272
Describe Purpose questions, 199
Evaluate Reasoning questions, 84, 220–221
Imagine Example/Analogy questions, 331–332
Interpret Meaning questions, 88, 114
Make Deduction questions, 239–240
Paraphrase Detail questions, 153–154
practice question set, 84–89
Predict Outcome/Explanation questions, 89, 290–291
Recognize Opinion questions, 133–134
Strengthen/Weaken Argument questions, 84, 313
Summarize Text questions, 86, 169–170
Responder(s)
as Anticipate Response question component, 265
author as, 266, 268, 271–273
finding clues about, 265–266
identity of, 266, 268, 271–273, 281
non-author, 268, 272, 273
Response(s)
as Anticipate Response question component, 265
Anticipate Response questions requesting, 268–269, 281
degree of justification of, 269–270
finding clues about, 266–267
See also Anticipate Response (skill)
Review All function (Section Review), 373, 379
Review flagged function (Section Review), 373, 379
Review Incomplete function (Section Review), 373, 379
Reviewing CARS errors, 98–104
delaying, 98
HIFI technique, 100–102, 104
post-phrasing technique, 102–104
WIMI technique, 98–100, 104
Review Section button (Section Review interface), 373
Roman numerals
Anticipate Response questions with, 270
Make Deduction questions with, 238
Paraphrase Detail questions with, 151, 153
Predict Outcome/Explanation questions with, 287
triaging questions containing, 70
RWT questions. *See* Reasoning Within the Text questions

S

Scattered questions
Anticipate Response, 270, 272
Describe Purpose, 197, 199, 207
Evaluate Reasoning, 218–222
Imagine Example/Analogy, 329–330, 339
Make Deduction, 238
negative phrasing and negations in, 70, 80, 151–153, 197, 207, 218–222, 238, 311, 321, 329–330, 339
Paraphrase Detail, 151–153
Predict Outcome/Explanation, 287
process of elimination for, 70, 151–152, 311
Roman numerals in, 70, 151, 153, 238, 270, 287
Strengthen/Weaken Argument, 311, 321
triaging, 70
Science sections of MCAT
CARS section vs., 8
chat questions in, 38
elaborative interrogation in, 13
Flag function in, 376
prediction matching, process of elimination, and guessing in, 75
Scope
of claim, in Strengthen/Weaken Argument questions, 307
of element, in Strengthen/Weaken Argument questions, 305–306
of subject, in Recognize Opinion questions, 129–130, 141
of summary, in Summarize Text questions, 167–168, 178
Second-guessing answer, 99, 101*t*
Section interface (MCAT), 371, 371*f*, 378
Section Review interface (MCAT), 370*t*, 373, 373*f*, 379
Semicolons, as keywords, 19, 109
Sentence factors in passage choice
complexity, 12, 15
length, 12, 15
Should not, as keyword phrase, 27
Simple inferences, answer choices containing, 152, 161
Single detail questions, 150
Single paragraph questions
Evaluate Reasoning, 221
Summarize Text, 168, 170
Situation(s), in Anticipate Response tests, 264
finding clues about, 266–267
identifying, 271, 272
questions requesting, 269, 281
similarities between, 267, 273
Skillbuilder activities
Anticipate Response, 274–280
CARS Prep phase for, 94
described, 7, 8
Describe Purpose, 201–206
Evaluate Reasoning, 222–229
Imagine Example/Analogy, 333–338
Interpret Meaning, 115–122
Make Deduction, 241, 243–248
Paraphrase Detail, 155–160
Predict Outcome/Explanation, 291, 293–298
Recognize Opinion, 135–140
Strengthen/Weaken Argument, 314–320
Summarize Text, 171–177
Skillbuilding phase (Phase 1) of CARS Prep, 94–95, 104
Skipping passages, in Navigator window, 372
Social media, 97
Social sciences disciplines, passages from, 5, 5*t*, 8
Solutions, investigating potential. *See* Investigate potential solutions step of TRIM Method (Investigate step)
Speculation, wrong answer that require, 314
Spreadsheets, for reviewing CARS errors, 98–100, 98*t*, 104
Stamina, errors due to lack of, 100, 101*t*
Stated details, answer choices containing, 152, 161
Strategy evaluation, on WIMI spreadsheet, 100, 104
Strengthen/Weaken Argument (skill), 91, 301–321
affirmative vs. negative relationships, questions about, 311, 321
applying Kaplan TRIM Method to, 84, 312–314, 321
causal relationships in questions testing, 21
in confirmation of diagnosis, 302
described, 78, 301–305, 321
element requested in questions, 308–309, 321
Evaluate Reasoning questions vs. tests of, 219
in evidence-based medicine, 303
example question stems, 308–312
frequency of questions testing, 78, 301, 303
identifying source of claims, 305–306
if true questions to test, 81
keywords in tests of, 24, 312
location clues in questions, 311–312, 321
location of new information in questions/answers, 309–310, 321
and other RBT skills, 78
practice questions and answers, 342, 343, 345–347, 349–350, 359, 361, 364–365, 367
predicting missing pieces, 307–308
recognizing logical relationships, 306–307
sample question, 302–304
Skillbuilder for, 314–320
Strikethrough tool (CBT MCAT), 370*t*, 375–376, 379
Structured CARS prep, 94–98, 104
Diagnosis and Troubleshooting phase, 95, 104
objective metrics for, 98
Skillbuilding phase, 94–95, 104
Timing and Endurance phase, 95–98, 104
Structure mismatches, wrong answers due to, 333

Summaries
- question stems that begin, 168
- scope of, 167–168, 178
- of single paragraphs, 168, 170
- in Strengthen/Weaken Argument tests, 305, 306

Summarize Text (skill), 91, 163–178
- applying the Kaplan TRIM Method to, 86, 169–171, 178
- converting passage distillation to main idea, 49, 165–167
- described, 77, 163–165, 178
- in diagnosis of complex illness, 164
- example question stems, 167, 168
- frequency of questions testing, 77, 163
- information in question stems, 168–169, 178
- and other FOC skills, 77
- practice questions and answers, 181, 183–185, 187, 361, 367–368
- sample question, 164–165
- scope of summary in questions, 167–168, 178
- Skillbuilder for, 171–177

Support
- assessing, in Evaluate Reasoning tests, 218–219, 230
- educated guesses about, 221
- Evaluate Reasoning questions on absence of, 220–222
- identifying evidence and conclusion from relationship with, 213–214
- in Strengthen/Weaken Argument questions, 306

Surface-level reading. *See* Content level of active reading (Level 1)

Surface questions, 6, 8, 70, 90, 114
- *See also* Foundations of Comprehension (FOC) questions

T

Targeted practice
- in post-phrasing, 103
- with question skills, 76

Target keywords
- defined, 24, 29
- examples, 25*t*
- in traffic light system, 19, 24

Targets
- in counterarguments, 23–24, 29, 214–215, 304
- identifying, 304, 306–308

Text, summarizing. *See* Summarize Text (skill)

Therefore, as keyword, 23, 35

Thesis statements
- passages without, 14, 15, 194
- in Strengthen/Weaken Argument tests, 305–306

Time, Contrast keywords for passage of, 19

Timed practice
- alternate timers for, 97
- for CARS section, 95–97
- chat questions and, 38
- rephrasing/predicting and, 74

Timer function (CBT MCAT), 374, 379

Timing and Endurance phase (Phase 3) of CARS Prep, 95–98, 104

Tone, misinterpreting, 99, 100*t*

Topics
- of opinions, 129–130, 133, 134
- of passages, 5, 12, 15, 100*t*, 166

Topic sentences, passages without, 14, 194

Traffic light system for keywords, 19, 20, 24, 28

Trees Over Forest error, 99, 101*t*

Triage decisions
- about passages, 10–12, 11*f*, 15, 69
- about questions, 69–72, 76, 90, 114, 133, 153, 169, 198–199, 220, 238–239, 271, 289–290, 312–313, 331
- for Anticipate Response questions, 271
- based on AAMC question type, 70–72, 90
- based on apparent difficulty, 10–12, 11*f*, 15, 70–72, 90
- based on question skill, 76, 114, 133, 153, 169, 198–199, 220, 238–239, 271, 289–290, 312–313, 331
- for Describe Purpose questions, 198–199
- for Evaluate Reasoning questions, 220
- for Imagine Example/Analogy questions, 331
- for Interpret Meaning questions, 114
- for Make Deduction questions, 238–239
- for Paraphrase Detail questions, 153
- practicing to improve, 271
- for Predict Outcome/Explanation questions, 289–290
- for Recognize Opinion questions, 133
- for Strengthen/Weaken Argument questions, 312–313
- for Summarize Text questions, 169

TRIM Method. *See* Kaplan Method for CARS Questions

Troubleshooting. *See* Diagnosis and Troubleshooting phase (Phase 2) of CARS Prep

True, factual statements that are, 128

True, wrong answers that are not most likely to be, 241

Type the question step of TRIM Method (Type step), 69–72, 90
- Anticipate Response questions, 270–271
- Describe Purpose questions, 197–199
- Evaluate Reasoning questions, 219–220
- identifying specific question skill in, 72, 76, 113, 133, 153, 169, 198, 220, 238, 270–271, 289, 312, 330
- Imagine Example/Analogy questions, 330–331
- Interpret Meaning questions, 113–114
- Make Deduction questions, 238–239
- Paraphrase Detail questions, 152–153
- practice question set, 84–89
- Predict Outcome/Explanation questions, 289–290
- Recognize Opinion questions, 132–133
- Strengthen/Weaken Argument questions, 312–313
- Summarize Text questions, 169
- triaging based on AAMC question type, 70–72, 90
- triaging based on question skill, 76, 114, 133, 153, 169, 198–199, 220, 238–239, 271, 289–290, 312–313, 331

U

Unidirectional relationships. *See* One-way connections

Unseen question status, 372

Unspecified direction of impact, questions with, 307

V

Verbs, in Describe Purpose question stems, 194, 198, 200

Vocabulary required, as factor in choice, 12, 15

W

What are you talking about? question, 38, 42

Where are you going with this? question, 38, 42

Why are you telling me this? question, 37, 39–41

Why do you believe that? question, 37, 39–41

Why I Missed It (WIMI) technique, 98–100, 98*t*, 104

Wild guesses, 75, 91, 240

Word charge model, 26, 26*f*, 27

Worked examples
- active reading, 32–33
- chatting, 38–40
- chunking, 36–37
- highlighting, 52–54
- outlining, 46–49
- *See also* Skillbuilder activities

Wrong answer explanations
- Anticipate Response practice questions, 348, 351, 366, 368
- Describe Purpose practice questions, 256–259, 362, 368
- Evaluate Reasoning practice questions, 257–260, 363, 364
- FOC question practice set, 184–188
- Imagine Example/Analogy practice questions, 346, 349–351, 362–363
- Interpret Meaning practice questions, 185, 187, 367
- Make Deduction practice questions, 256, 257, 259, 260, 367
- mixed practice set, 362–368
- Paraphrase Detail practice questions, 184–186, 363, 366
- Predict Outcome/Explanation practice questions, 347–349, 364
- RBT question practice set, 346–351
- Recognize Opinion practice questions, 186, 188, 365, 366
- RWT question practice set, 256–260

Strengthen/Weaken Argument practice questions, 346, 347, 350, 365, 367
Summarize Text practice questions, 184–185, 187, 367–368
TRIM Method practice set, 84–89
Wrong answer pathologies
answers that could be true, but are not most likely to be, 241
and characteristics of correct answers, 80–81
defined, 79, 92
dictionary definition trap, 79, 108, 115, 123
Distortion, 80, 81, 86, 92, 99, 101, 135, 141, 154, 162, 291, 299, 304, 306, 314, 321
evaluating, in CARS error review, 99, 101*t*
examples of wrong concept, 333
extreme positions, 80, 81
Faulty Use of Detail, 79–80, 87, 92, 99, 101, 154, 162, 171, 178, 200–201, 207, 222, 230, 274, 282, 314, 321
irrelevant answers, 306
Mistaken Identity errors, 99, 100*t*
Opposite, 80, 84, 85, 87, 89, 92, 99, 101, 155, 222, 274, 282, 291, 299, 304, 314, 321
Out of Scope, 80, 88, 92, 99, 101, 274, 282, 289
post-phrasing variant to identify, 103
relying on outside information, 13, 234, 273
requiring additional speculation, 314
reversing one-way relationships, 20
structure mismatches, 333
in Summarize Text tests, 164–165
Trees Over Forest error, 99, 101*t*

Y

Yes, keyboard shortcut for answering, 370*t*

Z

Zoom tool (CBT MCAT), 370*t*, 376, 379

Notes

Notes

Notes

Notes

Notes

Notes

The Kaplan Method for CARS Passages

PREVIEW for difficulty

Estimate difficulty based on topic and structure

CHOOSE when to read it

Decide whether to read the passage *now* or *later*

READ each paragraph actively

Use keywords to interrogate the text and identify the most important ideas in each paragraph

DISTILL the meaning of the passage

Capture the most important info from each paragraph in your own words or the author's words and determine why the passage was written

The Kaplan Method for CARS Questions

TYPE the question

Read the question stem and glance at the choices to identify the AAMC question type and difficulty and decide whether to do it *now* or *later*

REPHRASE the stem

Simplify the phrasing of the question stem to determine the specific tasks required to answer it

INVESTIGATE potential solutions

Use your distillation and the passage, if necessary, to predict what you can about the answer

MATCH your prediction to an answer choice

Look for an answer choice that is synonymous with your prediction or eliminate choices that conflict with it

CARS Question Skills

- CARS Skills
  - Foundations of Comprehension 30%
    - Interpret Meaning 20%
    - Recognize Opinion 20%
    - Paraphrase Detail 40%
    - Summarize Text 20%
  - Reasoning Within the Text 30%
    - Describe Purpose 30%
    - Evaluate Reasoning 40%
    - Make Deduction 30%
  - Reasoning Beyond the Text 40%
    - Anticipate Response 15%
    - Predict Outcome/Explanation 15%
    - Strengthen/Weaken Argument 50%
    - Imagine Example/Analogy 20%

Wrong Answer Pathologies

Wrong Answer Pathology	Why It's Wrong	Why It's Tempting
Faulty Use of Detail (**FUD**)	It doesn't answer the question asked.	It uses accurate details from the passage.
Out of Scope (**OS**)	It brings in outside information that has no connection to the passage.	The outside info might seem relevant based on your knowledge or personal beliefs. Plus you're expected to use outside knowledge on every MCAT section except CARS.
Opposite (**Opp**)	It reverses the direction of what would be a correct answer.	A single word like "not" can completely change the meaning of the choice.
Distortion (**Dist**)	It's more extreme than is supported by the passage, or otherwise misrepresents ideas or connections between ideas in the passage.	It may have the same direction as the correct answer but just goes too far. A single word like "always" or "never" can make the difference.